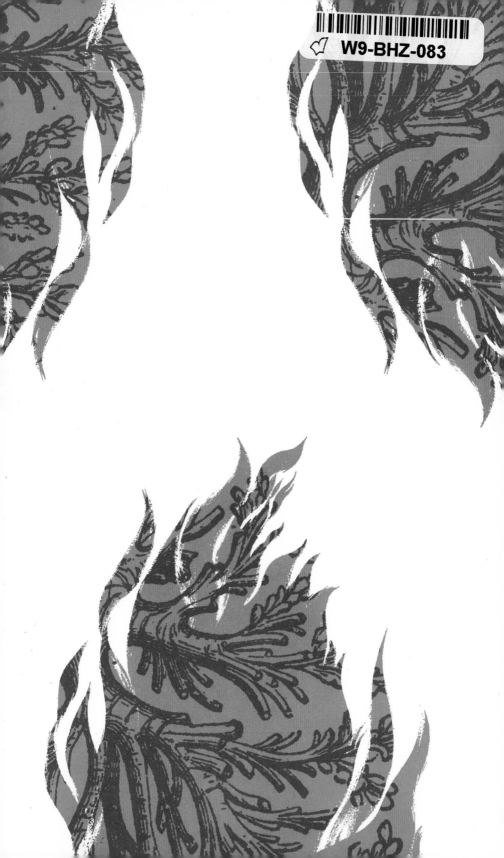

Also by Raj Patel

A History of the World in Seven Cheap Things
(coauthored with Jason W. Moore)

The Value of Nothing

Stuffed and Starved: The Hidden Battle for the World Food System

INFLAMED

INFLAMED

DEEP MEDICINE AND THE
ANATOMY OF INJUSTICE

RUPA MARYA and RAJ PATEL

FARRAR, STRAUS AND GIROUX
NEW YORK

Farrar, Straus and Giroux
120 Broadway, New York 10271

Grateful acknowledgment is made for permission to reprint the following material:
"Pando/Pando" from Streaming (Coffee House Press, 2014). Copyright © 2014 by Allison Adelle Hedge Coke.
"From the West Berkeley Shellmound to Moana Nui" by Fuifuilupe Niumeitolu.

Library of Congress Cataloging-in-Publication Data
Names: Marya, Rupa, 1975– author. | Patel, Raj, author.
Title: Inflamed : deep medicine and the anatomy of injustice / Rupa Marya and Raj Patel.
Description: First edition. | New York : Farrar, Straus and Giroux, 2021. | Includes bibliographical references and index. | Summary: "Raj Patel, the New York Times bestselling author of The Value of Nothing, teams up with physician, activist, and cofounder of the Do No Harm Coalition Rupa Marya to reveal the links between health and structural injustices— and to offer a new deep medicine that can heal our bodies and our world"— Provided by publisher.
Identifiers: LCCN 2021010075 | ISBN 9780374602512 (hardcover)
Subjects: MESH: Healthcare Disparities | Social Medicine | Social Justice | United States
Classification: LCC RA418 | NLM W 76 AA1 | DDC 362.1—dc23
LC record available at https://lccn.loc.gov/2021010075

Designed by Janet Evans-Scanlon

Our books may be purchased in bulk for promotional, educational, or business use. Please contact your local bookseller or the Macmillan Corporate and Premium Sales Department at 1-800-221-7945, extension 5442, or by email at MacmillanSpecialMarkets@macmillan.com.

www.fsgbooks.com
www.twitter.com/fsgbooks • www.facebook.com/fsgbooks

10 9 8 7 6 5 4 3 2 1

This is a work of nonfiction. Some names and details have, however, been changed, primarily to protect patient privacy.

This offering
for
our children
and
the practitioners of deep medicine,
past, present, and future

CONTENTS

INFLAMED

INTRODUCTION

I am talking of millions of men who have been skillfully injected with fear, inferiority complexes, trepidation, servility, despair, abasement.

—AIMÉ CÉSAIRE[1]

The body is also directly involved in a political field; power relations have an immediate hold upon it; they invest it, mark it, train it, torture it, force it to carry out tasks, to perform ceremonies, to emit signs. This political investment of the body is bound up, in accordance with complex reciprocal relations, with its economic use; it is largely as a force of production that the body is invested with relations of power and domination; but, on the other hand, its constitution as labor power is possible only if it is caught up in a system of subjection (in which need is also a political instrument meticulously prepared, calculated and used); the body becomes a useful force only if it is both a productive body and a subjected body. This subjection is not only obtained by the instruments of violence or ideology; it can also be direct, physical, pitting force against force, bearing on material elements, and yet without involving violence; it may be calculated, organized, technically thought out; it may be subtle, make use neither of weapons nor of terror and yet remain of a physical order.

—MICHEL FOUCAULT[2]

> She then told him: "The student has performed his austerities and faithfully tended the fires. Teach him before the fires beat you to it." But Satyakama went on a journey without ever teaching him. . . . The fires then said to each other: "The student has performed his austerities and faithfully tended us. So come, let us teach him."
>
> —CHANDOGYA UPANISHAD

AS THE WORLD BURNS

Your body is inflamed. If you haven't felt it yet, you or someone close to you soon will. Symptoms to look for include uncontrolled weight gain or unexpected weight loss, skin rashes, difficulty with memory, fever, trouble breathing, and chest pain. Inflammation accompanies almost every disease in the modern world: heart disease, cancer, inflammatory bowel disease, Alzheimer's, depression, obesity, diabetes, and more. The difference between a mild course and a fatal case of Covid-19 is the presence or absence of systemic inflammation.

Your body is part of a society inflamed. Covid has exposed the combustible injustices of systemic racism and global capitalism. Demagogues around the world kindle distrust and hatred. Governments send in the police to impose order, monitor lockdowns, enforce a return to work for those who comply and incarceration for those who do not.[3] From the United States to South Africa, India, Brazil, and China, people suffering oppression set tires and cars and gasoline alight on barricades. The petrochemistry of our protest reflects the materials that we have on hand. Everything we've made, we've made from fossil fuels: energy, food, medicine, and consumer goods.[4] The world has been organized to burn.

As a consequence, the planet is inflamed. Global temperature records are being broken, forest fires have turned from annual to perennial events, oceans are rising, and storms have become bigger and stronger. This is the epoch of endless fire. Human destruction is tearing apart the web of life, shredding the network of relationships between organisms and places in which our lives are embedded.[5] Inflammation is a biological, social, economic, and ecological pathway, all of which intersect, and whose contours were made by the modern world.

Inflammation is triggered when tissues and cells are damaged or threat- ened with damage. A complex and intricately coordinated response of the immune system, inflammation mobilizes resources to ultimately heal what has been injured. In a healthy, balanced system, once the mending has occurred, inflammation subsides. When the damage keeps coming, the repair cannot fully happen, leaving the inflammatory response running. A system of healing then turns into one that creates more harm.

As we explore inflammation in this book, we will sometimes use the language of the body in analogy. So: salmon are to rivers as hearts are to blood vessels. They both function as nutrient pumps in systems of circulation. We sometimes proceed by simile: dams are like vascular obstructions. We're not above metaphor. Trade routes, for example, are colonialism's arteries, moving people, capital, goods, and diseases around the world system, and connecting bodies, societies, geographies, and ecologies. The metaphor helps us to show that inflammation is systemic and that the systems are linked. But we aren't making a literary argument so much as a medical one. The inflammation in your arteries and the inflammation of the planet are linked, and the causal connections are becoming increasingly clear; your physiological state is a reaction to social and environmental factors. Racial violence, economic precarity, industrial pollution, poor diet, and even the water you drink can inflame you.

These connections are not new or even our own. Indigenous people have been articulating them for the past six hundred years, in an ongoing global resistance to the destruction of their ways of life. Abolitionists have been articulating them since 1619. From the

Global South, traditions of healing have survived successive waves of colonial destruction. Our work stands on the shoulders of movement workers and visionary thinkers from the past and our contemporaries, from the agroecological farmers of Amrita Bhoomi, in Karnataka, India, to the lived and theorized struggles for abolition of Angela Davis. We are duly inspired by Robin Wall Kimmerer's braiding together of science and story and the border-smashing articulations of Miles Davis and Frantz Fanon. Our analysis has been shaped by organizing with communities in struggle, and by the stories of patients who pointed the way to the connections we explore. We acknowledge and honor those people whose legacies of resistance have shaped our own understanding. To this foundation of knowledge that precedes us, we hope to contribute a political anatomy, one that can help identify the root causes of humanity's shared pathologies, in our bodies and in the world around us.

Consider the case of Shelia McCarley. She was born on the outskirts of Muscle Shoals, Alabama, on land that had once been Cherokee, a tributary of the Trail of Tears. Power lines strung along the Tennessee River during the New Deal era allowed industries to flourish and gave Alabamians work for a dignified wage. Meanwhile lax regulations permitted the industrial effluent to flow into the Tennessee River. McCarley grew up in Florence, drinking water drawn from the family well. On the weekends, she'd eat catfish pulled from the river with her own hands, fish that had lived and died in water tainted with mercury and "forever chemicals" like PFAS, or perfluoroalkyl substances.[6]

Found in everyday items like waterproof jackets, nonstick pans, and firefighting foam, PFAS are a family of five thousand "forever" chemicals, so called because they accumulate in our bodies and environment and never degrade.[7] They are behind a range of health problems including cancer, thyroid disorders, and immune system disruption.[8] Failure to regulate industrial production has led to their widespread presence in drinking water.[9] Corporations like 3M, which has a production plant on the Tennessee River, spent decades and dollars covering up the negative health and environmental impacts of these chemicals before finally agreeing to settling $35 million for putting PFAS into the water.[10]

When she was in her forties, McCarley left Alabama for California. Early in middle age, her health began to deteriorate. Her face became covered with rashes, her hair started falling out, and her joints swelled. Her body seemed to be attacking itself. At fifty-nine, she was transferred to University of California, San Francisco's Parnassus hospital; her chart declared she was suffering from an autoimmune disease called lupus.

But something wasn't right. She had some of the classical signs of lupus, like a rash and low counts in her blood cell lines, but the panel of tests that are diagnostic for the disease came back negative. Her illness was a mystery to the hundreds of health care workers who attended her at one of the world's most sophisticated hospitals. Rounds of steroids and other immune therapies did nothing. The most seasoned clinicians and investigators entertained rare and esoteric diagnoses but found no clear match-up with McCarley's course.

The one thing that every physician who saw her agreed on was this: the markers for inflammation in her body were as high as they had seen. It was as if she periodically went into septic shock. Sepsis affects an estimated 30 million people every year worldwide, killing 5 million of them, with the largest burden in the Global South.[11] The acute inflammation of sepsis is directly responsible for at least 20 percent of all deaths worldwide.[12] Typically in septic shock, a person's body sets off intense inflammation in response to an infection or trauma. Body temperature spikes to a fever to fight the offender. It can then plunge into hypothermia as the body fails to correct the offense. White blood cell counts peak and plummet. Blood vessels relax, leading to a dangerous drop in blood pressure. To compensate, the heart beats faster; sometimes people breathe faster, too, and become disoriented.

McCarley had a broad range of symptoms. She appeared to be infected, but no one could find an offending microbe. In the intensive care unit, she received drips of antibiotics and pressors, medication to stop her blood pressure from dropping. After a few days, she seemed better. In addition to quelling infections, antibiotics can also tamp down inflammation. As her symptoms lessened, she was taken off the antibiotics and removed from the ICU. Soon enough, her symptoms returned, so she was readmitted until she'd recovered enough to be released again. The cycle repeated: into the ICU and on a drip, symptoms abated; removed from the ICU, symptoms returned. All the while, there was no evidence of any infection or autoimmune disease.

By the fifth month, she began to despair. She was tired of being poked and prodded, of being offered a glimpse of recovery, only to have it snatched away when her symptoms returned. She asked her doctors to change her goals of care to no longer prolong her life and to allow her to die.

The treatment kept her alive, but eventually it broke her.

McCarley's autopsy revealed that over the course of five months, the marrow in her bones had been replaced almost entirely by activated macrophages. In a normal body, these white blood cells engulf bacteria, viruses, and our own sick or dying cells. But something had triggered her macrophages to go into overdrive—very likely the toxic exposures she grew up around in Muscle Shoals.[13] As the activated macrophages multiplied in her bone marrow, they pushed out other important cell lines, leaving no lymphocytes to respond to infection and no platelets to help clot blood. McCarley became vulnerable to infection and bleeding. She died from both, overwhelmed by inflammation.

To many of the nurses and doctors who still turn over her case in their minds, McCarley was killed by her body's own response to her environment, poisoned by the ongoing exposure to the modern world. But we will never know. Causal relationships are a hard-won scientific prize. It's impossibly difficult to isolate the reasons why McCarley's macrophages behaved the way they did. Over a sufficiently large population, however, it's possible to see patterns emerge. In 2012 a quarter of all human deaths were traceable to environmental factors in the air, water, and soil.[14]

Each toxin works on our body differently. The European Chemicals Agency suggests that there are over 144,000 human-made chemicals in the world today, few of which have been around for longer than a generation or two.[15] The body doesn't have that many tricks to rid itself of chemicals that cause harm. The fallback is to activate its own mechanism of damage control and repair.

But inflammation itself isn't a disease—it's a sign of a larger problem. From McCarley's devastated bone marrow to the clouded lungs of Covid patients,[16] the source of inflammation is more than a virus, or even the poisons with which we humans have contaminated our air and water. To understand why we are sick in the ways we are, we must understand more fully what's driving this phenomenon. What we need is a diagnosis.

DIAGNOSIS:
DIA (APART) + *GIGNŌSKEIN* (TO KNOW)

Every diagnosis, according to conventional Western medicine, is a story pulled apart, a narrative told out of joint.[17] The story begins in the middle, with a symptom. Doctors then weave a tale in flashback, one that began with a healthy body that next suffered some insult, trauma, or infection that fits a known pattern of disease. The story of diagnosis—at least the way doctors tell it—concludes with a treatment that may return the body to health at some point in the future, or at least allow the patient to manage the illness. But these kinds of stories don't always work.

Experiencing daily trauma at the hands of law enforcement, acute poverty, hunger, discrimination, forced displacement, and disproportionate exposure to toxins—it all makes people sick. If every diagnosis is a story, and every story begins with "once upon a time in a faraway place," the specific time and place matter.

Recall that in the Covid pandemic, not all patients were equal. Shuffle through the X-rays of Covid-infected lungs, and you'll see a steady rhythm of overactivated immune response; look from bed to bed in an ICU filled with Covid patients, and you'll see patterns emerge. Black, Indigenous, and people of color (BIPOC) were over-represented, their bodies subject to inflammation of all kinds, long before the SARS-CoV-2 virus ever settled into their lungs. Not only lack of access to health care, but systemic social and economic disenfranchisement rendered their bodies most susceptible to Covid when it hit. Their bodies were vulnerable, and they were at risk for increased exposure to the virus due to the desperate need for an income and whether or not their work was deemed essential.[18] In California, 80 percent of undocumented workers were considered part of the "essential critical infrastructure workforce" by the Department of Homeland Security.

Niria Alicia is a Xicana Indigenous woman who was born and raised in a farmworker community in the Rogue Valley of southern Oregon, in the ancestral homelands of the Takelma people. Both of Alicia's parents immigrated from Mexico to harvest the Bosc and Comice pears that are the valley's signature crop. While Alicia was born a US citizen, her mother was undocumented throughout her childhood, and her father only recently attained resident status. The community she grew up in is made up of farmworkers, hotel workers, restaurant workers, and landscape workers.

In spring of 2020, the pandemic swept the Northwest, and the economy cratered. Low-wage workers were the first to feel the pinch. The Rogue Valley working-class community mobilized networks of mutual aid to ensure everyone could pay their power bills and afford their groceries. But by September, poverty had become widespread and acute. That was when the fires started.

The local government sent out evacuation notices, but only in English and only to the whiter and wealthier city of Ashland, neglecting the poorer towns of Talent and Phoenix, where most of the immigrant community lived. One blaze, the Alameda fire, spread rapidly from North Ashland along a corridor of low-income housing, reducing Phoenix to ashes.

Alicia recalls, "The fire started in the morning. By nightfall, it had already torched some 3,000 structures and 75 percent of those structures are mobile homes owned by low-income white, senior, veteran, and Latinx people. An apartment complex can have six homes, but it is only considered one structure. They say some 3,000 households burned down. If we are considering the Latino community, we have large families. We live intergenerationally. That's likely 5,000 to 10,000 people who have lost everything."[19]

Most of the Latinx community[20] impacted by the fire had immigrated to the valley after being pushed out of their home countries by Washington-enforced neoliberal economic policy, political instability, or climate catastrophe. So like many who had experienced economic disaster, they didn't trust banks. "These workers and grandmothers literally kept their entire savings in cash in their homes," Alicia explains. The Alameda fire burned hot, with some estimates registering 1600 degrees Celsius: "One elder was hoping to find her five-gallon jars filled with all the coins she stashed intact when she rummaged through the wreckage. Instead she found a mess of melted metal." After the disaster, many undocumented people live chose to not apply to the Federal Emergency Management Agency (FEMA) for assistance. "When people realize that FEMA is a part of the Department of Homeland Security, they will be like 'I already lost so much. I don't want to be separated from my family.' So they don't access that help."

The fires delayed the autumn harvest and polluted the air. The average daily air quality index was above 500, levels hazardous to human health.[21] Now unhoused, picking grapes without socks and without N95 respirators, Alicia's community members accumulated the toxic impact of the fires in their bodies. Air pollution from wildfires can cause inflammation in the lungs and the blood vessels, leading to increased risk of heart attack and stroke.[22] It can also predispose people to worse outcomes from Covid.[23]

Throughout these hardships, the Immigration and Customs

Enforcement (ICE), or "La Migra" as the agency and its agents are unaffectionately known, continued their raids in the valley. "La Migra comes. They kick ass. And then they take names. My mom, who is a citizen, could be picked up and put in a jail, exposed to Covid. They have held citizens in these detention camps for months."

The root of a diagnosis is a knowledge of antecedent parts that make sense of the present in order to change the future. Without taking into account the myriad ways systemic injustice impacts the body, the standard medical narrative connecting the past, present, and future falls short, lacking the explanatory power to address and change the course of illness. An accurate diagnosis of Covid in the Rogue Valley must involve a complete history of the arrangements of power that led to certain lives being considered expendable, sacrificed to profits from pear trees planted on land acquired through colonial violence and theft.[24] Put a different way, an accurate diagnosis of the workers in Alicia's community would implicate the systems of injustice created during the colonial era, beginning with the exploitation and enslavement of the Takelma people and ending with a system of racial capitalism that treats migrant workers as disposable.[25] A story that fails to incorporate this history is one that can have no part in healing.

Today's medical and social sciences have a hard time navigating the connections between our health, our histories, and our societies. Academic silos are partly to blame. Hospitalists, historians, and sociologists rarely interact. But even this disconnect speaks to a deeper problem, woven into the origins of modern medicine. Most doctors— most humans, really—have unwittingly inherited a colonial worldview that emphasizes individual health, disconnecting illness from its social and historical contexts and obscuring our place in the web of life that makes us who we are.

In the nineteenth century, the growing field of physiology began to identify the linked systems affecting our health, locating disease in the physical reality of the body. As Michel Foucault wrote in *The Birth of the Clinic*, disease "is caught up in an organic web in which structures are spatial, the determinations causal, the phenomena anatomical and physiological. Disease is now no more than a certain complex movement of tissues in reaction to an irritating cause."[26]

The paradigm shift at that time lay in the recognition that diseases come from *somewhere within* the body's interconnected systems. According to Foucault, it was the job of the doctor to make this location visible and legible. Western medicine then trained physicians to look at an inflamed human body and connect symptoms of inflammation to the dysfunctions of an afflicted organ. In this book, we carry this theory of diagnosis a step further, locating the causal origin of disease in the multidimensional spaces around and beyond the individual body—in histories, ecologies, narratives, and dynamics of power. The inflammatory diseases we are seeing today are not the cause of the body's dysfunctional reactions. They are the body's correct responses to a pathological world. To understand what's driving inflammation, we must account for the things our bodies have been exposed to, in the places where our lives have been circumscribed. And to offer a treatment, we must show how we can escape.

The philosopher David Abram observes that "the body is itself a kind of place—not a solid object but a terrain through which things pass, and in which they sometimes settle and sediment."[27] To wonder why some things settle in some bodies and not in others is to begin to ask questions about power, injustice, and inequity, questions that are bound in modern medicine with questions of colonialism.

PILLAGE AND PLUNDER

Indigenous communities will tell you rather bluntly that colonialism is far from over. There are over seventy countries with Indigenous people whose lives are under threat by colonial expansion today. In 2018, 164 Indigenous people were killed in defense of their land against mining and agriculture enterprises.[28] Some of the world's most important economies, such as Australia, Canada, Brazil, and the United States, are settler colonies, and their projects to remove Indigenous communities' control over their land are ongoing.

Despite some annual rituals of contrition—Sorry Day in Australia,[29] Indigenous Peoples' Day spottily observed in some US states and cities, a cosmetic apology for genocide in Peru[30]—most countries have a state-sponsored policy of amnesia around the fate of Indigenous people. Since 1942 the United States, home to 573 federally recognized tribal nations,[31] has required schoolchildren to forget that number and each morning pledge their allegiance to "*one* nation under God."[32]

The litany of health disparities that Indigenous communities suffer presents a painful pattern. In Cameroon, members of Indigenous Baka communities will live on average until they are thirty-five years old—that's twelve years fewer than the country average. In Russia, Indigenous Nenet women are six times more likely to die in childbirth than the national average. In Australia, aboriginal infants die at almost twice the rate of settlers.[33] On the Pine Ridge reservation, Oglala Lakȟóta lifespan is sixty-six years old, while neighboring settlers in South Dakota can expect to live to seventy-five. Settlers living four hundred miles away live to eighty-six.[34]

Chances are that you are not among the world's 370 million Indigenous people. But colonialism affects you, too. Whether you're living in a settler colony in the Americas, in a part of the world controlled by European empires in Asia or Africa, or in Europe itself, the ideologies of modern colonialism are alive and well—and they are making you sick.

To be clear, colonialism isn't simply the physical occupation of land. It is a process, an operation of power in which one cosmology is extinguished and replaced with another. In that replacement, one set of interpretations about humans' place in the universe is supplanted. Patterns of identity, language, culture, work, relationship, territory, time, community, and care are transformed.[35] Colonialism has fundamentally altered our relationships with the web of life, and we are all living with its consequences. When Europe began its pillage of the Western Hemisphere in 1492, Indigenous cosmologies of reciprocity, relationships with and duties of care for water, land, and living beings were uprooted, replaced with a worldview animated by domination, exploitation, and profit.

In one of Christopher Columbus's diary entries, written on seeing the Western Hemisphere for the first time, he noted that he had seen all manner of unidentifiable living things and that he couldn't figure out how much they might sell for. There was, however, one commodity with which he was familiar, from his early years around the slave markets of Genoa: humans. On his first return from Arawak territories, he brought with him a hold full of slaves for the market in Seville.[36] It was the beginning of centuries of extraction and enslavement.

To understand how colonial cosmology has transformed and disrupted the web of life, consider the case of the beaver. Beaver was the most prized fur in Europe; its fur is naturally water repellent, and haberdashers across the continent used the underpelt to waterproof hats. What was once a practical item of clothing to keep you dry in the rain soon became a must-have fashion item across Europe. But by 1600 the European beaver was hunted to near-extinction.[37]

Enter colonialism. From 1822 to 1890, the United Kingdom imported 74 percent by value of all US fur exports.[38] Before Europe colonized the Western Hemisphere, there were 60 million to 400 million beavers in North America.[39] By 1900, they were all but extinct. Today there are around a tenth of their original number.[40] In some cases, Indigenous people were enslaved to serve the European demand for fur.[41] Disease introduced by Europeans also traveled along these trade routes.[42] In settlers' attempts to exploit Indigenous peoples for profit, they altered the bodies of these communities for generations.

The fall of beaver populations also changed the way rivers ran across the North American continent. The biodiversity that thrived because of the beaver's hydrological engineering plummeted. With their dams, beavers create successional habitats that provide slow-moving water sanctuaries for plants, insects, and other animals, such as salmon. As demand for pelts pushed trappers west across the North American continent, beaver pools disappeared.[43]

Rivers without their beavers flow straighter and offer less safe harbor, particularly during winter freezes. The annihilation of the beaver and its habitat reduced the number of potential salmon smolts in winter by 94 percent.[44] For Indigenous communities dependent on the salmon, this was devastating.

Rates of diabetes, cardiovascular disease, and depression skyrocketed in the Indigenous communities of Salmon Nation. Defined as "a nature state, as distinct from a nation state,"[45] Salmon Nation is the coastline and watershed spanning the fifty thousand square miles between the Yukon River in Alaska and the Sacramento River in California, where the Pacific salmon run.[46] The lives of Indigenous inhabitants are intricately intertwined with the health of the salmon, whose vitality is seen as a reflection of their own. The process that extirpated the beaver, changed the course of the waterways, and removed the fish from rivers is the same one that has left tribal people's bodies wracked with inflammation. The consequences of this colonial trade are still visible both by satellite and under the microscope.

Just as it altered the flows of water around the world, European colonialism brought flame. One member of the Belgian colonial forces in the Congo detailed, "As our party moved through village after village . . . a party of men had been detailed with torches to fire every hut . . . As we progressed, a line of smoke hung over the jungle for many miles, announcing to the natives far and wide that civilization was dawning."[47] The destruction of tropical forests, and of the cultures that live in those forests, isn't over. Australia has lost 40 percent of its forest cover since European invasion,[48] and battles over the future of extant land continues to be prosecuted between Indigenous communities and logging companies: one side sees the promise of profit, and the other sees life and culture being butchered by chain saws.

That one person's progress might be another's destruction has much to do with the intellectual life of European colonization. With a new continent to plunder came new ideas to license the theft. The fifteenth century saw the simultaneous inauguration of European empire and the ascendency of a scientific worldview that objectified and diminished life and the natural world.[49] The psychic technology crucial to justifying the expansion of empire was the invention of the diametrically opposed concepts of "society" and "nature." Humans who were capable of allegedly rational thought—usually white, Christian, landowning men—comprised "society." The rest of the planet—non-Europeans, women, animals, rivers, and plants—were defined as "nature," purely physical things without minds.

The seventeenth-century philosopher René Descartes, who spent much of his life in the Dutch Republic during its Golden Age of imperial conquest, codified an intellectual framework through which colonists could split the world into thinking and unthinking things. From his *Meditations*: "I think, therefore I am." Grounding existence in the experience of the self, Descartes concluded, "I am a thinking thing," and "I am not this body."

That he wasn't just dreaming about his body, that his perceptions of it were indeed real, was vouchsafed by God.[50] With a guarantee like that, the world was his to master. The separation of mind and matter allowed for, indeed demanded, the cleavage of the world—into material things and thinking things, into domains of the physical and the spiritual. This dualism of mind and body is fundamental to colonial cosmology and permeates every institution created through colonialism—especially medicine.

In the colonies, Europe's imperial projects specifically targeted the foods and medicines of colonial subjects to make them easier to dominate. Through campaigns that merged official medical knowledge and armed force, European missionaries and medics waged war on Indigenous shamans and healers. Physicians were a part of the violent colonial project, bringing new medicines and conceptualizations that dissected Indigenous peoples apart from their ways of knowing and consequently from their health. Campaigns against witchcraft and the ignorance of colonized people were lessons in the brutal imposition of a colonial worldview.

Colonial cosmology sees *things* where *persons* once were. What once was alive with personhood—a forest, a river, a mountain—becomes inanimate, disconnected from ecologies, open to exploitation. In the United States, this mindset is enshrined into law. Attempts to confer legal rights of personhood to Lake Erie were struck down by the courts, while laws that bestow on corporations the rights of people continue unchallenged. And there's a reason: it's easier to scoop the heart out of a mountain when it's a resource than when it's a living relative.

Many people don't realize that the same will to power that is ravaging Indigenous communities around the world is making the planet and most of its inhabitants sick. But what's worse, the medicine we rely on to heal from these insults is itself rooted in colonial cosmology. The history of modern medicine *is* the history of colonialism. It's no wonder we're not feeling any better.

BUT MODERN MEDICINE IS GREAT

We're often told that we've never had it so good.[51] Even amid the Covid pandemic, medicine points toward cures. Life expectancies are on the whole increasing, maternal mortality is falling, and childhood stunting looks like it might be a thing of the past. But this celebration of the past two hundred years is possible only in the same way that a banker, plummeting off a ledge, is able to say "so far, so good."

Look closer, and the story gets more complex. In the UK, severe cuts to the safety net, over the last thirty years, have led to a plateau on life expectancy since 2009.[52] In the United States, life expectancy has fallen for three consecutive years since 2015, and this was before Covid reduced life expectancies for white, Black, and Latinx people by one, two, and three years respectively.[53] Maternal mortality rates in the United States are dismal, and in New York City, in this century, you are twelve times more likely to die after having a baby if you happen to be a Black woman than if you are a white one.[54] Globally, the number and proportion of hungry people is increasing and has been since 2015.[55] The Covid pandemic points to a systemic vulnerability in global health and health care systems.

Defenders of modern medicine can concede these points and still celebrate that, for instance, we no longer have to suffer smallpox, a disease that was once endemic in Europe and Asia and that was brought to the Western Hemisphere through colonization. The story of smallpox's elimination is, in miniature, the story of colonial medicine.

Edward Jenner is often credited as "the father of immunology" for having developed the smallpox vaccine.[56] Famously, people working in dairies, often women, already knew that a bout of cowpox conferred immunity to smallpox.[57] But it took Jenner to introduce the idea into the circles of medical knowledge—for this "old wives tale" to get the imprimatur of medical authority. He conducted experiments on young working-class boys, infecting them with cowpox and waiting to see if they then contracted smallpox. He wrote up his findings in the right kind of media, and medical knowledge was produced. Such was the success of his work that other European countries embarked on extensive vaccination campaigns.

The cowpox needed to be brought over in living human bodies. For this purpose, uninfected orphaned boys were taken from Spain and a chain of infection created between them, so that at any given time, at least one had productive cowpox boils. Four of the sixty-two boys died in the sea voyages of the 1803–13 campaign. Tens of thousands of people were vaccinated, and thousands of lives were saved. In the process, modern medicine eliminated existing pathways of knowledge and built temples to its own.

To be clear: we are supporters of peer-reviewed science, and we reference it widely throughout this book. Our concern is that the modern medical industry patches up bodies broken by the same system through which medicine itself was produced. It takes work to ignore the gradients of power across class, race, gender, and histories of genocide, enslavement, and theft. Modern medicine is, we'll argue, premised on the will to power, a systematic domination not just of some humans by others but of the domination of humans over other beings in the web of life. Let us call this practice of domination "colonial medicine." By ignoring the injustices that have produced it, and in which it participates by commission and by omission, colonial medicine is complicit in the damage it purports to heal.

A good example of this colonial sleight-of-hand is clear in a glass of water. The demand to stop fluoridating municipal water supplies is, in the United States, sometimes derided as paranoid. Sodium fluoride has been proven to reduce dental caries when applied to teeth. Caries are painful and can have long-term health effects. Low-income children are particularly prone to dental caries. If you remove fluoride from water, as Juneau, Alaska, did in 2008, the average number of cases of dental caries in children increases, in that case from 1.55 to 2.52 five years later.[58]

So is it a crime, as is so often represented in common sense, against poor children to stop fluoridation? We don't think so. It's possible to understand why children in low-income households have poor dental health, and to want to tackle that problem without subjecting a wide population to chemicals that have, surprisingly, a very thin epidemiological history.[59] While fluoridation may have emerged in the 1940s as a low-cost public health intervention to manage working-class dental problems, today it is a billion-dollar subsidy for the fertilizer industry, in which hydrofluorosilicic acid is a by-product. This industrial waste has found a lucrative afterlife in water supplies around the world.

Recent findings of neurological changes in children exposed to fluoridated water are surprising only because no one thought to look before to see what would happen if humans took a chemical that had been proven to protect teeth only when brushed onto them and then spat out, and started drinking it every day.[60] Resisting fluoridation doesn't mean condemning poor children to pain and future dentures:

it's understanding how industrial chemical companies make it easier to think about dosing an entire city rather than spend money on free dental care for the poor.

If fluoridation skeptics have a point, might a similar case be made for Covid skeptics? A survey in March 2020 suggested that nearly 40 percent of people in the United States thought the threat of Covid was blown out of proportion (54 percent of Republicans held this view versus 20 percent of Democrats), and 23 percent of rural people in the United States don't trust public health officials.[61] Almost everywhere, the pandemic has been politicized, and monetized, but this is nothing new. The World Health Organization identified "vaccine hesitancy" as a major public health threat in 2019, before the pandemic.[62] Leading the world in suspicions around vaccines are countries like France and Japan, where worries about medical safety are suffused with a distrust of the prevailing political class and the veracity of government information.[63]

How, then, can we condemn Covid deniers and still find fault with modern medicine? Like them, we're skeptical of authority and suspicious of those seeking to profit off a disaster.[64] The difference lies precisely in that the community constituted by saying no is, in our case, one that has a far longer history. We're not individual small-government conservatives of Reagan's vintage, or fearmongers of the Deep State. Along with Indigenous healers, we have a more nuanced understanding of health, power, and the colonial state. Our skepticism and refusal are rooted in science, not in a rejection of it. This is why our book doesn't pull away from the science we need to understand the biology, chemistry, physics, and ecology of inflammation. For those who haven't had the opportunity to read science beyond high school, we offer this book as an invitation to gain skills that have been denied you by a society that is increasingly skeptical of any kind of peer-reviewed science and that walls education away from the masses.

Our path through vaccine skepticism recognizes the history of mistrust and abuse that communities—particularly BIPOC people—

have suffered at the hands of medical and state power, and we offer a collective solution.[65] We embrace a vision of liberation grounded not in rugged individualism but in collective decolonization.[66]

DEEP MEDICINE

There is a medicine that is mindful and active in resisting colonial cosmology. Fighting the damming of rivers, the invisibilizing of Black pain, the clear-cutting of forests, the incarceration of minorities, the monocropping of foods, the poor health outcomes of Black and poor people, the land theft and genocide of Indigenous people, the wage gap, and the attempts to control women's reproductive power is all part of the healing arts that we call "deep medicine." It's a practice that any healer can begin immediately. It starts with the act of repairing those relationships that have been damaged through systems of domination.

In 2008 a young radiology resident, Yehonatan Turner, felt frustrated reading CT scans without knowing anything about the patients as people. He started including a photo of patients' faces alongside their scans and then studied the impact on radiologists, who could see the person whose images they were analyzing. All radiologists involved with the study reported feeling more empathy toward the patients after seeing the photograph, and in turn, the interpretations they gave were more "meticulous."[67] Rehumanization can begin with something as simple as looking at a photograph.

Human bodies are rendered alien from doctors through the rituals of education in biology. Most humans get some version of this biological miseducation in high school, and it is how most of us are taught to relate to the web of life. The school system teaches us to amputate our concern for other living beings and for the land itself. Animals are just meat, land is just a commodity, work can be bought and sold, humans are a resource, and everything else a means of production. The result is our license to use animals in any way we see fit and to be able to trade in land. This is how life and territory are orphaned from humans.

Rehumanizing, then, means seeing not only the human behind a CT scan but the more-than-human behind the picture of any individual. Our bodies have evolved in systems of deep relationships with the sun, soil, water, tides, seasons, archaea, bacteria, viruses, animals, plants, fungi, and the rest of the teeming world. Each of those depends on relationships with one another. The study of ecology is becoming indispensable to the study of medicine because humans are not just a single animal, but a multitude, an ecology of beings living on us, in us, and around us.

Studying the ways in which systems interact to create health or illness is the leading edge of a revolution of understanding in medicine. The reductionist understanding of disease in singular terms, such as one gene encoding one faulty protein or one drug targeting one receptor, can get us only so far. We evolved as systems within systems. There is nothing singular about us.

Today, instead of simply looking at the impact of one single gene, geneticists are looking at multi-omics, global assessments of processes and molecules that can give a more accurate picture of what is happening in a living being in states of health or disease.[68] Systems-level understanding is yielding important new understandings in medicine and in the very concept of health. Our anatomical systems are embedded in more systems—ones that humans have engineered and that make up our surrounding ecologies. At this space of intersection, the medical imagination is limited. Computing the total world of exchanges between the webs of life around us is a massive undertaking. Understanding how they interact to create harmony or dissonance is critical to mapping the future of health and life on the planet.

Decolonizing medicine begins with the project of rehumanization and reconnection, linking scans to people's faces; patients to their families, their cosmologies, communities, and histories; peoples to their lands and mountains and waters; and relatives to one another across the vast web of life. It is a process of imagining a "we" that is bigger than the sum of you and me. It involves a far wider community than Facebook can ever offer. It is the process of healing what has been divided and conquered. Resistance to colonial medicine is grounded in radical imagination: radical not as in somehow inconceivable or unattainable, but as prison abolitionist Angela Davis describes, as in "grasping things at the root."[69] Decolonizing is training our gaze on the origins of suffering in order to uproot them. It is the ambition to build a community of respect for the "animacy of life itself."[70] In a pandemic, it is recognizing that the source of the problem is not the vaccine or the billions that are made from it, but the fundamental disconnection from fellow living beings that allowed the disease to flourish in the first place.[71]

Disconnection lies at the heart of the origins of Covid. Indigenous communities have always taken animal lives, in ways that have respected and been grateful for those lives. But through decades of deforestation and habitat loss, we've forced those animals closer together. Animals that might have encountered each other only rarely are encountering one another far more often. Herein lie the origins of the interspecies jumps that likely produced Covid and that will produce the next pandemic: 60 percent of human infectious diseases come from pathogens that jump from other animals.[72] The industrial systems that turn animals into commodities make it easier for this to happen.[73] In 2009 H1N1 came from industrial pig production, possibly from the US-Mexico border. Covid mutated new infectious variants in the confines of Danish mink farms.[74] The global common denominator is a human supremacy over life that cannot fathom a greater intelligence than our own.

In Lakȟóta territory, elders will tell you that the damming of Mni Sose (the Missouri River) was the first moment in the cascade of events that led to now-endemic rates of diabetes. Traditionally, foods and medicines were gathered in the cottonwood forests at the banks of the river. But damming the river flooded these forests, and as this rich, sustaining ecosystem was lost, so too were the memories and traditions of how people had nourished and healed themselves for thousands of years. The people became increasingly sedentary and relied on food and medicine brought in by colonial forces through colonial structures that persist today. Rates of diabetes skyrocketed and have remained elevated ever since.

The Itázipčho and Oóhenuŋpa Lakȟóta elder Candace Ducheneaux believes the diseases that afflict the industrialized world are diseases of colonization. "The heart disease, lung disease, obesity, depression, diabetes, cancer, Alzheimer's, and auto-immune diseases which are so commonplace now never existed before the colonizers came," she says. Analysis of the remains of Indigenous people from the time before European invasion confirms her assessment. The excavated bones of precolonial ancestors show the presence of infectious disease, most commonly from *Staphylococcus* or *Streptococcus*. They reveal that anemia was common; abraded knees point to widespread degenerative joint disease. But the bones show no signs of diabetes.[75]

If you find yourself more convinced by studying skeletal remains than by listening to the oral histories of Indigenous people, you're a participant in a colonial system of organizing truth. Reconstructing history through bones misses much that oral histories capture. Yet in a colonial world, stories passed down by Indigenous elders cannot be considered true until they are validated by the empires that colonized them.

Colonialism has altered our relationship to knowing and understanding. It has altered the relationships that Lakȟóta people—and all people—once had with the world around them. It has policed what can be regarded as science, and who can be peers in review. More than that, it has severed a relationship to the past, to a cosmology that helped point to vital relationships between beings.

Colonialism has changed the architecture of how we live, imposing objectifying and extractive structures on cosmologies thousands of years old. It has changed how stories are told and which ones are told and which ones are forgotten. These structures persist and continue to wreak havoc on individual bodies, on our societies, and on the planet. Its signature is damaged relationships, and the outcome is inflammation. Nowhere is this clearer than in the practice of colonial medicine, which focuses on the individual to keep the systems invisible. Our individual healing is connected to healing our society, and our healing of the ecosystems upon which our lives depend. To engage in this holistic vision is to practice deep medicine.

THE ANATOMY OF INJUSTICE

Practitioners of modern medicine are not trained to be healers. They are trained to be biomedical technicians. When the causes of poor health lie outside the patient, in the environment or in society, doctors are frequently at a loss. Hunger, for instance, isn't considered a disease that falls under doctors' purview—a sign of how broken modern medicine has become. Doctors are trained not only to look exclusively at the patient as a solitary individual—shorn of context or structure, stripped of life in all its complexity—but to treat that individual as a broken machine, as a dysfunctional and occasionally noncompliant robot bearing a symptom. This is a relic of colonial thinking.

We have laid out this book as a subversive political anatomical survey, taking individual bodily systems and showing how ancient and modern science connects that body to the web of life through histories and relationships of power. Each chapter isolates one system of the body—immune, circulatory, digestive, respiratory, reproductive, skin, endocrine, and neurological—as seen through Western medicine. We want to take this familiar, disconnected understanding of health and make it strange by extending the borders and limits of those systems, weaving into them silenced histories, invisible ecologies, molecular movements, and mythologies. As such, we outline a cartography of illness, drawn by lines of power, in hopes of uncovering a path to a future where health in its broadest terms might be possible.

We use oral histories, historical source material, and peer-reviewed literature from several branches of knowledge to build our understanding of the interactions between the body, society, and the planet. While some of the studies we draw from speak directly to causation, many of the more recent data we cite outline powerful associations. These associations are often the first step in pointing scientific inquiry down the paths to more detailed conclusions around cause and effect.

For every example of colonial inflammation, we offer deep medicine, ways of thinking through how we might find one another through the work of decolonizing and through building communities of care. Since the diagnosis is systemic, our prescriptions are too. We don't offer encouragement to shop organic, to buy supplements, or to use apps for mindfulness. Decolonizing is not something that can be done alone. But it is already happening in communities where land is being rematriated, where solidarity economies of mutual aid and support are being established, where communities are renewing their relationships with local ecologies and retelling their stories, some of which have been silenced for centuries.

For Indigenous communities in North America, the act of connecting young people back to their ancestral lands is cutting suicide rates without the use of Western medicine or pharmaceuticals.[76] Having a sense of belonging improves health outcomes. Cultural continuity and dignity are in themselves determinants of health.[77] These benefits are available and relevant not to Indigenous people alone. They are a path for all of us who must learn to relate differently than in the prescribed ways—and with the proscribed identities—that colonialism has created for us.

For many, this won't be an easy book to read, because it *can't* be an easy book to read. Colonialism has made the institutions through which we daily become who we think we are. Historically it fashioned schools, hospitals, prisons, corporations, borders, charities, militaries, farms, and homes, whether in settler societies, postcolonial countries, or in colonial metropoles. Confronting that is difficult work, particularly because treating the inflammation we are collectively facing requires us to understand the dimensions of pathological thought that brought us here.

For some, especially those who are most impacted by colonialism's violence, certain sections of the book may feel traumatizing. The same may be true for those whose privilege comes through that violence. It was hard to write this book because it required taking an unflinching look at how we've been made by those histories. But with communities of care, it's possible to build a better world through that discomfort. Read together, out loud, if that helps. We're calling not for individual shame and therapy but for its political opposite: a collective reckoning, transformation, healing, and justice.

Decolonizing invites us to stretch our diagnoses back to a time when the concept of *the self* mattered less than the relationships upon which our lives depended, from the microbes inside us to the world around us. It calls on us to develop new methodologies of diagnosis, ones that center other ways of telling our stories and other ways of knowing that connect us to entities beyond our skin. Instead of pulling apart to know, we are bringing together to understand. This kind of diagnosis situates our damage and our healing more clearly in the past, present, and future.

We are grateful to you, our ancestors, our families, the ancestors of the stolen land on which we ourselves write and to their descendants who are still here, to the healers and holders of science before us and the web of life through which we have been able to write this book. We hope that your journey along this path will be as revealing as ours was as we wrote these words, and that by the book's end you will find yourself, as we have, a far more plural being.

1

IMMUNE SYSTEM

I AM BECAUSE YOU ARE

Biology is about recognition and misrecognition.

—DONNA HARAWAY[1]

The role of the physician is to translate "medically unknown symptoms" into social problems.

—NANNA MIK-MEYER[2]

What do you call second-class citizenship? Why, that's
colonization. . . . They try and make you think they set
you free by calling you a second-class citizen. No, you're
nothing but a 20th century slave.

—MALCOLM X[3]

The body has an ancient and powerful mechanism to heal itself: the inflammatory response. Inflammation occurs when the body's innate immune system responds to damage or a threat. Inflammation can be acute or chronic, localized or systemic, but it involves a whole host of cells and molecular messengers participating in a complex, choreographed set of interactions. The goal is repair and recovery—restoration of the body's optimal working conditions, a state called homeostasis.[4]

The acute inflammatory response is a time-limited event. Activity increases sharply in the face of a threat or injury and then resolves when the threat has passed and the damage is repaired. Once healing is complete, specific regulating molecules turn off the response.[5] Sometimes, though, the response doesn't switch off, and the result is a chronic systemic inflammatory state. When that happens, the body's healing mechanism is transformed into a smoldering fire that creates ongoing harm. The result is a crucial breakdown in the immune system's ability to repair damage and restore homeostasis.

Acute inflammation can begin with an infection, when innate immune cells recognize molecular signatures found on the surface of bacteria, fungi, or viruses called pathogen-associated molecular patterns. These signatures haven't changed much over millions of years of evolution, and because humans have evolved in tandem with these organisms, our innate immune cells have developed ways to recognize them. Acute inflammation can also be triggered by cellular injury. In this situation, damage-associated molecular patterns, which consist of cellular debris, are released in response to physical or chemical injury.[6]

Following activation by these molecular patterns, tissues and immune cells release a host of signaling proteins called cytokines. Some of these messengers amplify inflammation—they're called pro-inflammatory—and other, anti-inflammatory ones abate it. Pro-inflammatory cytokines—interleukin-1β (IL-1β), interleukin-6 (IL-6), and tumor necrosis factor-α (TNF-α), for example—keep the inflammatory response cooking. They stimulate the release of other inflammatory mediators, such as C-reactive protein (CRP) from the liver. These are some of the key biomarkers currently used to track acute inflammation.[7]

The acute and chronic inflammatory responses share some important characteristics and molecular mechanisms, but they also differ in essential ways. While acute inflammation is triggered by molecular patterns both from pathogens and from damages, chronic inflammation is prompted in the absence of infection. It is set off by damage-associated molecular patterns and other SOS signals from living cells that are under duress.[8] As such it is often referred to as "sterile" inflammation. Hormones and nerve signals that respond to psychological stress can set off these SOS signals.[9] So can air pollution and other characteristics of modern life. When the inflammatory response is sustained from repeated triggers, molecules generated by innate immune cells in response to these SOS signals create collateral damage. Add to that damage from an entire lifetime of exposures that generate more inflammation, and the body never has a chance to repair.

Acute inflammation can occur at any age, as we know from the toddler with an ear infection or the teenager with a skateboarding injury. But chronic inflammation happens only with advanced age. The older you get, the more likely you are to suffer from it; not only that, it ages you disproportionately. Your birth certificate might claim you're middle-aged, but you could clock decades older on the inside. This close relationship between aging and inflammation has led to the clever neologism "inflamm-aging."[10]

Central to this relationship is cellular senescence, the process by which aging cells permanently stop dividing but remain metabolically active. Under certain conditions, some senescent cells go on to express the senescence-associated secretory phenotype.[11] This functional change transforms them into vigorous producers of the pro-inflammatory cytokines and other molecules that drive systemic inflammation. Mounting evidence indicates that senescent cells with this phenotype are involved in the onset and progression of the age-related diseases of chronic inflammation, such as cardiovas-cular disease, diabetes, chronic kidney disease, chronic obstructive pulmonary disease (COPD), osteoarthritis, and Alzheimer's.[12] These cells may be driving the runaway inflammation of severe Covid in the elderly[13] and the pathology in autoimmune diseases, such as rheumatoid arthritis.[14]

But not all aging cells develop this phenotype as they become senescent. Ones that do have accumulated a lifetime of cellular dam-age due to a variety of exposures.[15] While both endogenous and ex-ternal factors can drive the development of chronic inflammation, a study documenting 210 healthy twins found that external factors—environmental and social—had the biggest influence.[16] Damaging ex-posures are the game changer, converting our aging cells into ones that do us harm.

The sum of lifetime exposures to nongenetic drivers of health and illness, from conception to death, is called the *exposome*.[17] The exposome encompasses chemical, social, psychological, ecological, historical, political, and biological elements that determine whether aging cells will become drivers of chronic systemic inflammation.[18] The exposome of modern industrial societies is rife with triggers for inflammation-related diseases. Modern diets contain more processed foods and less fiber, both of which can alter the gut microbiota pop-ulation and function, leading to changes in the immune system that can create inflammation.[19] When we are physically active, skeletal muscle releases anti-inflammatory cytokines called myokines,[20] but modern lifestyles increasingly limit the occasions for strenuous ac-tivity. Some cities are entirely unwalkable, necessitating travel by car. There's a reason that doctors are forever telling you to eat more fiber and get more exercise.

The exposome of modern life differs radically from that of In-digenous and traditional people who maintain critical relationships with the living systems upon which their lives and health depend.[21] While systemic inflammation and its accompanying diseases have increased dramatically across industrialized societies,[22] they remain rare in traditional ones, such as the Shuar hunter-gatherers of the Amazon,[23] the Hadza of Tanzania,[24] the Tsimané foragers who tend the forests of Bolivia,[25] the horticulturalists of Kitava, Papua New Guinea,[26] the subsistence farmers of rural Ghana, and even the Irish Travellers before they were recently forced into settled modern housing.[27] Members of these groups are exposed to a variety of microbes and infections, but they do not show the same chronic systemic inflammation that drives modern noncommunicable disease.[28]

The immune system is toned by the exposome, much the way a muscle is toned by exercise or a guitar string is made taut by turning a tuning peg. Immune systems toned by damaging exposomes seem to respond to an insult like Covid with overwhelming inflammation, like a string being pulled too tight. Severe Covid is overexpressed in socially oppressed groups.[29] Early in the pandemic, in the Zhejiang Province of China, severe cases were more often seen in agricultural workers and less frequently in people who were self-employed.[30] This trend repeated around the world.[31] An exposome that counteracted damage, making room for more care—like giving workers a guaranteed income so they could stay home with their families during the pandemic—would allow for a more measured immune reaction in the face of a real or perceived threat.[32] The interaction of the exposome with the genome gives rise to the disparities we see in health and illness across different demographics. While genetics play a part, the exposome's impact, we argue, is more immediate and, importantly, more alterable.

Were we writing a simple how-to book, we might point to ways you as an individual could address the pro-inflammatory exposome of the industrial world. For example, disruptions in circadian rhythms caused by the blue light from a phone at night lead to an increase in inflammation-driven diseases such as diabetes, depression, high blood pressure, and obesity.[33] So you could simply download an app that turns blue light to yellow at night. Or you could take melatonin, which has potent anti-inflammatory properties.[34] But many exposures aren't optional. They are systemic. Those who are working the night shift,[35] experiencing job stress, debt, and economic precarity,[36] enduring trauma from surviving genocide or police killings,[37] living with industrial waste,[38] noise,[39] and wildfire pollution[40] are people for whom exposure is rarely a matter of choice. The combined impact of the modern exposome is a shift in the inflammatory response, from one that heals to one that harms.

This damage is a consequence not of individual choices but of the mandates of a certain social, economic, political, and environmental ecology. To see these connections, and then repair them, is not to pine for a preindustrial lifestyle. It is instead to reject the logic of personal responsibility when so much of what shapes our health is beyond individual control. Once you see it, it's impossible to make peace with a world that causes this systemic harm—not without wanting to change it. This activation is what the philosopher Alain Badiou calls "exile without return," a practice we must apply to our medical approach. One must banish oneself from an empire of institutionalized medicine built on injustice and build a better way of healing, along with others committed to the same vision.[41]

Ideas of expulsion and belonging are ones that medicine deals with rather centrally. When you say you're shrugging off a cold, or fighting an infection, you're invoking a language of self-defense, together with an understanding of what should remain within the bounds in your body and what should not. No branch of medicine deals more directly with those issues of territory and belonging than immunology.

THE *IMMUNES* STRIKE BACK

The word *immunity* derives from a legal quirk of the Roman Empire. *Munus* in Latin kicked off the English word *municipality*. *Munera* (the plural of *munus*) were the duties that Roman citizens were obliged to perform.[42] As the Roman Empire expanded, it extended a kind of second-class citizenship to nonmunicipal cities within the boundaries of its empire. Foreign residents of these *civitates liberae et immunes* were not properly Roman in the same way as Rome's nonslave male inhabitants. They were thereby exempt—*immune*—from the duties that made them fully Roman.

It is unclear whether Rudolf Virchow, one of the founders of modern medical immunology, knew of this history, but he certainly understood what it felt like to be *immune*, to be within a world yet estranged from it. During the Revolutions of 1848, Virchow was both a citizen of Berlin and not properly of the Berlin in which he found himself. He was armed and ready to fight the old world so that the new world might be born. The Prussian forces "shot at us from a great distance, out of range for a pistol," he reported from atop the barricade.[43]

Virchow wasn't alone. The Revolutions of 1848 reverberated throughout Europe and the world. From Finland and France to Chile and Brazil, restive urban workers recognized their second-class citizenship and rose up to demand justice—equality, better working conditions, a political and social voice. Within the literature that informed the uprisings, *The Communist Manifesto,* which first appeared in German in February 1848, is perhaps the most widely known. It is no coincidence that just a few years earlier, in 1845, one of its authors—Friedrich Engels—had written an epidemiological work, *The Condition of the Working Class in England.*[44]

In order to write it, the twenty-four-year-old Engels had excused himself from "the dinner-parties, the port-wine and champagne of the middle classes," to spend time in conversation with Manchester's working class.[45] He used ethnography, epidemiology, geography, and class analysis to account for why he found "the rate of mortality four times as high in some streets as in others, and twice as high in whole classes of streets as in other classes."[46]

Clearly, Virchow had read Engels.[47] In 1848 he and his colleague Rudolf Leubuscher editorialized in their new journal *Medical Reform* that "medicine is a social science, and politics nothing but medicine on a grand scale."[48]

Virchow was born into a farming family, but one well-connected enough to secure his admission to the best medical college in Berlin, where he proved an exceptional student.[49] In 1848, at the age of twenty-six, he was appointed to a governmental commission to investigate an outbreak of typhus in Upper Silesia—what is now modern Poland and Czechia—a region that had been annexed by the Kingdom of Prussia and was under the domination of its German-speaking aristocrats.[50] While he was there, he saw how disease and hunger ran together, in "a devastating epidemic and a terrible famine."[51] His diagnosis was a social critique:

> The worker has been permitted to demand the means of his subsistence, he has been guaranteed work to enable him to acquire the means, there were those highly praised Prussian schools to provide him with an education appropriate to his class and, finally, the sanitary police were entrusted with the task of supervising his living conditions. And what an army of well trained civil servants were available to enforce the laws. They intruded into private affairs, watched over the most intimate social relations, and assiduously patronised any attempt on the part of "the subjects" to improve themselves. The law was there, the civil servants were there, and yet thousands of people died of famine and epidemics. The laws were useless, for they were nothing but words on paper. Similarly the actions of the civil servants merely resulted in words on paper. . . . The civil servants had not been appointed by the people to serve their interests. Rather they were appointed by the police state and to serve the interests of the state. Thus, the civil servants were either the oppressors of the people or mere typewriters.[52]

A radical new political vision was needed to address the impact of Prussian imperial rule on public health. Lack of education in the native language, "the Catholic hierarchy," and "the great landed proprietors" were the silent vectors of the typhus epidemic.[53] And the doctor's prescription: "education in the Polish language; self-government, separation of church and state; shifting of taxes from the poor to the rich; improvement of agriculture; development of cooperatives; and the building of roads."[54]

Like epidemics, famine is neither natural nor inevitable. The widespread hunger that Virchow witnessed in Upper Silesia was a policy failure driven by external events, ones that swept across Europe. The market economy was being brutally enforced throughout the continent. In England's first colony, Ireland, a lack of genetic diversity had left the potato crop vulnerable to infection by a fungus. From 1845 to 1849, a million Irish citizens died from famine. And yet in 1846 Ireland exported 500,000 pigs and 30,000 tons of grain to England, where prices were higher. The Irish died for want not of food but of money to buy it.

When local government officials in Cork proposed paying Irish laborers higher wages for a public works program that would allow them to buy food for their families, *The Economist* scolded them for the error of suggesting

> to pay them not what their labour is worth, not what their labour can be purchased for, but what is sufficient for a comfortable subsistence for themselves and their family. Do they not see that, on this principle, they must pay a man not in proportion to the value of his labour but in proportion to the size of his family—that they must pay the decrepit and imbecile married man with ten children at least 2 [shillings] per day, while the able, diligent, frugal, and fore-looking bachelor may be put off 4 [pence] or 6 [pence]? Do they not see that to do this would be to stimulate every man to marry and to populate as fast as he could, like a rabbit in a warren—in other words that to apply this to Ireland would be to give brandy to a man lying dead drunk in a ditch?[55]

To put it bluntly, as *The Economist* did in 1846, "they have been kept at home and taught to rely more than ever on others and less than ever on themselves." Rather than be tempted by such policy, Ireland's colonists should adhere "to the principles which have been deduced from many facts by scientific men and confirmed by experience."[56] Suffering was the stimulus the poor needed to enter the labor market. Any attempt by the government to interfere with the laws of laissez-faire would merely prolong the economic injury, rather than allowing it to heal.

The same liberal economics that plagued the Irish also harmed the Silesian colonial subjects. The Silesian textile industry was in steep decline and got no support from the Prussian Empire, despite a workers' uprising in 1845.[57] The convergence of an El Niño cycle, which disrupted weather patterns,[58] incubated crop diseases and drove up food prices across the continent, combined to expose deeply entrenched inequities between the German-speaking elite and the Polish periphery of Prussian society—a political, social, and economic system that made the famine possible.[59] When Virchow returned to Berlin that spring, he found a world on fire. The city was one of several across Europe where the urban poor had reached a breaking point. Decades of political organizing had raised workers' hopes and expectations, so when the combination of climate shock and disease precipitated a global food price spike, they were ready to take to the streets.[60]

Throughout Europe, states crushed the Revolutions of 1848. Virchow himself was exiled from his post at the Charité Hospital for his participation in the uprising.[61] And while in his later years he might have resigned himself to the counterrevolution,[62] his biological research would continue to be animated by ideas of action and reaction, justice and exploitation, belonging and betrayal. He hypothesized that infectious diseases like tuberculosis and typhus were caused not by the bacterium itself but by the body's reaction to the bacterium. He also speculated that because the cells of different people reacted in different ways, the diseases presented with varied expressions. Virchow believed that social conditions more than anything else primed the body for these expressions: oppression would lead to more pronounced manifestations of disease, and justice would enable healing.[63]

Given his deep commitments to equality, Virchow was suspicious of racial categorizations and the hierarchies of supremacy they supported. At the dawn of the German nation-state, the political right championed scientific racism under the banner of Darwinism. This is why Virchow was a fierce anti-Darwinian.[64] In a bid to disprove the scientific racism of the 1870s, he oversaw a study of 6,758,827 German schoolchildren, which measured the skull sizes of Jews and Aryans and showed that there was no such thing as a pure German race.[65] (The Nazis would attack his work decades later.) But Darwin continued to cast a shadow over the study of the body's defenses, including the question of how the body knows to muster a defense in the first place. In the conclusion of his epochal book *On the Origin of the Species by Means of Natural Selection, or the Preservation of Favoured Races in the Struggle for Life*, he summarized the process of natural selection like this: "from the war of nature, from famine and death, the most exalted object which we are capable of conceiving, namely, the production of the higher animals, directly follows."[66]

When we think of the immune system, most of us think of war: our bodies defending against and destroying a foreign invader. It's a startling, even unsettling militaristic image—one that can be traced from Darwin to a Russian scientist who attacked a starfish with a rose thorn.

METCHNIKOFF AND THE MACROPHAGE

In his autobiography, Ilya (Élie in translation) Metchnikoff, the Russian zoologist whose inquiries were foundational to modern immunology, recalls a fateful day in 1881:

When the whole family had gone to a circus to see some extraordinary performing apes, I remained alone with my microscope, observing the life in the mobile cells of a transparent star-fish larva, when a new thought suddenly flashed

across my brain. It struck me that similar cells might serve
in the defense of the organism against intruders. . . . I said to
myself that if my supposition was true, a splinter introduced
into the body of a star-fish larva, devoid of blood vessels or a
nervous system, should soon be surrounded by mobile cells
as is to be observed in a man who runs a splinter into his
finger. This was no sooner said than done. There was a small
garden to our dwelling . . . [and] I fetched from it a few rose
thorns and introduced them at once under the skin of the
beautiful star-fish larvae as transparent as water.[67]

When he put indigo on the tip of the offending thorn, he could
see small cells from within the larva's skin cluster around it and engulf the droplets of dye on the thorn's surface, "eagerly devouring"
the intruding enemy.[68] How, Metchnikoff wondered, did the starfish
know that the thorn didn't belong inside its body, and why did it
react the way it did? He wondered whether it was possible to devise
a general theory of this reaction, looking not only at the redness
and bleeding that signal an immune reaction in humans but more
broadly at the web of life.[69]

These investigations, inspired by the starfish, were the basis of
a series of remarkable lectures, "The Comparative Pathology of Inflammation," that Metchnikoff gave at the Pasteur Institute in 1891.[70]
Alive with curiosity and scientific insight, he began the first lecture
with the observation that infection is "a struggle between two
organisms"—a nod to Darwin's *On the Origin of Species*.[71] Metchnikoff
proposed to do for infection what Darwin had done for the struggle
between species: "The phenomena of the active struggle among animals . . . being much more prominent, have attracted the attention
of naturalists for years, whereas those of infection, which are far less
on the surface, have been but rarely and insufficiently studied."[72]

After announcing his ambition in the first lecture, he turned in
the second to look at the smallest units of life. He saw a Darwinian
struggle between individual single-cell creatures, which engage in
complex chemical and biological warfare to preserve themselves and

fend off attackers.[73] In the third lecture, he moved from single-cell organisms to simple multicellular animals and plants.[74] Although they could heal and regenerate, he found that plants showed no signs of inflammation.[75] Their cells couldn't engulf and devour enemy organisms because the cell walls were so thick, a result of having evolved for a static and defensive life. In other organisms, however, he saw a capacity for motion that allowed their cells to eat the various intruders he introduced to them. Cellular digestion, then, according to Metchnikoff, was the difference between a thick, woody knot on a wounded plant and a similar scar that formed on a person's skin. Although these healings might look superficially similar, scar tissue in animals requires a star actor that doesn't exist in plants: the phagocyte.[76]

Phagocytes are, literally, cells that eat. Phagocytosis involves engulfing things, such as bacteria or dead cells. Metchnikoff saw phagocytes as central to inflammation. When watching a hydra grow a new head, he observed "the regenerative side of inflammatory processes, but not the phenomena of inflammation itself or at least not the accumulation of phagocytes at the injured spot."[77] In other words, you know when inflammation is happening because the phagocytes show up. For Metchnikoff, inflammation was *defined* by the presence of "a phagocytic reaction on the part of the animal organism" to foreign parasites.[78] Note that he wasn't terribly interested in the *healing* part of inflammation. He didn't say in his lectures whether his starfish larvae lived to be pierced another day.

For Metchnikoff, there was no cease-fire, no armistice, no deescalation: merely one phagocytic victory upon another, *ad mortem*. Inflammation was a flare of conflict and a sign that well-regulated patrolling of the body's perimeter was taking place. This is how Darwin's metaphors of perpetual war were directly translated into our conventional understanding of the immune system, a violent interpretation of our healing processes that still haunts modern medicine today.

Metchnikoff's seminal research identified what we now call the *innate immune system*, which reacts immediately to ancient molecular patterns that signal damage or infection. Inflammation and phago-cytes are part of this first-responder branch. There are several im-mune cells that engulf things, but the hungry phagocyte that captured Metchnikoff's imagination is called the macrophage. It is a key player in wound healing and in chronic inflammation.

But the immune system has another branch, one that illustrates a less violent scene of healing: the *adaptive immune system*, also called the *acquired immune system*. It is more specialized in its actions and stores memories of prior infections.[79] After inoculation against a vi-rus, for example, the adaptive immune system learns that when it encounters that same pathogen, it should generate T cells to remove infected cells, and it expands B cells to make antibodies that bind to and neutralize any free-floating virus. When the worst has passed, a few responding T and B cells remain in circulation, "remembering" that exposure pattern, ready for future encounters. The adaptive im-mune system develops specific biological responses and maintains recognition of prior exposures over an individual's lifetime, through antibodies and memory cells.

The innate immune system has also developed ways of recogniz-ing organisms, through pathogen-associated molecular patterns. That memory is instilled before birth and transmitted across generations. In other words, the innate immune system serves as a community resource. Having built up recognition mechanisms over eons, it es-tablishes a transgenerational molecular vocabulary that allows it to respond to various requests for attentive care, regardless of an indi-vidual's prior exposures.

Adaptive immune cells work closely with the innate immune cells, and various phagocytes—dendritic cells, macrophages, and neutrophils—are the bridging communicators.[80] The adaptive immune system's precise response is a function of the delicate interplay be-tween cytokines and other cellular signals from the innate immune system, which dictate which cells will carry out particular tasks—from clearing intracellular organisms to eliminating cancer cells to eradicating parasitic worms that might have made their way into the body.[81] It's less a war of dominion than a dance with multiple partners and multiple directors, each taking and giving cues to the other. It is set across the entire body, choreographed with the purpose of maintaining optimal functioning conditions.

The adaptive immune system and the innate immune system work together to shape immunity types, which are characterized by specific cytokine profiles and actions. Type 1 immunity finds and eliminates microbes that manage to steal into our cells, such as bacteria, protozoa, and some viruses. Type 2 immunity induces cells and antibodies to protect against helminths and venoms. Type 3 immunity incapacitates extracellular bacteria and fungi. Importantly, these different types are determined by how prior exposures and the surrounding environment tone the immune system.[82]

When the immune system is improperly toned—for example, by too much of a toxic exposure or by not enough beneficial microbial exposure—types 1 and 3 immunity can cause autoimmune disease, and type 2, allergic diseases.[83] Children growing up on a small farm where no pesticides and mostly hand tools are used develop protection from developing allergic disease,[84] but those growing up in California's Salinas Valley, where farmworkers are exposed to robust levels of organophosphate pesticides through industrial agriculture, develop an increased risk of allergic disease.[85] The difference is due to the environments that shape their type 2 immunity.

Lupus, asthma, inflammatory bowel disease, atherosclerosis, multiple sclerosis, and diabetes are all examples of inflammatory diseases that occur when these various types of immunity are functioning incorrectly.[86] We are still learning how the shaping of these immunity types leads immune cells to react in different ways, but over the past century and a half, the science is proving that Virchow's insights about systemic factors were prescient. The invisible human structures created by society, as well as the invisible nonhuman community—microbes and helminths and other creatures—who live among us, shape our immune modulation.[87] Future research may demonstrate an immunity type that is characterized by the body's reaction to the grind of social oppression. Covid has provided us with an unparalleled opportunity to deepen our understanding here.

Social forces precondition, for example, how bodies react to the SARS-CoV-2 virus. The same infection is expressed differently in different groups of people because of how the immune system has been toned over time, through lifetimes and ancestries of social oppression. Severe manifestations of Covid occur in people with impaired activity of type I interferons.[88] Interferons get their name because they are a kind of cytokine that interferes with viral replication,[89] and they can avert a massive inflammatory response in the face of viral infection.[90] Genetics account for some of the variation in circulating levels of type I interferons, but it doesn't paint the whole picture.[91] Chronic social defeat—a technical term describing repeated and inevitable loss in moments of social conflict—suppresses type I interferon activity and overexpresses pro-inflammatory cytokines.[92]

Severe Covid is also mediated by the senescence-associated secretory phenotype, which, in addition to appalling conditions in nursing homes, may explain why elderly patients have had it so rough in the pandemic.[93] But this phenotype is also generated through accelerated aging brought on by cellular damage, the causes of which we will explore fully and which include phenomena such as stress, trauma, and environmental toxicity.[94] The exposome of oppression, made concrete through the architecture of our society, preconditions the immune system for catastrophic reaction to Covid infection and helps explain one aspect of why death rates were so high in historically oppressed groups, ravaging poor, Black, Indigenous, and Latinx communities in the United States.[95] Covid has revealed the violence that our society inscribes on certain bodies, those that colonial powers have alienated and deemed to be foreigners and foes.

It is no wonder that modern medicine has imagined the immune system to be a war machine, poised to crush our enemies. The metaphor mirrors Cartesian ideas about the borders between "self" and "other," that colonial cosmology that opens the door to violence and domination. Metchnikoff's writing, like Virchow's, was shaped by the politics of his day, which in turn were the politics of the modern state. As the physician and historian Alfred Tauber put it, for Metchnikoff, the phagocyte "acted as an autonomous agent to serve as the body's police, conferr[ing] conformity to the integrated whole."[96] What he conjured is the modern border patrol agent, a roving database of possible threats, capable of discriminating between foreign and domestic ones. And if ever a body appears not to belong, the dutiful phagocyte of colonial medicine will act as judge, jury, and executioner.

THE "BROKEN WINDOWS" THEORY OF IMMUNOLOGY

Through the first half of the twentieth century, as Europe reluctantly granted independence to its colonies, *immunes* became immigrants. The former colonists admitted their erstwhile colonial subjects to the metropole—including our own parents.[97] There they were never embraced as locals, but merely tolerated.

In 1949, soon after India's independence and the formalization of apartheid in South Africa, a scientist from another former British colony made explicit the "self" and "other" tacit in Metchnikoff's work. The Australian immunologist F. Macfarlane Burnet published the second edition of his *Production of Antibodies*,[98] spurred by the 1928 Bundaberg Tragedy. In a freak accident, twelve out of twenty-one children given a diphtheria vaccine in Bundaberg, Queensland, had been killed. The subsequent inquiry pointed to *Staphylococcus* bacterial contamination as the culprit—which was an odd finding indeed. Our skin is teeming with *Staphylococcus*, and we don't usually die from it.

Macfarlane Burnet stuck to a Darwinian interpretation of this medical mystery. He suggested that over evolutionary time, the predator-prey relationship can in some cases arrive at a stalemate. Otherwise-fatal *Staphylococcus* achieves a state of immunological equilibrium, where the "self" of the body recognizes it as "other" but is able to tolerate rather than vanquish it.[99]

Once again, immunology developed in tandem with the politics of its time. According to Macfarlane Burnet, the body, like liberalism, called for a tolerance without parity, contingent on the recognition of a "self" and an "other." People deemed "other" would not be killed but merely tolerated—*immunes* in a perpetual state of nonbelonging.

If liberalism's problem is that "religious, cultural, or ethnic differences are sites of natural or native hostility, [t]olerance is conceived as a tool for managing or lessening this hostility to achieve peaceful coexistence."[100] But there's a difference between those doing the tolerating and those being tolerated. As the philosopher Wendy Brown puts it, from the perspective of the modern imperial hub, "we *have* culture while they *are* a culture."[101] The flip side of liberal tolerance is that it upholds colonial supremacy.

Today, one of the enduring problems facing immunologists is that humans don't come preloaded with immunity to everything. Even with phagocytes and the acquired immune system, the body doesn't know how to attack every possible threat. Rather than stamping everything foreign as automatically bad, the immune system behaves more subtly, embracing a truth that many politicians don't: most foreigners are friends, not foes. The biologist Polly Matzinger, who arrived at her trade via an unusual route, understood this as few of her fellow scientists did.

The daughter of a French potter and a former nun, and a World War II resistance-fighter-turned-painter-and-carpenter, she came from a creative and restless family. Her youth involved stints as a jazz musician and a *Playboy* Bunny. Living in Davis, California, she frequented a bar that was a favorite drinking spot for local professors. One day she overheard a conversation about animal mimicry, and she asked, "Why has no animal ever mimicked a skunk?"[102] Taken with the originality of the question, one of the professors encouraged her to become a scientist.[103]

In an interview with *The New York Times*, she shared her experience in graduate school:

> We learned that the immune system fights anything that isn't part of our bodies. But that didn't make sense to me. I wondered why mothers didn't reject their fetuses, why we didn't reject the food we eat, or the stuff in the air we breathe. But my professors all said, "Don't worry about it."
>
> So I stopped worrying. This is a cowardly habit that we scientists can fall into. If we really can't answer a question, we sometimes stop asking it.[104]

Early in her career, she wrote seminal papers that were so innovative, she knew she would not be taken seriously as a young woman publishing solo. So she arranged for some of her early papers to be coauthored by her colleague Galadriel Mirkwood—her dog.[105] Within a decade of finishing grad school, she was working at the National Institutes of Health, asking that question about identity and rejection once again. Her research pushed up against the "sheer number of things to which we must be tolerant—all the potential peptides made by 55,000 different bodily proteins, plus more than 1012 potentially different B and T cell idiotypes—while maintaining the ability to respond to foreign antigens."[106]

Matzinger challenged the idea that the human body is as interested in "the self" as nineteenth-century liberalism was. It is a dynamic assembly of many different species, from our own cells to the millions of organisms who live on and inside us, whose presence is critical for development and health. The "self" of immunology is more porous and fluid than the one in liberal political science, able to be shaped by social, economic, and political injustices. Matzinger herself wrote, "The immune system does not care about self and non-self[;] its primary driving force is the need to detect and protect against danger."[107] In other words, it is "more concerned with damage than foreignness."[108]

But just as Metchnikoff's work was informed by the prevailing imperial politics and metaphors of his time, Matzinger's work drew on the social and political cosmologies of the post–Cold War United States, which included the rise of neoliberalism and its updated attitudes toward social control. She invited readers to

> imagine a community in which the police accept anyone they met during elementary school and kill any new migrant. That's the Self/Nonself Model [of immunity].
>
> In the Danger Model, tourists and immigrants are accepted, until they start breaking windows. Only then do the police move to eliminate them. In fact, it doesn't matter if the window breaker is a foreigner or a member of the community. That kind of behavior is considered unacceptable, and the destructive individual is removed.
>
> The community police are the white blood cells of the immune system.[109]

Like Metchnikoff's and Virchow's analogies, Matzinger uses ideas about the police in the body politic, another unfortunate example of how colonial carceral logic seeps into modern medicine. But her analogy describes a very different conception of police function, reflecting a new social order that preaches tolerance and moves us away from the citizen-foreigner dichotomy. In the "broken windows" theory of policing, it is the presence of *disorder*—a broken window that remains unfixed in a low-income neighborhood—that is equated with danger. Likewise in the Danger Model, only entities causing or threatening actual harm in the body trigger the immune response.[110]

Matzinger agreed with her predecessors that the immune response is complex, contextual, and multifactorial. Where she differed was in her identification of the triggers. Therein lies the explanatory power of her model. She found that the immune response "is called into action by alarm signals from injured tissues, rather than by the recognition of nonself."[111] A damaged cell will release damage-associated molecular patterns triggering inflammation.[112] For example, an abundance of uric acid, a highly inflammatory molecule produced by cellular damage, creates the clinical syndrome known as gout. Phagocytes that bridge the innate and adaptive immune systems take up these alarm signals and present them to T cells to activate a further, more engulfing inflammatory immune response.

The Danger Model also describes how a nonself entity, such as a virus, can become a beneficial agent of transformation for the self. Cells have developed mechanisms to resist viruses, but there are no living species without viruses. And viruses can bring about adaptive biological change. They are estimated to cause almost 30 percent of the adaptations in proteins that humans have in common with other mammals.[113]

Viruses that fly under the radar long enough to incorporate their genetic material into host cells can give rise to new phenotypes that may confer a survival advantage. Viral-derived genes are crucial to the evolutionary development of the human placenta. A viral gene encoded a protein that allowed the virus to fuse to host membrane cells, facilitating infection. When that viral genetic material got inserted and stabilized into the human genome, its function was repurposed. That same protein's fusing capability now promotes a layer of cells that merge the placenta and the uterus.[114]

The recognition that immunity is a process of negotiation and damage management, rather than a complicated kind of passport control at the border of self and other, has profound implications. Matzinger's model builds on Virchow's intuition. Illness is not simply caused by a foreign entity: it is the body's response to damage that may or may not be precipitated by that entity. The immune system is not just a war machine, as many still tend to think it is. Viruses can become us, a part of who we are. Humans are not little states with their own border patrol but assemblies in a web of life.

It's important to recognize, however, the limits to Matzinger's analogy. It still follows the colonial framework of "self" and "non-self," drawing on the liberal concept of tolerance to explain how they relate. Liberalism, while preaching tolerance, creates an entire class of disenfranchised people that it deems to be "other." In some cases, liberal tolerance actually justifies this disenfranchisement. At first blush, broken window policing may seem more tolerant, but it has been used to justify the overpolicing of *immunes*—low-income, Black, brown, and Indigenous communities. Only the mere presence of disorder gives the police license to enter a home, too often to fatal effects. The point here is not to position Matzinger's broken window immunology as infallible but to show how modern medicine always reflects the colonial politics of its time.

Medicine has come to understand the emergence of disease through the metaphors of war and tolerance because these were the liberal and neoliberal political metaphors at hand. Virchow was right when he understood "medicine as social science on a grand scale." What happens, then, when we're ready to see medicine in general, and the immune system in particular, not as a theater of war but as a composition with the rest of the web of life? What does that song actually sound like?

THE ART OF HEALING

As you speed through the pages of this book, the paper slices into one of your fingers. Cue the orchestra. Wound healing is a symphony in four overlapping movements: hemostasis, inflammation, proliferation, and maturation. *Hemostasis* can be understood by the word's Greek roots: *heme*, meaning "blood," and *stasis*, meaning "stoppage." It is the body's attempt to stanch bleeding. When paper slices skin, the rupture of blood vessels exposes circulating platelets to the protein collagen, which forms the stretchy matrix of connective tissue that sits right under the vessel wall's inner lining. This contact starts the process of blood clotting,[115] setting off the coagulation cascade, a biochemical counterpoint between platelets and chemical messengers, that leads to clot formation and laying down the matrix upon which repair cells can work. Assuming the coordinating duties of conductor, cytokines released by platelets motion the orchestra to the next movement, which opens with a crescendo in the inflammatory response.[116]

In this second movement, which is fast and bombastic, neutrophils are the first white blood cells to set the urgent melody. These are phagocytes that harmonize the innate and adaptive immune responses. They are chemically drawn to the injury by the mediators that the platelets released. These mediators also make the blood vessels in the area leakier, facilitating the migration of more white blood cells—and incidentally swelling the skin around the cut. Neutrophils make even more inflammatory cytokines, such as IL-1α and IL-1β, amping up the inflammatory response by calling in other white blood cells to layer the harmony, by way of consonance, dissonance, and ultimately resolution. Neutrophils start this harmonic exploration as they begin eating up bacteria.

Macrophages and leukocytes are the next white blood cells to join the inflammatory movement, with macrophages taking the lead.[117] They stop bacteria in their tracks by releasing molecules called free radicals, such as reactive oxygen species. These free radicals cause damage to the bacteria and to our own cells. Macrophages also release nitric oxide, which also causes local blood vessels to dilate, bringing more blood-borne assistance by way of other immune cells to the site of injury. That's when the bass drops. When nitric oxide synthesis is impaired as it is in diabetes, wound healing is also impaired.[118] As they play their part, macrophages also clean up the stage, phagocytizing dead bacteria and other debris and using enzymes to remove and digest dead tissue from the wound. They also regulate the creation of the scaffolding upon which the new skin will grow. At the same time, they call on and invite the participation of cells that will proliferate to make the new skin and cells that will stimulate the growth of new blood vessels.[119]

The third movement of wound healing is proliferation. New voices emerge, bringing the promise of repair. Fibroblasts, endothelial cells, and epithelial cells set the mood here. They are coaxed by the cytokines and growth factors released by platelets and macrophages to lay down the substances needed to heal the skin.[120] While the inflammatory movement was full of tension, with broad strokes, the theme of this movement is precision. Fibroblasts migrate to the wound site, where they produce collagen just until enough has been laid down—indicating the precise, remarkable biological control of wound repair.[121] Endothelial cells, which constitute the inner lining of blood vessels, create new blood vessels—a process called angiogenesis. Likewise, epithelial cells, which form the skin's outer layer, start proliferating at the wound's edges to cover it up in response to the same inflammatory cytokines and growth factors.[122]

The final movement, the denouement, is maturation. Here the theme of the prior movement is broken down, and a stronger but slower variation is elaborated—*adagio*. The original clot is dissolved, and the collagen that was initially laid down is replaced with another version that increases the wound's overall tensile strength. Granulation tissue, which makes up the wound healing bed, is replaced with a scar. Then the movement continues over months, with remodeling occurring on the cellular level, in a beautiful call-and-response between the cells and the extracellular matrix that they create and that surrounds them. After three months, the scar reaches its maximal tensile strength, just 80 percent that of unwounded skin.[123] The immune cells go quiet, the wound repair process switches off, and the healing is complete.[124]

A WOUND THAT NEVER HEALS

The body's capacity to heal wounds is part of its ingrained intelligence, evolved over millennia in tandem with its surroundings. But the modern world has thwarted these mechanisms of healing, turning them into ones that do more damage. This is no more evident than in the inflammatory disease whose etiology is becoming clearer and whose rates are growing worldwide—cancer.

In 1863, Virchow hypothesized that cancer occurs at the site of chronic inflammation, where irritants and the inflammation they cause encourage cells to proliferate out of control.[125] His intuition was spot on. The microenvironment in inflamed tissue supports the transformation of normal cells into cancerous ones, in a process called neoplastic progression. When cellular proliferation is sustained and occurs with the ongoing presence of inflammatory cells, growth factors, and DNA-damaging agents, cancer happens. In this context, instead of normal wound repair with the inflammatory response turning off, cells sustaining DNA damage continue to proliferate, taking advantage of the growth factors that tissue injury brings.[126] Cancer cells then hijack wound healing's inflammatory machinery to serve their own growth. The inflammatory response, instead of healing a wound, continues to cause injury. Cancer is, in essence, a wound that does not heal.[127]

Let us explain how this works. When the immune system functions in its optimal state, it can detect and eliminate nascent cancer cells before they become a problem.[128] This process is called immunosurveillance and is indispensable in the defense against cancer. Immune cells survey tissues for signs of cellular DNA damage, and when they find it, they can arrest the cell's replication by forcing it into senescence, or activating apoptosis—the cell's programmed death function. But as we know, when cells are forced into senescence, some will go on to develop the senescence-associated secretory phenotype, prompting more inflammatory cytokines. These in turn contribute to the microenvironment of inflammation in the tissue where a tumor grows.[129] In chronically inflamed tissues, cancer cells can escape this immunosurveillance and continue to grow undetected.[130] This is when cancer becomes clinically evident, growing from a few aberrant cells to a mass you can feel or detect on a CT scan.

As tumors grow, they develop more techniques to evade the immune system's detection. They also produce pro-inflammatory cytokines, recruiting and hijacking a diverse population of immune cells for their own self-preservation.[131] One type is the macrophage, which, under the influence of cancer cells, expresses a cytokine that curbs the antitumor response of T cells, in essence training the immune system to tolerate the cancer.[132] These macrophages secrete compounds that promote angiogenesis, making new blood vessels. Now the tumor is tapped into the body's nutrient supply and into its liquid network of blood vessels and lymphatics, which malignant cells can use as a superhighway. This is how cancer spreads, or metastasizes.[133]

Just as Virchow noticed, many malignancies start at a site of infection or chronic inflammation, which is why conditions associated with chronic inflammation come with an increased risk of cancer: colorectal for inflammatory bowel disease,[134] esophageal for acid reflux,[135] prostate for prostatitis.[136] After tobacco smoking, infections are the leading cause of preventable cancer, responsible for over 15 percent of malignancies worldwide.[137] Persistent infections can induce chronic inflammation.[138] The human papillomavirus can lead to chronic inflammation of the cervix,[139] and certain strains are responsible for 80 to 90 percent of all cases of cervical cancer worldwide.[140] The hepatitis B virus brings about hepatitis (inflammation of the liver), and if that infection becomes chronic, you're 13.7 times more likely to develop liver cancer.[141] The bacterium *Helicobacter pylori* generates gastritis (stomach inflammation) and peptic ulcers, which can lead to gastric cancer.[142]

To resolve a persistent infection, white blood cells produce reactive oxygen and reactive nitrogen species, part of their normal response to an organism that sets off the inflammatory response. But these free radicals cause cellular and DNA damage in our own tissues too.[143] This cycle of cellular insult and then repair, which involves increased cellular proliferation, generates an environment of marked genetic instability. As cells replicate to repair damaged DNA, our genes can get copied with errors introduced. These mistakes slip by uncorrected, giving rise to genetic mutations. Some of these mutations allow a cell to grow without regulation.[144]

Infecting viruses can also simply insert cancer-causing genes into the host's DNA. Likewise, immunosuppressive viruses, such as HIV, can undermine immunosurveillance, allowing cancer to escape detection.[145] Cancer also subverts apoptosis, keeping tumors growing in spite of their load of damaged DNA. As the disease progresses, tumors often outgrow their blood supply, resulting in further tissue damage. This sets off more inflammation.[146]

If DNA damage is the spark that starts the fire of cancer, inflammation is fuel for that fire. And cancer itself is an inflammatory state.[147] Even in tumors without a known direct causal link to inflammation, such as breast cancer, inflammation is present.[148] Treatment of colon cancer and certain other cancers with nonsteroidal anti-inflammatory medications, like aspirin, consistently decreases cancer rates and deaths.[149] Because cancer thrives in this kind of milieu, immunotherapy now targets not only the tumor itself but also the inflammatory microenvironment.[150]

FIGHTING FIRE WITH FIRE

While inflammation appears to be a largely pro-tumor phenomenon, certain kinds can have an antitumor effect, meaning that immune and inflammatory cells can actually destroy tumors. T cells and macrophages survey and get rid of aberrant cells,[151] and they can be trained to enhance their cancer-fighting properties.[152] The skin condition psoriasis, for example, often features intense inflammation but presents no increased risk of cancer. This inflammation mobilizes macrophages in a way that promotes their anti-tumor actions.[153]

"Good inflammation" activated by the innate immune system to protect against cancer was something that William Coley noticed in the late nineteenth century. He was a surgeon treating sarcoma, a fast-growing and fatal bone tumor. He observed that people who developed severe postoperative wound infections caused by the bacterium *Streptococcus* at the tumor site had spontaneous and sustained tumor regression.[154] So he injected a few of his other sarcoma patients with *Streptococcus*, to see how that might impact the tumor. The cancers he was treating did regress, but the infection ended up killing the patients. Later he mixed a slurry of heat-killed bacteria *Streptococcus pyogenes* and *Serratia marcescens*, creating a concoction he called Coley's Toxin.[155] This time the formulation didn't kill anyone. And according to his case reports, it promoted tumor regression.[156]

In spite of this reported success, Coley did not standardize his formula, and his record keeping was disorganized, making it hard to generalize his findings to other treatment settings. Perhaps most important, Coley's Toxin struggled to find favor at a time when pharmaceuticals were being developed from recently discovered petroleum. At the turn of the twentieth century, up to 95 percent of all oil refining in the United States was controlled by J. D. Rockefeller. The Rockefellers shaped the path of medical research by generously funding scientists who were developing drugs from petrochemicals as the magic bullet for cancer treatment.[157] The medical institution derided Coley's work with microbial extracts as lacking clinical evidence. But some diehards remained convinced that the immune system could be stimulated or enhanced to cause tumor regression. In 1962 a clinical study of Coley's Toxin found a dramatic response in twenty of ninety-three patients.[158] A follow-up report on Coley's work, compiled by his daughter, Helen Coley Nauts, also showed the concoction's effectiveness. Of the thousand patients he had treated, five hundred had complete regression of the tumor.[159]

More recently, on the principles Coley followed, *Mycobacterium bovis* Bacillus Calmette-Guérin (BCG) has become the mainstay of treating superficial bladder cancer. In fact, it is one of the most effective examples of cancer immunotherapy. BCG introduced into the bladder induces "good inflammation," mobilizing the body's own T cells and macrophages and their cytokines to fight the cancer.[160] Not only does

BCG stimulate the immune destruction of cancer cells, but it leaves their memory in T cells, suppressing recurrence. For more advanced cases, BCG delays progression to metastasis and improves survival rates.[161] Another example of immunotherapy is the use of IL-2, a cytokine that expands certain T cell populations in a specific subset of patients with metastatic melanoma, a deadly skin cancer. Lifespans increased for people with what was formerly seen as an untreatable disease.[162]

Interestingly, some acute infections appear to *lower* the risk of cancer and increase the odds of cancer regression. Childhood mumps has been associated with a lower incidence of ovarian cancer,[163] and the measles and mumps vaccine available today can boost the immune system's response to cancerous cells.[164] The measles virus has anticancer properties, which can be put to better service in people who have already been vaccinated.[165] Infant illnesses, such as a cold before the age of one year, are known to prevent acute lymphoblastic leukemia, by priming the immune system to prevent this cancer from forming later in childhood.[166]

This priming may explain why *Helicobacter pylori* infection rates are high but gastric cancer rates are low in Black Africans, while both infection and gastric cancer rates are high in Black Americans.[167] The environment that most Africans encounter is on average microbially richer than that of the Global North. It appears that bacteria, viruses, and parasites tone immunity in a way that protects against cancer, even in the face of a bacterium known to cause it. People of African descent on the Pacific coast of Colombia also have high rates of *Helicobacter pylori* and low rates of gastric cancer.[168] Helminths and other parasites are common there and likely contribute to this immune priming.[169]

That said, as Virchow knew, the exposome matters. The exposome of many Black Americans is microbially denuded and contains numerous systemic triggers of chronic inflammation: intergenerational trauma, trauma from police killings, daily acts of discrimination, debt, and water and air pollution.[170] All these exposures push the body out of homeostasis, and taken together, they cause its alarm systems to ring nonstop. The immune system endeavors to rebalance in the face of this damage, like a dancer who missteps and tries to find their center of gravity again. Social oppression preconditions the bodies of Black people in the United States, so that when *they* encounter the bacterium *Helicobacter pylori*, they are far more likely to develop gastric cancer.[171]

A hundred years after the medical establishment derided Coley's work, the field of immunotherapy now holds some of the most promising advances in cancer treatment. Like her father, Helen Coley Nauts was a strong advocate for such research. She too was disparaged by experts in the field, such as Cornelius "Dusty" Rhoads, the first director of the Sloan-Kettering Institute, now the Memorial Sloan Kettering Cancer Center. Rhoads became infamous for a leaked private letter in which he wrote about transplanting cancer into his Puerto Rican patients in an effort to exterminate them.[172]

The scandal didn't slow his career. The Rockefeller Foundation funded him generously, and more specifically, its spin doctor, Ivy Lee, supported him. Lee had been handling media crises for the family ever since the 1914 Ludlow massacre, when twenty-four people—including children—were killed in a labor riot that broke out at a Rockefeller-owned mine.[173] She managed to get preprint access to articles about Rhoads's letter and altered the language to make it sound like his racism was only "a joke."[174] Pictured on *Time* magazine's June 27, 1949, cover, with the title "Cancer Fighter,"[175] Rhoads became conventional chemotherapy's biggest cheerleader. He favored repurposing mustard gas, from a chemical weapon derived from petroleum to something doctors infuse into a patient's bloodstream.[176] Metchnikoff's view of the immune system as a kind of war machine endures: killing is much easier to conceptualize than healing. Undeterred, and convinced by her father's findings, Nauts established the Cancer Research Institute in 1953, which continues to support cutting-edge investigations into immunotherapy.[177]

Advances in this field have made common outcomes that were unheard of just twenty years ago. A man with metastatic melanoma lives disease free ten years after diagnosis. The tumors of a woman with renal cell carcinoma vanish after treatment stops. What sounded fantastical back when many currently midcareer physicians were in training is now one of the most promising areas of drug development for the treatment of cancer. Unlike chemotherapy, which directs a seek-and-destroy approach toward tumors, immunotherapy targets the immune system at various points to unleash its own ability to eliminate cancer cells.[178] We know by now that the choreography of the immune system can be either hindered or supported. When we support those processes, by stopping the ongoing damage causing inflammation and by enhancing this innate healing ability, we allow the dance to happen in its most health-enhancing way.

Checkpoint inhibitors were some of the first, most effective immunotherapy drugs to hit the market. They hone in on specific molecular sites that act as brakes on T cell activation and proliferation. In the absence of malignancy, these brakes create immune tolerance and prevent autoimmunity.[179] When they are inhibited, the brakes are released—cytotoxic T cells and natural killer cells become free to unleash their wrath on cancer.[180] Checkpoint inhibitors now extend survival in metastatic melanoma patients past what prior standard treatment offered.[181] Clinical trials of these drugs demonstrate remarkable tumor regression in different kinds of cancers.[182]

While these drugs hold great promise, there's a catch. Enhancing the immune system's cancer-eliminating functions is associated with lots of collateral damage in the form of—you guessed it—inflammation: enterocolitis, hepatitis, pneumonitis, myocarditis, dermatitis, and autoimmune kidney damage, to name a few.[183] In some cases, inflammation of the pituitary, thyroid, and adrenal glands have necessitated lifelong hormone replacement.[184] In rare cases, inflammation of the brain has occurred, proving fatal.[185] As research progresses and treatments become more targeted, these side effects are under better control, but the very nature of these drugs is to release the same function of T cells that drives autoimmunity.[186]

Another problem is that the most effective checkpoint inhibitor therapy treatment course for advanced melanoma literally costs four thousand times its weight in gold: approximately $295,566 per patient. With 589,430 patients dying from metastatic melanoma annually in the United States, the bill for their treatment would come to $173,881,850,000. Even with adjusted doses and schedules, these drugs are still exorbitantly expensive, costing as much as $1 million per patient per standard treatment course.[187]

Modern chemistry promises to take cancer away, but it's hard to ignore that industrial chemistry also causes cancer. Cancer rates are 2.5 times higher in what we call "developed" nations than in poorer countries.[188] In China, North America, and Europe, where cancer rates are the highest in the world, the disease ranks as the leading cause of death for people ages thirty to sixty-nine.[189] As poor countries push for so-called development, their cancer rates are rising too, even when controlling for things like improved detection and population aging.[190] India's Cancer Train, which transports sick peasant farmers from the fields of Punjab to the cancer hospital in the neighboring state of Rajasthan, is a sign of this catastrophe.[191] The agricultural Green Revolution of the 1960s that brought increased crop production also brought loads of synthetic pesticides and fertilizers, which leached below the surface, poisoning the water brought up by pumps at village wells.[192] Those working closest to the ground are most susceptible to the carcinogenic effects of these chemicals.

Lorenzo Hidalgo was thirty-six years old when he was diagnosed with one of the most aggressive forms of colon cancer his doctors had ever seen. A child of undocumented immigrants, he was born and grew up in a farmworker community, where his father worked in the fields and his mother raised the children. For ten years, Hidalgo was employed as a gardener and frequently applied the herbicide Roundup to suppress weeds on the grounds, when he was instructed.

Physically fit and an active runner with no prior history of illness, he knew that something was wrong when he developed an unusual, aching pain in his groin and in his back. CT scans revealed a mass in his colon and masses in his liver, bones, and lungs. Biopsies showed that a rapidly proliferating form of colon cancer had spread throughout his body. In the last few weeks of his life, the mass in his colon bled heavily, and he became dependent on blood transfusions, unable to leave the hospital lest he exsanguinate. Ultimately, the transfusions could not keep pace with the bleeding, and Hidalgo died exactly four months after he first felt the pain.

Today, Roundup is the world's most popular weed killer.[193] Marketed by the Monsanto Corporation in the 1970s, it was touted as far safer than the herbicides it replaced. But rising rates of young people dying from colorectal cancer began in the mid-1990s, at the same time as the release of seeds genetically engineered to tolerate Roundup.[194] Glyphosate is the active ingredient in Roundup, and its use increased fifteen-fold from 1996 to 2014.[195] In 2015, the International Agency for Research on Cancer (IARC), the World Health Organization's cancer unit, designated it as "probably carcinogenic to humans," fueling lawsuits that, to date, have yielded $11 billion in settlements.[196]

A 2013 study conducted at the Chulabhorn Graduate Institute in Thailand found that because glyphosate can act like estrogen, it causes hormone-dependent human breast cancer cells to grow.[197] This research was one of over a thousand publicly available studies that informed the IARC decision, and one that contributed to a rich debate about the future of pesticides in Thailand.[198] The Thai National Hazardous Substances Committee voted in October 2019 to ban glyphosate, along with chlorpyrifos (associated with neurological developmental delay in children)[199] and paraquat (banned in Europe since 2007).[200]

Bayer purchased Monsanto in 2018, and rushed to defend its new asset. The company approached the US Department of Agriculture's undersecretary for trade and foreign agricultural affairs, a former employee of Dow Agrosciences. The US trade representative gathered intelligence on the relevant Thai government officials, information that was supplemented by dossiers provided by yet another agricultural conglomerate, Archer Daniels Midland. Ultimately, the Thai government backed down from the glyphosate ban, though the government succeeded in prohibiting chlorpyrifos and paraquat. (All three chemicals are available for purchase in the United States.) Despite the industry's best efforts, dozens of countries currently or soon plan to have restrictions on glyphosate.[201]

Stopping glyphosate use is especially important because it induces epigenetic changes in DNA, suggesting a pathway for generational toxicity, as if its effects on individuals weren't bad enough.[202] Epigenetic changes are alterations to our genome that do not affect the DNA sequence but do impact genetic expression. They impact what DNA is expressed and how it is expressed. These changes are how damaging exposures—from environmental chemicals to violence—become written onto, not into, our DNA.[203] Studies on identical twins raised in two different environments are offering insights on how epigenetics are influencing disease.[204] Twins share the same genetic material but can manifest disease differently, influenced by environmental exposure. And those environmental differences can be subtle, even within the same womb, where fetal placement or umbilical cord size might be different. With the Zika virus in Brazil, twins were born where one had the infection and the other was spared. Infection risk in utero with these twins was an epigenetic phenomenon.[205]

The addition of methyl groups onto DNA was the first identified epigenetic modification and is the change brought by glyphosate.[206] These DNA tags can alter cellular functioning and inhibit the expression of certain genes.[207] This is one way cells that have the same genes, such as a nerve cell and a muscle cell, synthesize different proteins with different functions. While DNA methylation is a normal part of cellular differentiation, it can be caused by environmental chemicals in parts of the genome where methyl groups interfere with healthy functioning.[208] When methyl groups occur in our germ-line DNA—how glyphosate can impact sperm—those alterations are transmitted to future generations. Health problems were not seen in the rats exposed to glyphosate or even in the first generation of offspring. It was the great-grandchildren of exposed rats that had increased rates of prostate disease, obesity, kidney disease, and ovarian disease, caused by methyl groups added into genetic regions involved in these conditions.[209] We are living with the impact of exposures our great-grandparents experienced. And our great-grandchildren, too, are at risk from the exposures we face. Consider, then, the wisdom of the Haudenosaunee people, whose Seven Generations Principle holds the present generation accountable to the forthcoming community that their actions will impact.[210]

Glyphosate is in our food, our water, and the dust under our feet—just one example of how global capitalism affects human health. Because it is so widely used, you would very likely find it in your urine if you went looking. A random sample revealed glyphosate in 93 percent of the people tested.[211] Data collected over twenty-three years, starting in the early 1990s, shows a 1,200 percent increase in levels of glyphosate and its metabolite in urine of people over fifty in California.[212] Consuming an all-organic diet can drop urinary levels by 76 percent in just six days.[213] But organic food is more expensive. When the market determines our exposure, our health apartheid will inevitably get worse. Lower-income communities have little choice but to eat foods that are chemically contaminated.

Glyphosate is one of many harmful chemicals that have become prevalent in our lives, unbidden and dangerously underregulated. The consequences of a toxic planet for the human immune system aren't surprising.[214] In the Global North, children are increasingly diagnosed with cancer.[215] Treatment is catching up with illness, and the number of children who die from the disease is falling. Inevitably, however, gradients of power govern incidence and recovery: low-income children are more likely to die than their richer peers,[216] and people of color and the poor are more likely to be exposed to environmental hazards and other systemic triggers for chronic inflammation.[217]

In the story of cancer and chemistry, the harm comes from exposure, and exposure inversely follows gradients of social power. Disproportionate harm is wrought on liberalism's second-class citizens: the working class, women and children, the disabled, the colonized. But revolution requires new perspectives. If you look down from Virchow's perch on the barricades, you'll see that it is from communities of these very *immunes* that deep medicine emerges. Great change has always come from incensed citizens ready to agitate for it. If you're struggling to think of an analogue to Rome's *Civitates liberae et immunes*, you needn't look too far. In the United States, look only to one of its largest colonies: Puerto Rico.

HISTORY IS WRITTEN IN THE BODY

Puerto Rico is the Western Hemisphere's oldest continual colony, known as Borikén to its Indigenous people. Columbus arrived on the island during his second voyage in 1493. The Spanish subjugated and enslaved the island's inhabitants to work colonial plantations and gold mines. Violence and disease took a drastic toll on the native population. The story written in the official census reports goes like this: in 1778 there were 2,300 Indigenous inhabitants on the island and by 1802, the original people of Borikén were extinct.[218] Modern-day descendants were told they were largely of Spanish ancestry. But the whispers of grandmothers on the island tell a different story, and a study of mitochondrial DNA confirms their claim. A survey of people across Puerto Rico found that the majority have Indigenous DNA. The next most common ancestry is African, and coming in last is Caucasian.[219]

The Boricua healer, ceremonialist, and two-spirit activist RaheNi Gonzalez reclaims the identity "Taíno," a moniker used by colonizers to refer to the Indigenous people of the region. They reflect on the history of their ancestors and how that manifests in Puerto Ricans today. "A lot of people denied their indigeneity on the island, because of colonialism. So people pushed their Indigenous heritage away as racism made social hierarchies. Indigenous identity went underground. But it was always there. In my family, we have people with European features like blue eyes, people with Indigenous features and long straight black hair, and family with African features with dark skin."

Those structures of racism persist today, as Puerto Ricans live like *immunes* in their own homeland. Having prevailed in the 1898 Spanish-American War, the United States annexed control of Guam, Puerto Rico, and the Philippines, establishing a second wave of colonial rule. The new conqueror's legal system tried to solve the ensuing riddle: what do you call lands that you've conquered and would very much like to keep as part of your country, without calling them colonies or granting the humans living there anything like citizenship? In its 1901 Insular Cases, the US Supreme Court ruled that these islands were "foreign to the United States in a domestic sense"—that is, they were outside the United States because they had not been among those states that had united to form the country, but nonetheless they were encompassed by US sovereignty. Residents were US nationals but not US citizens.[220] Not quite self and not quite other.

Today Puerto Rico has yet to recover from the devastations of US rule. Congress wields tight fiscal control over the islands' debt repayment regimes, through a Financial Oversight and Management Board.[221] While Puerto Rico's money matters to its colonists, the bodies of the island's inhabitants don't. In a 2016 study of Medicare users, comparing Hispanics on the mainland to Hispanics in Puerto Rico, those on the island received a significantly worse level of care when evaluating across seventeen different performance goals, such as blood pressure control and access to appropriate medications.[222] Good medicine is hard to come by, as is good food.

When Gonzalez travels home to the island, they have a hard time finding healthy things to eat. They are sensitive to chemicals in industrial food offerings, and Puerto Rico's markets are flooded with food they can neither eat nor afford. "Most of what's available there is processed food and junk food. When you find a cauliflower that costs you $3 in Oakland, it costs you $8 on the island, thanks to the

Jones Act. Before colonialism, we used to be healthy people, with good diets of fish and yucca. Now I have a hard time eating in my own ancestral territory."

In 2017 Hurricane Maria tore through the island. The official death toll was 64; a Harvard study estimated a mortality of 4,645.[223] But to the US government, Puerto Rican death appeared to matter as little as Puerto Rican life. Gonzalez felt that the hurricane woke the people up from their slumber.

> When Hurricane Maria came, it shook the island up, and it shook everyone awake. How the US failed to help us showed how alone we really are. People went months without stable access to power, food, and water. It forced my people to step up and show up for themselves. People, especially the younger people, started organizing and growing their own gardens, all over the place to feed themselves and the community. They are getting in touch with their Taíno roots, the language, the rituals. They are remembering the old names for the plants. It's an awakening.

Across the island, agroecological projects are cropping up. Before the hurricane, Puerto Rico imported about 80 percent of its food. "After the hurricane," says Sylvia De Marco, who works the land in Huerto Semilla, an agroecological garden in the heart of San Juan, "even people who didn't care about food started to care. It really opened people's eyes: that we have to depend on our soil, not shipping containers."[224]

Restoring the island's agriculture will mean healing from structures and policies that dismantled Indigenous ways of tending the land and growing food. And that will involve healing from the trauma that colonialism brought and that persists today with US domination. Gonzalez relates, "When the colonizers came, they found good, loving, healthy people. We lived in balance with our surroundings and ate well. What does it do to watch your loved ones murdered, raped, and enslaved? The impact of that trauma lasts through the generations."

Aoife O'Donovan is a researcher who hails from the world's other oldest colony, Ireland. She is elucidating the biological pathways of trauma on the body that Gonzalez intuits. In fact, the impact of trauma really does last through generations, and its trace is scribed by inflammation. Post-traumatic stress disorder (PTSD) is a mental illness characterized by depression, anxiety, and a state of hypervigilance caused by exposure to traumatic events. Evidence is accumulating that trauma and PTSD impact the immune system and are strongly associated with inflammatory diseases. Trauma is an element in the exposome that tunes the immune system to sound out the full range of systemic inflammation.[225]

O'Donovan views stress and inflammation as adaptations that have important short-term benefits but terrible long-term impacts. The connection between trauma and inflammation appears to be transmitted both genetically and nongenetically. "It makes evolutionary sense," says O'Donovan. "If I'm living in a traumatic and stressful time, my children should be born ready to deal with the challenges in the world around them." Some of that priming happens in utero.[226] And it also happens when parents around the world do what they always do with their children—tell them stories.

Storytelling is a critical part of the exposome. Stories shape our understanding of the world around us and our place in it. Elders describe for children what is dangerous and what is safe in the environment around them. Stories are how cosmologies are created, recreated, and passed on, and they have real biological impact. If you are told stories from a very early age that the world is a terrible and dangerous place, the stress of that will literally get under your skin and shorten the lifespan of your cells.[227] Black children in the United States are given "the talk" about the very real dangers of police violence that they face—a lifetime risk of being one in one thousand murdered by law enforcement.[228] While this communication is of the utmost importance in preparing Black children for the police terror they face, it can also lead to shortening of the life cycle of their immune cells.[229] In such ways, a story literally gets translated into the molecular language of our cells. The problem here is not the story but the social reality of racist police violence that makes internalizing the story an act of survival.

The mechanism by which a harmful reality creates damage in our cells is the acceleration of our cells' aging process.[230] Cellular aging is determined, in part, by the length of the ends of our chromosomes—called telomeres. Telomeres are noncoding repetitive segments of DNA that form protective caps on the ends of our chromosomes.[231] In normal aging, with cell division, a bit of the telomere is lost.[232] After a telomere is shortened to a certain length, cell division stops forever, and the cell enters senescence.[233] A cell's telomere is its molecular clock, dictating how many divisions it has left, or how much longer it will live. The shorter a cell's telomeres, the fewer cell divisions it will have, and the faster it will reach senescence. The older we get, the less telomere length we have.[234]

There is an enzyme that reverses this course, called telomerase. It is active in embryonic development and, in adults, in stem cells and activated immune cells. Telomerase adds more telomere back, prolonging the time before a cell enters senescence. Throughout life, telomere length appears to be a dynamic phenomenon.[235] Telomerase has been dubbed the "fountain of youth" enzyme, and current research is investigating what activates it, in hopes of extending the duration of healthy cell functioning. As with every aspect of the immune system, this same benefit, given an unhealthy milieu, can be used for harm. When a cancer develops, it exploits this enzyme to give its cells immortality.[236]

While telomeres are shortened normally through cell division, they erode abnormally through a damaging exposome—by environmental toxicities, oxidative stress that causes DNA damage, and trauma.[237] In one study, women with the highest level of perceived stress had telomeres shorter by ten years than women with relatively low stress.[238] Black men who report unfair treatment by police, experienced either personally or through the stories they're told, have shorter telomeres than people who do not experience this trauma.[239]

Trauma can prune telomeres in childhood, when a child is exposed to stressful events.[240] This is one plausible mechanism by which adverse childhood events, such as being exposed to violence in early life, lead to inflammatory diseases such as cardiovascular disease and diabetes in adulthood. Remember that a telomere is like a clock, and it appears to get set in childhood. Once the clock runs out, those immune cells become senescent. If the senescence has been forced by telomeres damaged through exposure, these cells then drive systemic inflammation.

When a pregnant woman experiences severe stress, the unborn baby experiences telomere shortening, which makes violence against pregnant women an urgent public health issue. Zoom out, and you'll see that ancestral stress and trauma trigger changes in the descendants who did not experience the exposure firsthand, mediated through epigenetic changes.[241] Many of these changes are reversible. With care, telomeres can lengthen again.[242] But even if these alterations are dynamic, the fact that they happen highlights how a socially oppressive exposome can damage people's health for generations to come.

Back in Borikén, Gonzalez asked what it does to the body to witness so much trauma. We now see how history becomes embodied, written inside our cells, carried in our molecules. Inheritance transports the biological weight of the past through the present, into the future.[243] Genocide, and the PTSD that ensues, leaves deep wounds, and the immune system keeps those stories alive in the body. Consider how the trauma of US rule impacts the people of Puerto Rico today; the prevalence of autoimmune disease there is high, with the highest lupus rates in the world.[244]

After decades of chasing down genetic markers for lupus, researchers are turning more of their attention to the environmental causes of autoimmune disease.[245] Along with toxins in the air, they must also consider how history and lines of power shape the immune response along these inflammatory pathways. The healing process must involve restructuring the world to make it a safe place for survivors to flourish—in other words, deep wounds require deep medicine.

CULTIVATING COMMUNITY IMMUNITY

There are things that can lower inflammation in the body and diminish the danger signals set off by a dysregulated immune system. As we've said, eating better can help: the "Western diet" is implicated in all kinds of autoimmune trouble.[246] One large-scale study found that French people who said they consumed organic food had lower cancer rates than those who didn't.[247] And eating less—30 percent fewer calories than normal, called caloric restriction—while maintaining a healthy level of nutrients can revitalize the immune system.[248] Deciding to restrict one's caloric intake or to eat pesticide-free fruits and vegetables may indeed be medically wise. That 2 billion people in the world don't get to make that choice doesn't invalidate the science.[249] But it does clearly show that immunity is not a problem that can be solved merely at the level of individual choice.

Taking some actions for your own health may improve the prospects of those around you. As we all emerge from more than a year of lockdown, this ought to be familiar. Zoologists use the term *social immunity* to refer to what happens when an immune response is beneficial not just to the individual mounting it but also to others in the community. Many animals have discovered the benefits of living in close proximity. Cooperation in groups leads to more efficient care of the young, more abundant food procurement, and more effective defense against predators.

But when an infectious disease takes hold, it can spread rapidly among those sharing close quarters. Animals as diverse as honeybees, lizards, and primates have developed practices that confer immune protection to the whole group. Social insects offer antimicrobial secretions to one another, practice social distancing and quarantine, collect and dispose of waste, and protect nests from infected individuals.[250] It's tempting to see here a harmonious and perfect representation of what humans ought—but fail—to do to contain an outbreak. But insects will also kill both infected and healthy neighbors to prevent the spread of disease among their community. We are very glad that humans rarely do this in a direct way. And yet institutional neglect and structural violence make the outcomes functionally similar.[251]

In Durban, South Africa, a city of 3.4 million people, around 1 million residents live close together in informal shack settlements.[252] These settlements have "VIP" toilets—ventilated improved pit latrines—but their deep pits are rarely emptied of feces. S'bu Zikode, a student who lived in one of the settlements near the University of KwaZulu-Natal, found children playing in a dump one day. As he approached them, he saw white flecks around their mouths. "I thought they'd been eating rice," he told us. But looking closer, he realized that the children were playing in seething piles of parasites. "What I witnessed that day was devastating and something that shocked me, something that was hard to share because it was just unbelievable." It moved Zikode to start organizing for better toilets, access to water, and the creation of a childcare facility. His struggle is part of a global one; shack settlements house over a billion people around the world.[253] Nearly 4 percent of all deaths worldwide today could be prevented with better water and sanitation.[254]

S'bu Zikode helped start an organization called Abahlali base-Mjondolo (from the Zulu for "residents of the shacks"). It exists to protect the dignity and livelihoods of people who are waiting for the South African dream to reach them.

Shack settlements were land occupations in the 1970s, 1980s, and 1990s—spaces within the segregated cities of apartheid South Africa in which Black people lived without permission in white neighborhoods. After apartheid, the African National Congress–led state assured residents that these spaces were only temporary waiting rooms, to be evacuated during the transition between apartheid and the new South Africa, born in 1994. Since then, however, the shack settlements have grown and now act as permanent housing. There migrants from beyond the city, and sometimes the country, live and even die while waiting for a better life.

Abahlali baseMjondolo has antagonized the ANC by drawing attention to the degrading conditions in which shack dwellers are made to live and the betrayals they've endured. Despite these circumstances, systems of mutual aid flourish. Newcomers to the shack dwellers movement undergo a conscious process of political education. The protocols that make social immunity work in these settlements rest on the philosophy of *ubuntu*. Zikode explains it like this:

> We are human beings *because* of others. When we have induction workshops, we teach not just about leadership but about how one becomes a better human being. If you get that right, you are actually avoiding a number of misconceptions that follow. Because [being a member of Abahlali baseMjondolo] is not about you. It's about a culture of taking responsibility for a nation. A culture of individualism is much more used in this capitalist system, where, you know, it's all about you.

Abahlali's understanding of "nation" isn't defined by the colonial dichotomy of self and other, by a mandate for belonging or not belonging based on unequal distribution of power. Instead, belonging is about whether you are part of the community. In 2008 and 2015, waves of xenophobic attacks in South Africa targeted hundreds of alleged foreigners,[255] but not in the settlements affiliated with Abahlali baseMjondolo.[256] Rather than participate in the communitarian violence and identity politics peddled by the ruling party, Abahlali

shack dwellers recognize that citizens and noncitizens are all equal
as *abahlali*, "residents":[257]

> If you live in that settlement, you are part of that settlement.
> So you are protected not only from being attacked, not only
> from hate, but from all forms of discrimination. If we were
> an organization of service delivery, we would fight over lim-
> ited resources or services. But we do not do that. Before
> we engage in the politics of service delivery, we engage in
> a politics of *ubuntu*, a politics of humanism that defines us.

One of the protocols of *ubuntu* is taking the time to greet others. Each person asks every person in the room how they and their
family are, and they are asked these questions in turn. It takes a
while, but the alternative, Zikode points out, is worse. To casually
ask "What's up?" and not care about the answer is to succumb to the
misconception that you are who you are solely because of yourself.
An inquiry about someone and their family is a diagnostic act, a way
of probing to make sure that relations are thriving, an opportunity to
make sense of how someone is now because of what they are going
through elsewhere.

The extent to which relationality matters in *ubuntu* is hard to
overstate. In English, the "I" in "I am because of others" is a fixed
entity—but in *ubuntu*'s conception, the "I" is more fluid, more plural:
"I am/becoming because of others."

The state treats the shack dwellers as *immunes*, nominally free but
not fully of society. This is why movements within such settlements
go out of their way to affirm these people's dignity and personhood.
As the armed revolutionary Virchow understood, being a second-
class citizen means knowing that a better world must be brought into
existence. It means recognizing the current state of emergency and simultaneously imagining a radically different future. It means knowing that the self contains multitudes. The feminist scholar Donna

Haraway describes "the split and contradictory self" as "the one who can interrogate positionings and be accountable, the one who can construct and join rational conversations and fantastic imaginings that change history."[258] James Baldwin threatened "the fire next time." *Immunes* know that the time is nigh for fire, and it's time to get to work.

2

CIRCULATORY SYSTEM

SALMON ARE THE PUMP

The hundred rivers of the earth are like the streams of blood [*xuemo*] in man. Just as the streams of blood flow along, penetrating and spreading, and move and rest all according to their natural order, so it is with the hundred rivers.

—WANG CHONG[1]

You ask me to plow the ground! Shall I take a knife and tear my mother's bosom? Then when I die she will not take me to her bosom to rest. You ask me to dig for stone! Shall I dig under her skin for her bones? Then when I die I can not enter her body to be born again. You ask me to cut grass and make hay and sell it, and be rich like white men! But how dare I cut off my mother's hair? It is a bad law, and my people can not obey it. I want my people to stay with me here. All the dead men will come to life again. Their spirits will come to their bodies again. We must wait here in the homes of our fathers and be ready to meet them in the bosom of our mother.

—SMOHALLA[2]

D r. Heather Certain was forty-four years old when she had her heart attack. She had none of the traditional risk factors—no high blood pressure, no high cholesterol, no history of smoking, no diabetes or family history of cardiovascular disease. She was an avid runner, clocking an average of twenty miles a week, an easy nine-minute miler. Fifteen years out from her medical training, she was working as a hospital-based physician, or hospitalist, in Madison, Wisconsin.

For three weeks, she had had a stuttering chest pain that came and went. She chalked it up to acid reflux. Because we have been taught to look out for heart attack symptoms characteristic in men, it is common for women and their doctors to overlook their rather different presentation: fatigue, arthritis, sleep problems, and acid reflux.[3] Women often seek help later than men, and clinicians don't address their concerns as quickly because they don't attribute the symptoms to something as serious as a heart attack. But when about a quarter of all heart attacks, regardless of gender, result in sudden death before the patient arrives at the hospital, this poses a problem.[4]

Over the course of a week, Certain's pain became more intense and persistent. After she attended a high-intensity exercise class, she took two antacids and then two more. The pain got worse. She told her husband to take her to the emergency room. On the way there, the pain became crushing, radiating to her jaw, her left shoulder, and her back. She was unable to get out of the car by herself. The emergency room staff took her into the hospital and performed an

EKG, which showed the dreaded tracing that is characteristic of an acute blockage of one of the arteries delivering blood to the heart. She was taken to the catheterization lab, where her heart entered a fatal cardiac rhythm. Twice the paddles were applied to her chest. Twice she was shocked back to life.

Cardiologists threaded a catheter through the radial artery in her wrist all the way upstream to her heart. They poured dye into her vasculature and took pictures. They saw a complete blockage of the left anterior descending artery. This blockage is invariably fatal without intervention. It's sometimes called "the widow maker," but that's an anachronism: since 1984 in the United States, more women have died annually of cardiovascular disease than men.[5] For people over forty-five years old, within a year of having a first heart attack, 26 percent of women will die compared to 19 percent of men. Within five years of having a first heart attack, 47 percent of those women will die, compared to 36 percent of men.[6]

One factor influencing these dismal results is the gender of the treating physician. Women who are treated by a male physician are less likely to survive a heart attack. Male and female heart attack patients fare the same when they are under the care of female doctors.[7] For hospitalizations from any cause, people are more likely to survive when they have a female internist. In the United States, if men practiced medicine like women in hospitals, at least thirty-two thousand lives would be saved each year.[8] In general, female physicians communicate better, spend more time with their patients, and tend to follow clinical guidelines more closely than their male colleagues.[9] Certain was lucky to have a female doctor.

After the procedure, she was sent to the ICU with a balloon pump in place to support her dangerously low blood pressure. Later that evening, the rounding cardiologist told her with a smile, "Don't worry. You should be back at work in two weeks."

"Really?" thought Certain, listening to the sound of the pump supporting her heart's every beat. The thought of returning to seeing fifteen hospitalized patients a day made her chest tighten.

This reaction was key to understanding the cause of her heart attack. In recovery, Certain mused with her fellow hospitalists, ruling out cause after probable cause of her illness. Finally they came to a consensus, diagnosing a condition that was so ubiquitous, it hardly seemed worth mentioning, one that made up as much of the backdrop of her life as the sky: stress.

For hospitalists, the causes of constant stress are obvious. These internal medicine doctors are the workhorses of the hospital system. They take care of three out of every four hospitalized patients.[10] "We are on the bottom of the hierarchy of physicians, with not much support," Certain said. In the United States, hospitalists don't earn as much as their other hospital-based colleagues, only two-thirds of what ER doctors earn.[11] Income concerns factor into working-life stress, in large part because of the debt accrued in medical school.

Burnout—whose signs range from cynicism to emotional exhaustion to decreased productivity—is pervasive and rising. Since the 1970s, when care workers first noticed that professionals like them, from teachers to nurses, showed similar psychological stress indicators, a diagnostic index has been used to measure burnout.[12] In the health care sector, those levels have been rising internationally, and that was before the traumatic bursts of stress associated with Covid in health care systems around the world.[13] At baseline, up to 68 percent of physicians report feeling burned out, which is considered an independent risk factor for cardiovascular disease.[14]

In increasingly business-oriented, profit-based health care systems, financial considerations can put a physician's allegiance to their employer at odds with their moral obligation to their patient. Imagine the dilemma faced by San Francisco physicians during the pandemic, when unhoused, chronically ill patients who were ready for hospital discharge had no safe shelter to go to. Had the physicians refused to discharge them from the hospital so they would be safe, the cost for the health care system would have been exorbitant, depleting resources needed for sick patients. But sending them out to the streets as Covid rates were rising was an affront to their oath to do no harm.

The moral injury that results from these conflicts between what you know is right and what your work demands of you is an important driver of burnout.[15] If you've been annoyed that your care provider looks at a computer screen more than they look at you, rest assured that your care provider dislikes it too. The electronic environment and the clerical demands placed on health care workers are also significant contributors to burnout.[16]

Add to job stress the burden of financial worry, and you have a potent mixture. The average new doctor in the United States starts their medical career with $240,000 in student debt. Debt is such a constant part of life for physicians, it's hardly named as a recognized source of stress. But debt may be breaking our hearts. And if it's bad for medical doctors, whose professional credentials offer them the status and basic financial security that help protect against stress,[17] you know it's going to be worse for everyone else. Doctors earn more than nurses or personal care workers, and in Brazil and the United States, doctors earn *far* more than any other health care worker. But no matter where you look, one factor remains true worldwide: relative wage rates in any given branch of health care fall when the number of women working in that specialty goes up.[18]

FLOWS OF SILVER, FLOWS OF DEBT

Consider the political philosopher Thomas Hobbes's classic account of the social and political order, *Leviathan*, written during the English civil war and published in 1651. The illustration, which he helped design, shows the Leviathan rising above the land, holding symbols of secular and divine power. This imposing biblical figure is composed of over three hundred people. In Hobbes's view, the whole is the sum of its parts, and he uses the circulatory system as a metaphor for the binding connections in the body politic, "whose veins receiving the blood from the several parts of the body, carry it to the heart; where being made vital, the heart by the arteries sends it out again, to enliven, and enable for motion all the members of the same."[19]

As life is sustained by the circulation of blood pumped by the heart, Hobbes believed, society is nourished by a system of trade in which "all commodities, movable and immovable, [which] are made to accompany a man to all places of his resort, within and without the place of his ordinary residence; . . . In so much as this concoction, is as it were the sanguification of the commonwealth: for natural blood is in like manner made of the fruits of the earth; and circulating, nourisheth by the way every member of the body of man."[20] The free flow of commercial transactions, he noticed, keeps the commonwealth healthy. Imbalances in the body politic lead to "sedition, sickness; and civil war, death." An astute diagnostician, he understood the link between inflammation and great inequalities of wealth:

> There is sometimes in a commonwealth, a disease . . . when the treasure of the commonwealth, flowing out of its due course, is gathered together in too much abundance, in one, or a few private men, by monopolies, or by farms of the public revenues; in the same manner as the blood in a pleurisy, getting into the membrane of the breast, breedeth there an inflammation, accompanied with a fever, and painful stitches.[21]

Public health studies agree with Hobbes: concentrations of power and capital have created unequal flows of goods and services that have left an epidemic of inflammation, physical and metaphorical. For many people, life is nasty, brutish, and short not because they are outside the protections of the modern state and the circulations of wealth that it manages, but because they are enclosed within its unjust social and political order.

In the Covid era, we've all come to appreciate rather directly how disease travels from person to person and from place to place. That flow has a shape, a vascularity. There are conduits and borders and impermeabilities and directions and choke points.

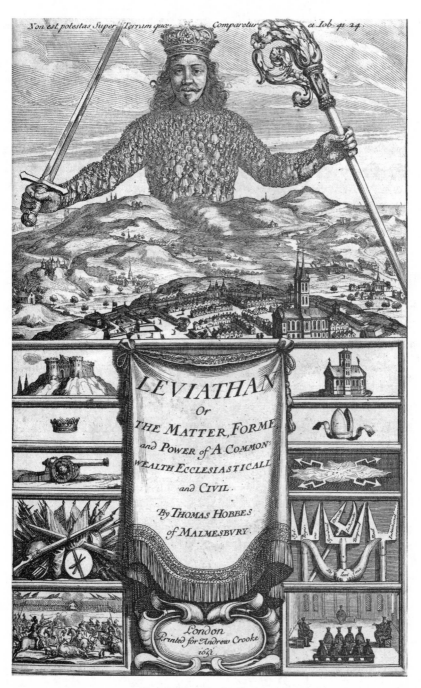

Frontispiece to *Leviathan*

Disease often follows trade routes. And like the circulatory system, these flows of people, goods, and money are interconnected in complex ways that bear on the health of bodies and societies. Take the introduction of cholera to Europe in the 1830s. The pathway of that disease can't be explained simply by pointing to contemporaneous travelers between Asia, Russia, and Germany. The movement of goods from Asia was bought with flows of money from Europe. The value of the coins was in the silver that was extracted and shipped from the Western Hemisphere, the colonization of which was funded by the abundant treasures about which Hobbes was so concerned two hundred years earlier. Then as now, the biggest hoarders of treasure were not the entrepreneurs or royals but the banks that had developed new financial systems to fund imperial conquest.

Europe's militaries were paid for by government borrowing. In the century after 1470, Spain was able to grow its ranks of soldiers tenfold not simply through the goods it stole from the Western Hemisphere but because the promise of future plunder made the country more creditworthy.[22] Empires, in order to exploit their colonial dominions, need vaults of money and credit to pay for weapons and soldiers. Private banks provided this concentration of wealth. In exchange for collateral and interest, private banks in Genoa, Venice, and elsewhere in Europe financed the circulation of armadas, conquistadors—and disease.

Debt made colonial invasion possible. It was also the social technology through which Indigenous communities were worked to death, tasked with the duties of repaying Genoese loans with South American silver. Spain's colonies in Peru and Mexico were, in the early colonial era, the source of 80 percent of the world's silver.[23] In Mexico City, Lima, and Seville, the names of the reigning Spanish monarchs were stamped on the first global currency, the silver peso or Spanish dollar. As the money flowed from the silver veins of Mexico and Peru through Europe to China, other flows choked the Indigenous civilizations. Central to these exchanges was a liquid that never left Peru and Mexico, but without it the exports of money would have ceased to pulse: mercury.

Crush silver ore with mercury, salt, water, and copper sulfate, and the silver forms a dense amalgam that sinks in water and is purified by boiling away the mercury. Over the colonial period, the largest mine in Peru, in Potosí, sent 23,000 tons of silver to Spain. To produce it, thirty-two thousand metric tons of mercury was turned into vapor.[24] (In 2005 the combined anthropogenic mercury vapor on Earth totaled 1,930 metric tons.)[25] The mercury and the work to retrieve it for mining in Potosí were provided by the city of Huancavelica, two thousand kilometers (1,243 miles) away. As Nicholas Robins explains in an important history, *Mercury, Mining, and Empire*, the human cost was immense.[26] The fevers, tooth loss, tremors, and drooling associated with mercury poisoning were known at the time—less so were the neurological symptoms of hallucination and insomnia.[27] But it *was* known that those unfortunate enough to be caught in a blast of mercury vapor would die agonizingly.

Why, then, would anyone agree to work in a mercury or silver mine? It wasn't a question of agreeing: the colonial government forced them. Spanish law frowned upon enslaving Indigenous people directly. Slavery had been justified in Europe, Africa, and the Middle East by accusing the enslaved of crimes against Christendom. In the Americas, where inhabitants could reasonably claim never to have heard of Christ, it was harder to argue that local faiths had deliberately traduced Christianity. Colonial administrators rose to the legal challenge by claiming that the locals could achieve spiritual salvation through work.[28] By repurposing an Incan system of tribute labor, the *mita*, a succession of governors were able to keep silver flowing east and their consciences clear.

Under the *mita*, one seventh of all adult men had to move at their own expense to the mines and donate their labor to the Spanish crown.[29] Unlike slaves, *mitayos* were paid—but poorly, with only a modest stipend, to keep them in debt and thus in servitude. The

Spanish were exploitative and the work conditions were lethal. According to one 1645 report, "Of 100 Indians that come to Potosí not even forty return to their town."[30] One reason was that the high turnover in *mitayos* propelled the spread of diseases to which Indigenous Peruvians were highly susceptible: due to influenza and smallpox, the population fell from a pre–European invasion level of 9 million to 600,000 by 1520. Facing a labor shortage, the colonial administrators extended the age range of workers, from children to the elderly, and even this didn't make up for the losses due to working conditions and disease.

There were ways to avoid the *mita*: men could flee their own community for another, where they would be exempt from *mita* service but wouldn't be able to access land. With nothing to sell but their labor, and still required to pay tribute to the church and the crown, they would soon find themselves in servitude and in debt. Death offered no escape: if the debtor died, his family would inherit his obligation.

Mita was debt, and debt was death. As the anthropologist David Graeber observed, the creation of debt, together with police to enforce its collection, was all colonizers had to do to trigger a cascading series of exploitations and injustices.[31] Insufficiently salaried work required colonized people to submit their labor to the colonizers in perpetuity. Desperation was as crucial to the new global economic infrastructure as railroads and ships and international trade. They were engineered simultaneously.

For their part, the colonizers offered some basic supports to ensure that workers would return to the job if they got sick. There was health care of a kind, but it was distributed unequally. Potosí's colonizers had the San Juan de Dios hospital, which was so well funded that its patients "could be dressed with silver and gold."[32] The hospitals to which Indigenous workers were admitted were poorer and staffed by fewer personnel. The segregation of Indigenous from colonizer was a central part of the colonial project, of course. It offered a visible lesson in the fruits of Christian civilization that might, with

enough application and faith, be available to the descendants of Indigenous workers.[33]

Not unreasonably, Indigenous communities distrusted that the
system that had poisoned them in the mine would heal them in
the hospital. They were right. Mercury vapor didn't respect hospital
boundaries. In Potosí and particularly in Huancavelica, the air, soil,
and water around the mines were so contaminated that hospitals
were less places of healing than places to die. The difference between hospitals for rich and poor lay in the quality of the bed upon
which the last rites were administered.

In the 1700s, a century after Hobbes published *Leviathan*, the *mita*'s
terms of servitude grew more onerous, its pool of recruits stretched
even wider, and the church's greed for tithes and the state's for taxes
deepened. Sporadic uprisings gave way to the Great Rebellion in Peru
from 1780 to 1783, which struck back at the empire but ultimately
failed, inciting new waves of colonial oppression. The Spanish prosecuted their war on Indigenous communities through forced relocation, deculturation, the enforcement of Spanish-language learning,
the criminalization of Indigenous medicine, religious conversion, and
family separation.[34] This colonial toolkit circulated across colonial
frontiers along with the coin that its application produced.

Although Peru gained its independence in 1824, its colonial scars
run deep. The *mita*'s legacy endures through inequities in landholding and systemic differences in poverty between the communities
that fell under it five hundred years ago and those that didn't.[35] The
story of mercury production in Huancavelica and Potosí, and its deep
connection to the debt-fueled first wave of globalization, is written in
the soil and water, a permanent toxic legacy. And it is written in the
bodies of Indigenous peoples to this day.

Debt remains central to coercing work, to ensuring the circulation of capital, and to making governments in poor countries open
up their lands to those in rich ones who would extract from them.[36]
The end of direct colonial rule left the institutions of colonialism
intact. The banks—those pumps of international credit and debt—

still needed to be paid, and the national police and army were still ready to act as local debt collectors. If governments defaulted on their loans, the national bourgeoisies would suffer; the local elites took the reins of colonial debt administration, even if the bank head-quarters remained in the Global North.

Postcolonial governments have followed the prescriptions of multilateral institutions like the World Bank and the International Monetary Fund. Loans are made in US dollars or their equivalent. In order to repay, governments have to sell goods and services that might earn those dollars. Thus, by borrowing and fearing the conse-quences for nonpayment, postcolonial countries have transformed themselves. Local industries have been decimated in favor of dereg-ulated export manufacturers. Forests have been leveled into fields for tropical cash crops for the international market. Rivers have been dammed to irrigate those crops. As the writer Eduardo Galeano put it, the earth's veins have been laid open, so that minerals might be pulled from the soil. A colonial ecology is one of fire. Control over these resources has been fought through coups and dictatorships, through the burning of villages and harvests and books.[37] Insofar as landscapes remain free from extractive damage, they are fenced off as tourist attractions, for visiting foreigners wielding their dollars, euros, and renminbi.

Like the global financial system, national economies are built around debt. They are in many respects circulatory systems for con-centrating wealth and power, and for producing and reproducing a colonial social and political order. The rich can borrow almost in-definitely and default repeatedly. They use their money to capture the levers of government to expand even further their interests. In contrast, the poor—states and individuals—will pay dearly and in perpetuity for default and find themselves under the yoke of insti-tutions designed to keep them this way. International banks, backed by government policy and a system of international debt and credit that redistributes wealth to the top, are mostly engineered to pass the stress test in times of crisis. The rest of us, however, are destined to carry the burdens of these stresses, and to fail the test. As Hobbes sharply observed, in these inequities "breedeth there an inflammation."

DEBT AS A CHOKE POINT

It's sometimes hard for outside observers to see quite how stress manifests itself, especially when we're trained to look at the baubles of the modern world as signs of success and progress. John Peck, the executive director of the Wisconsin-based Family Farm Defenders, runs into this problem when city students come to his members' farms for summer camp. As he explains, "Here's a farmer whose annual income is about $30,000, but in their barn they have $2 to $3 million worth of equipment. One of these tractors is worth half a million dollars. So the kids will climb up into this tractor, and there's GPS, and the kids go, 'Wow, this is worth more than any car I will ever own, more than a Lamborghini.' True, the farmer has all this equipment and all this land worth millions of dollars, but his income from that is still only $30,000."

Embedded in a global circulatory system of finance capitalism, industrial agriculture, and food exports, small American farms have million-dollar tractors in the barn and nothing on the table. Over 80 percent of US farms have revenue of less than $100,000, and in 2019 the income for the poorest was $2,696.[38] For a farmer, Peck explains, that means "he qualifies for food stamps. He has no health care, and he's dependent on getting a fair price for his product from the giant processor, and the bank who's owning a lot of this equipment really. So your land is collateral. Now, we have massive foreclosures happening in farms. I'm on the suicide hotline for Farm Aid. So I get calls from all over the Midwest, and farmers are feeling like they can't make it. They call me to try to get help, and I talk to them. Farmers have internalized the mythology that it's always their fault if they don't do well. And then . . ."

John breathed deeply. "My neighbor committed suicide when I was growing up. He committed suicide at the breakfast table because the bank was going to foreclose on their farm. He thought it was his fault. And so [I'm] trying to talk farmers through that and saying, 'No, there's other alternatives'—but you know, farms are people's homes too, so when they foreclose on a farm, there's a homeless farm family, and now who owns that land? Now, it's bank land, right?"

Suicide rates are higher in rural than in the urban US; farmers experiencing hopelessness when faced with foreclosure are certainly a leading risk group.[39] For those who have already lost their family land, for those who often find work on other people's farms, the situation may be more dire than for their employers. The data, however, are silent. We know much more about farmers' health than about farmworkers' health. Those who circulate from field to field in the United States, India, Europe, or indeed anywhere are poorer than those for whom they work, and their health status has systematically been less of a medical and political priority.[40]

There is, however, a marker in the blood for those willing to look. Some studies have found a dose-response effect between levels of debt and odds of suicide: the greater the debt, the greater the level of mental distress.[41] Poor mental health is strongly linked to high personal unsecured debt (debt that isn't tied to a mortgage or a car).[42] Payday loans, for instance, trap borrowers in particularly brutal repayment structures, charging far higher levels of interest than, say, mortgage loans. A typical payday loan of $300 can result in a final total payment of $800—an APR of 400 percent, a truly extractive level of interest.[43]

The anxieties associated with repayment are linked to feelings of helplessness and loss of control over one's life, all of which are linked to elevated levels of the marker of inflammation: C-reactive protein.[44] Worse, the fear of default is compounded by the fact that once borrowers have successfully repaid a payday loan, they'll likely need to take out another. In a fifteen-year study involving nearly forty thousand people in the UK, individuals with higher levels of C-reactive protein were four times more likely to kill themselves than those with low inflammatory markers.[45]

The suicide risk associated with stress and inflammation can be viewed as the acute impact of debt. The chronic impact is cardiovascular disease. One study found that having more debt was associated with a 1.3 percent increase in diastolic blood pressure, which is the bottom number of a blood pressure reading. While this may seem like a small effect, it is clinically significant: an increase of 2 mmHg of diastolic blood pressure is associated with 17 percent greater risk of high blood pressure and 15 percent higher risk of stroke.[46]

Since the 1980s in the United States, overall household debt has tripled.[47] Between 1989 and 2006, US credit card debt rocketed from $211 billion to $876 billion.[48] Canada and Europe see the same trends.[49] With working-middle-class wages stagnant, many people need more than they can earn. But people are not simply living outside their means with poor budgeting habits, as conservative critics often claim. Those with the most severe credit card debt often have had recent job loss or health problems, indicating that something much bigger than their own bank accounts is broken.[50] When a person suffers a heart attack, they enter the medical system, which can create more financial stress. A 2019 analysis of financial data from Canada shows that after a cardiovascular event such as a heart attack or stroke, people tend to bring in less income in the long term, further exacerbating medical debt.[51] In a survey of US heart disease patients from 2013 to 2017, roughly 45 percent said they had financial hardship from medical bills incurred during the treatment of their illness.[52]

Income volatility, which has been reaching new peaks since 1980, leaves its traces in our hearts. An increase in income over six years leads to a lower risk of cardiovascular disease over the following seventeen years, while an income drop over six years is associated with a higher risk of cardiovascular disease over the following seventeen years.[53] A sudden unpredictable loss in income between the ages of thirty and forty-five independently causes a doubling of cardiovascular risk in the subsequent ten years. Some of this may be due to behavioral changes, such as missing doctors' appointments and skipping medicines because of their high cost in the for-profit US health care system. But clearly those who experience income loss are, like farmers facing foreclosure, exposed to extraordinary stress and feelings of hopelessness—psychological states that affect our bodies at a molecular level.[54]

These effects do not fall equally. In the United States, middle-class Black people earn 70 cents for every dollar that middle-class white people earn, and systemic injustices in banking, housing, and taxation mean that those households are able to turn into assets only fifteen cents for every dollar of wealth held by middle-class whites.[55] The gap between what they earn and what they need generates chronic stress, which, as we will see, activates the sympathetic nervous system and adrenal hormones.[56] This economic stress combines with the toxic exposome of police violence, historical trauma, daily acts of discrimination, environmental health hazards, and poor food availability to create a potent pro-inflammatory threat that aims like an arrow straight to the heart. This unequal distribution of inflammatory triggers may explain why Black people have the highest rates of cardiovascular disease in the United States.[57]

AN INTRODUCTION TO THE BIOCHEMISTRY OF STRESS AND INFLAMMATION

Stress and inflammation co-evolved to return our bodies to homeostasis. If homeostasis were a tightrope walker walking across a cable, the stress response would be a moment of lost balance, and the inflammatory response would be the corrections made to restore balance and keep the walker moving. The activation of these responses means that the body is not in its optimum working condition. Something has been damaged or is under threat of being damaged. The molecular messengers for stress and inflammation are causally connected, and the intersections of these two responses is an area of active research that will open the door to greater understanding of many diseases impacting modern humans. As the pathways continue to be clarified, we may come to understand them as two parts of the same system.

Biologically speaking, stress is a state of real or perceived threat to homeostasis.[58] It is provoked by psychological, environmental, and physiological stimuli that create a cascade of hormones, neurotransmitters, and cytokines working together to restore homeostasis. The stress response is a tightly choreographed interaction between the immune, endocrine, and nervous systems. It addresses actual or potential damage and is intimately integrated with the inflammatory response. Over the course of human evolution, the nature of our stressors has greatly changed. Instead of the acute stress of a bear running after us, we are more exposed to chronic stressors, such as making house payments so we don't end up on the street or going for a jog while Black in a racist society.

Stress activates the hypothalamic-pituitary-adrenal (HPA) axis and the sympathetic nervous system, which are both under regulatory control of the hypothalamus, a gland that sits in the brain at the intersection of the immune, endocrine, and nervous systems.[59] The HPA axis is an endocrine superhighway that runs between the brain and the adrenal glands, priming the body to address stress by way of steroid hormones that the body makes, such as cortisol.[60] The sympathetic nervous system's fibers can stimulate every tissue in the body, preparing for fight-or-flight responses mediated by the hormones norepinephrine and epinephrine, also known as adrenaline.[61] These two arms of the stress response together affect the executive, cognitive, fear, reward, and sleep/wake centers of the brain. They also impact the gastrointestinal, reproductive, cardiovascular, respiratory, immune, and endocrine systems.[62] Stress is felt in every nook and cranny of the body.

In the face of acute psychological stress, pro-inflammatory markers, such as IL-1β and IL-6, rise, as does C-reactive protein.[63] This suite of molecules acts together, where IL-1β from immune cells stimulates the release of IL-6 from immune cells and other cells, which stimulates the release of C-reactive protein from liver cells, which then goes back and amplifies the systemic pro-inflammatory actions of IL-6.[64] This mobilization brings about the biological resources to prevent damage, to mitigate it, and to prepare to repair it if needed. An exposome punctuated with moments of acute stress—like police shooting an unarmed, unhoused community member in front of your home—will cause a sharp bump in these molecules.

The cytokine IL-6 sits at a critical intersection of neural, metabolic, and regenerative processes.[65] Its levels spike when the acute inflammatory response is triggered. This is why researchers and clinicians track it as a marker of inflammation. Generated immediately at a site of infection or trauma, IL-6 sends out warning signals throughout the body.[66] This same cytokine has both anti- and pro-inflammatory actions. The dominant action depends, as Virchow described, entirely on context.[67] It dictates the transition from acute to chronic inflammation and from localized to systemic.[68] When stress is systemic, IL-6 has a profoundly pro-inflammatory action, serving as a continuous alarm signal to the body.[69]

The cycle of alarm feeds back on itself. The hypothalamus responds to increased circulating cytokines by stimulating the adrenal glands to release cortisol. This acts on cortisol receptors inside cells to terminate the inflammatory response, serving as a negative feedback loop. In chronic stress, however, these receptors resist the constant signal of elevated cortisol levels and consequently fail to stop the inflammation.[70] Constant activation of the stress response leads to pathological manifestations, such as low-grade inflammation and decreased immune response in the face of viral infections.[71] This is one way chronic stress can make us more vulnerable to colds and other viruses such as Covid.[72]

Sustained stress can change the balance of immune cells, shifting from an anti-inflammatory profile to one that drives more autoimmune and cell-injury patterns.[73] The stress of facing a late debt payment can cause this kind of change.[74] Chronic stress appears to be additive, imprinting its impact on the body in the form of inflammation even from early childhood.[75] The presence of stress during childhood leads to an exaggerated stress-induced inflammatory response as a person ages.[76] Although the causal link has not yet been discovered, telomere erosion from oxidative stress inside cells and the development of the senescence-associated secretory phenotype are likely involved in early priming. In situations where stress is unrelenting, it is associated with chronic modest elevations of C-reactive protein and IL-6, which currently define the clinical phenomenon of low-grade inflammation.[77]

When chronic stress is the background noise of life, it impacts our cells, our DNA, and our children. By making epigenetic alterations to the genome, stresses such as work burnout, economic precarity, hunger, and systemic discrimination can create heritable changes in our DNA.[78] When a mother is stressed during pregnancy, the unborn child's DNA can get tagged with a methyl group in a genetic region that makes them more vulnerable to harmful impacts of stress themselves. That DNA change can then be transmitted to that unborn baby's offspring, and some changes can persist down multiple generations.[79] Again, this is not to essentialize the dysfunction but to call for transformative measures that overturn manufactured causes of stress, such as debt and racism. Psychological stress also drives oxidative DNA damage, and that damage is a cause of premature cellular aging.[80] Depression, a stress-related disorder, also causes immune cells to exact oxidative DNA damage.[81] This oxidative process erodes telomeres, which as we saw in the previous chapter are the endcaps of our chromosomes that serve as a cell's biological timekeeper.[82] All these pathways lead to premature senescence, which triggers the pro-inflammatory senescence-associated secretory phenotype.[83] This cellular damage appears to be an important cause of the chronic systemic inflammation that can cause cardiovascular disease.[84] Up to 30 percent of the US population has this kind of low-grade inflammation.[85]

Certain behaviors can mitigate these pro-inflammatory processes and create a buffering effect, both psychological and physical. Practicing compassion meditation in the face of a stressful event decreases the rise in IL-6.[86] Engaging in regular physical exercise alters brain chemistry to help counteract the damaging effects of stress.[87] But most modern people turn to popping a pill to treat their ailments, because meditation or exercise won't help them when the flows of wealth and power have been designed to keep them stressed, especially if they're poor or working class. Across countries, relative poverty is associated with higher rates of depression.[88] The prescription rate of antidepressant drugs has been rising internationally too, and the United States leads the planet.[89] Over one in ten Americans now use antidepressants, a rate that increased 400 percent between 1988 and 2008.[90] This burst of prescription coincided both with soaring consumer debt and with multibillion-dollar direct-to-consumer marketing for blockbuster antidepressants—and the pharmaceutical industry more than made its money back.[91]

While pharmaceuticals are powerful tools, they can cause even more stress for those who cannot afford them. Tocilizumab, a drug that blocks IL-6's inflammatory actions, has been shown to improve depression and anxiety in people who are taking it for rheumatoid arthritis.[92] But a standard weekly treatment course costs $18,460 per year.[93] The median US household income was less than $70,000 in 2019 and has certainly fallen since.[94] When a leading cause of personal bankruptcy is medical debt,[95] it's no surprise that levels of C-reactive protein are elevated in a significant portion of the population.

All this stress is enough to give someone a heart attack.[96] For the 40 percent of patients with cardiovascular disease who, like Heather Certain, have none of the traditional risk factors such as diabetes, high cholesterol, a history of tobacco smoking, or a family history of cardiovascular disease, stress and inflammation are causing heart disease.[97] In fact, laboratory tests that measure levels of C-reactive protein and other inflammatory markers in the blood provide a more complete risk assessment for cardiovascular disease than those that measure cholesterol.[98] While quitting smoking, going vegan, medi-tating, and getting more exercise can help decrease the chances of suffering from cardiovascular disease, these changes in personal behavior won't stop the collection agencies from calling. Enclosure in the capital flows of finance capitalism, and its deep colonial his-tory, literally transforms the movement of blood and hormones, neu-rotransmitters, and cytokines in our bodies.

CARDIOVASCULAR DISEASE AS AN INFLAMMATORY DISEASE

Cardiovascular disease became the world's top killer only relatively recently. As early as 1900, infectious diseases, such as pneumonia, were the leading causes of mortality in the United States. With the rapid development of antibiotics, rates of fatal pneumonia fell. Around the same time, both life expectancy and rates of cardiovascular disease increased.[99] Conventional wisdom claims that because we are living longer and no longer dying of infection, we are now increasingly dying from cardiovascular disease. But it's not so simple. While antibiotics saved us from dying of infectious disease, scientists are now wonder-ing if those drugs might be complicit in the onset of the unabated in-flammation that leads to heart disease. The logical connection between antibiotics and heart attacks lies in the folds of our intestines. If you're wondering what our gut has to do with our heart, you're stuck in a fallacy in Western anatomy that separates our body into distinct geog-raphies, when in fact we are quite hopelessly interconnected. As we shall see in the next chapter, when the microbial community that lives in our gut is disrupted through antibiotics, inflammation ensues.[100]

In the medium and large arteries, inflammation can provoke either the development of atherosclerotic plaque or the erosion of the vessel's inner layer, which can ultimately lead to a blockage. Atherosclerosis—the hardening of an artery as it is progressively clogged by plaque—is something surgeons can feel when they run their hands along a vessel. Living with high cholesterol, high blood pressure, diabetes, obesity, a sedentary lifestyle, and tobacco smoking increase your risk of developing atherosclerosis. These conditions are also associated with chronic inflammation.[101]

When low-density cholesterol (LDL) molecules, which we have come to know as "bad cholesterol," infiltrate the innermost layer of an artery wall, the part that is closest to the blood flow, enzymes begin to break them down, releasing molecules that activate inflammation. This cascade recruits a host of other immune cells, which eventually form atherosclerotic plaque.[102] Such plaques can rupture, exposing clotting molecules that are normally hidden from blood directly to the bloodstream, which causes a blood clot to form. As it grows, the clot blocks further blood flow through the vessel, causing downstream tissue death. This is what leads to most heart attacks and strokes.[103]

In 2008 researchers proved that inflammation was an independent factor in the development of cardiovascular disease. They gave a cholesterol-lowering drug called a statin to people with normal cholesterol levels but risk factors for cardiovascular disease and evidence of systemic inflammation, flagged by an elevated C-reactive protein. This medicine also has anti-inflammatory effects. The statin reduced the number of heart attacks and strokes in people with normal cholesterol, but it wasn't clear if that benefit was due to lowering LDL, lowering inflammation, or both.[104]

The debate in cardiovascular medicine continued over whether LDL's effects on the arteries or systemic inflammation from other sources causes cardiovascular disease. In 2017 researchers demonstrated that targeting inflammation alone can decrease the risk of nonfatal heart attacks, strokes, and cardiovascular death in people who had already had a heart attack. They used an anti-inflammatory medication that acts on IL-1β.[105] When this cytokine was targeted in cardiovascular patients, even with no change in cholesterol levels, their risk of cardiovascular events dropped significantly. Systemic inflammation independently drives cardiovascular disease.

The causal connection also runs in the other direction. Cardiovascular disease causes inflammation. While the infiltration of arterial walls by LDL sets off the localized inflammation that results in atherosclerotic plaque, chronic systemic inflammation raises our circulating levels of LDL as well, creating a positive feedback loop.[106] Whatever causes the body to be inflamed will stimulate the processes that create cardiovascular disease, and the cardiovascular disease causes ongoing inflammation.

The vicious circle of heart disease and inflammation can be broken. While exercise and diet can help, they are not sufficient to address the cardiovascular impacts of chronic inflammation brought on by the stresses of overwhelming debt or running away from increasingly destructive wildfires. For that, we need to move upstream to unblock the flow of resources and even the flow of water. The importance of that work can be seen in the health of a creature who offers some of the best anti-inflammatory medicine through its flesh—salmon.[107] Historically, Indigenous people who ate large amounts of wild salmon had low rates of cardiovascular disease.[108] That changed when colonialism altered the ancient flows of water over land with dams and industry. The downstream consequences have been catastrophic. Attempts to resuscitate salmon populations through farming have left us with fish that are less healthy in themselves and less capable of offering us the historical anti-inflammatory benefit of wild salmon.[109] If waterways are the vasculature of the earth, then the fish that travel from river to ocean and back again are the heart, pumping nutrients inland through their journey to nourish so many things—the soil, the trees, their offspring, and our own bodies.[110] And if these fish are the heart, large dams are the blockages that cause the ecosystem's heart attacks.

DOWNSTREAM ECOSYSTEM DEATH

Humans have been rechanneling water for millennia, sometimes for agriculture, sometimes for trade (as in the Panama Canal), sometimes for indoor plumbing and sanitation systems (as in Mesopotamia more than five thousand years ago),[111] and sometimes just to show off: Sri Lanka was for centuries the site of the world's most voluminous dam, a fourteen-kilometer-long vanity project built by a tyrant, Parakrama-bahu. In modern times, the push toward large dam construction began in the Great Depression, accelerated by the circulation of images of the Hoover Dam, a boast of US dominion over nature.[112] Most of the world's major river basins have impounded waters, as the Earth's rivers are blocked by forty thousand large dams—funded by the largest public and private banks, demanded by planners and industrialists, made possible by the exigencies of state power.[113] These edifices have altered historic flows of water over land in a short period, causing widespread disruption to human settlement, entire ecosystems, and the climate—and also to our health.

The arrest of a river's flow changes the ecological relationship between the land and the water. Nutrients get trapped, allowing algae to proliferate. When algae blooms die, their decay consumes oxygen in the water, suffocating other aquatic organisms and making the water undrinkable. It also generates carbon dioxide and methane, one of the reasons why dams are increasingly recognized as agents of climate change.[114] Controlled releases from dams inject rivers with water that is too cool in the summer and too warm in the winter, throwing off thermal cues that animals need for their life cycles.[115] Because of the Glen Canyon Dam, sections of the Colorado River are now too cold for native fish to successfully reproduce.

A dam incarcerates not only water and nutrients but also the sediment that usually travels from the headwaters to the ocean. Rivers dissipate their tremendous potential energy in traveling from a place of high elevation to the sea through the friction between the fluid-sediment mixture at the river's edge.[116] In a dammed river, the downstream water lacks the suspended clay, silt, and sand that a wild river usually carries. So it takes on a much more destructive character, hungrily carving the banks. This is not enough to reach its full potential sediment load, however, so when it arrives at the ocean, it often doesn't carry enough to maintain the coastline.[117]

What dams arrest isn't just the flow of water, nutrients, and sediment. In a number of cultures, rivers are understood as mothers: in Thai, the Mae Nam Khong is the "mother of all rivers"; Emajõgi is Estonian for "Mother River." For Hindus in South Asia, the sacred river is the goddess Ganga Maiya, or "Mother Ganges."[118] Cree, Maori, and Nuu-Chah-Nulth traditions agree on the vitality and sacredness of water in connecting all life.[119] Colonial power over rivers and oceans was a form of damming, a redirecting of flows of money, goods, and people—and disease. The control of waterways by the modern state, especially in the United States, was an act of domination not only over water and land but also over people. The Bureau of Reclamation, charged with damming the West and claiming territory not just from nature but from the Indigenous people living on it, is part of the Department of the Interior, whose other major arm is the Bureau of Indian Affairs.[120] Orwell couldn't have named these agencies better.

SALMON ARE THE PUMP

Pacific salmon range over the Pacific Rim coastline from South Korea to Russia, over to Alaska and down the coast of California. After they hatch in freshwater inland pools, they move out into the ocean, where they grow from one to seven years old. Once mature and ready to spawn, they begin their homeward journey. This migration inland, often for hundreds of miles and climbing thousands of feet, pumps nutrients from the marine ecosystem deep into the land: old-growth fir trees contain nitrogen from oceans hundreds of miles away. In addition, salmon bodies bring marine nutrients to wolves, bears, insects, birds, herbs, shrubs, and even soil, through the excrement of animals who have eaten the fish.[121]

In the Pacific Northwest, salmon stocks have dropped to less than 5 percent of what they were at the time of the Lewis and Clark expedition in the early 1800s. Deforestation, mining, pollution, and dams have posed insurmountable problems for them inland, while overfishing has driven down their numbers out in the ocean. In 1969 one hundred thousand Chinook salmon returned to the Snake River in Idaho to spawn. In 1996 only one salmon was able to complete the journey.[122] Of all the obstacles that lie in the way of journeying salmon, large dams have had the most impact.

Chief Caleen Sisk of the Winnemem Wintu tribe, from the Shasta region of northern California, is intimately familiar with the damage done by a large dam. The Shasta Dam stands 183 meters (602 feet) high, and when it was constructed in the 1930s and '40s, in the name of progress, it flooded 90 percent of the traditional homelands of the Winnemem Wintu, displacing the tribe—and the salmon, who could no longer complete their 1,000-kilometer (600-mile) journey up to Shasta.

"These salmon are on the endangered species list. If there were a list for culturally devastated people, we'd be on that list, because there's only 126 of us left, that are following and speaking for the salmon," says Chief Caleen. She spoke to us from her home on the remaining Winnemem Wintu land, a 17-hectare (42-acre) park in Shasta County.[123]

The long relationship between the Winnemem Wintu and the salmon is detailed in a creation story that begins with a spring that bubbles fresh water at the foot of their mountain. Chief Caleen recounts:

> In the beginning, Creator made all the spirit beings, and these spirit beings were inside of Bulim Phuyuq, Mount Shasta. They were in there for a long time, and then Creator came back, and he says, "I've built a place outside here. I want you to take physical form and take care of it." The spirits each picked who they would be. Eagle went out and Worm went out, and Butterfly went out and Bear went out. Each spirit named itself. Coyote and Wolf and Elk and

Moose. Finally, there was this one little spirit-being walking around the sacred fire inside of Bulim Phuyuq, scratching his head, wondering, "What should we do? What will I be?"

And he'd think of something and then say, "No, no— Salmon already did that." Finally, he decides that it's going to be Human. And he names himself Human as he comes out of the spring and goes down to the meadow. As he does that, the Creator looks at him and says, "Oh, that one's going to need a lot of help." So he calls back the mountain spirit and calls back the water spirit and the fire spirit, and as he's doing this, Salmon hears about what's going on. And so he's curious, and he comes back into the mountain and he offers to help. Most of all, he offers to give his voice to the Human so that they can try to fit in alongside the rest of life.

And so, from that time, humans rely on the salmon and the salmon take care of us. It's not like we have to go hunting for them. They swim right back to us to take care of us. They feed us. They make our mountains better. They feed everything else that we need in our environment. They are the most giving animal, from the time that they are eggs to the time that they are adults to the time they're eggs again. They are always feeding something. They are feeding the bugs, they're feeding other fish, the coyotes, the wolves, the cats, the birds, the whales, and also the humans.

Salmon are a keystone species, without which entire ecosystems would collapse. Trees that grow closer to creek beds with salmon grow larger and taller than trees farther away, thanks to the nutrients from the decomposing bodies of the fish.[124] Salmon flesh is also particularly good at abating inflammation, with its high omega-3 fatty acid content. These fatty acids, found in fish and certain plant oils, decrease the risk of sudden cardiac death, decrease the risk of the clot formation that precedes a heart attack or stroke, slow the development of atherosclerosis, and reduce inflammation.[125] Fish oils high in omega-3 fatty acids prevent oxidative damage, which keeps telomeres lengthened. This is one proposed mechanism of their superpower. Omega-3 oils from fish literally slow down the biological inflammaging clock.[126] But with fewer and fewer mature salmon returning to their spawning sites, they are less able to nurture the forests and the people. Even before the Shasta Dam went up, the Winnemem Wintu noticed that the fish returning home had decreased in number and were not as healthy as before.

In the 1850s commercial fishing by colonial settlers on the West Coast had no limits but racial ones: Chinese fishermen were not allowed to harvest salmon. In the first few years of the Gold Rush, over twenty thousand Chinese followed the flow of money to California, becoming by far the largest immigrant group. It didn't take long for white Californians to blame them for lowering their profits, so they structured society to force the Chinese out. Commercial fishing was one of the first of such exclusions—a form of racist enclosure of the water commons.[127]

By 1885, within a few short decades of California's formation, six canneries in the Sacramento River delta were packing ninety thousand cases of salmon per year until the run dried up from overfishing.[128] The Gold Rush decimated salmon breeding grounds. Gravel beds in streams where fish would bury their eggs were overrun with excess rocks and trees as well as pollutants like mercury as hydraulic cannons blasted into mountains to quench the miners' greed. An estimated 1.5 billion cubic yards of debris ended up in the waterways, permanently damaging salmon habitat. That's enough material to build a mile-wide highway from Seattle to San Diego.[129]

In the late 1800s, instead of halting commercial fishing and environmentally degrading processes to allow salmon populations to recover, the government promoted the establishment of hatcheries and farms. One agent of this change was Livingston Stone, a pastor-turned-piscatologist who traveled to the McCloud River, at the base of Mount Shasta, where salmon were known to weigh 10 to 20 kilograms (20 to 50 pounds). He met the Winnemem Wintu to learn about the life cycle of Chinook salmon.

"At first he didn't believe that the Pacific salmon die after they spawn and feed the next generation with their decomposing bodies," said Chief Caleen. "But then he saw we were right. He learned about how the fish lay their eggs. He learned about spawning. But then he left. And he didn't learn the songs and the dances and how to light the fires along the river so the salmon could find their way home."

What he did instead was to open the nation's first federal fish hatchery, in 1872, on Winnemem Wintu land: the Baird Hatchery, in operation until it too was flooded by the rising waters of the Shasta Dam.[130] To stock it, hatchery workers captured fish after they made their way up the river.[131] They clubbed the female salmon over the head and slit their bodies open so tens of thousands of eggs per fish could be stripped out. The workers squeezed the males for their milt, which contains spermatozoa. Then scientific spawning occurred in large bowls. When the new salmon hatched, they were released into the river. This process was developed in the late 1870s by Stone and continues today.[132] Since this time, Chinook salmon eggs have been shipped from the McCloud River all over the world, as far as New Zealand.

But fish hatcheries have failed to bring back robust salmon populations in their native localities where dams and refineries operate.[133] This is because they are intended to provide symptomatic relief, while the root cause of the disruption to flows of salmon goes unaddressed. The damage to the river, the fish, the Indigenous communities, the trees—all of it—remains. It's an ecological debt whose principal is untouched. Conservation strategies are a way to shave off some of the interest.[134]

While hatchery incubation methods can generate greater rates of juvenile salmon release than their equivalent in the wild, the resulting genetic diversity is much lower, and the survival strategies of hatchery fish in the ocean are consequently restricted. Fewer than

1 percent of hatchery salmon return home to spawn. With less genetic diversity, hatchery fish and farmed fish are also more prone to disease,[135] such as piscine orthoreovirus, which leads to inflammation of skeletal muscle and the heart.[136]

Farming salmon is unhealthy not only for the fish but also for humans. An evaluation of farmed and wild salmon from around the world showed that farmed salmon contain greater concentrations of organochlorine contaminants such as PCBs and dioxins.[137] Instead of eating other fish and krill like their wild relatives, farmed salmon are often fed corn, soybeans, and rapeseed oil. As a result of their diet and confinement, farmed salmon produce far fewer omega-3 fatty acids than their wild cousins do, making them less able to turn down our bodies' inflammation.[138] In fact, farmed salmon raised on vegetable oil have increased levels of pro-inflammatory omega-6 fatty acids in their bodies that end up in our bodies when we eat them.[139] Through incarceration and prolonged mistreatment, colonial systems have managed to turn one of the best naturally available medicines—wild salmon—into a source of more sickness.

The stories of interference in the ancient relationships between land, water, humans, and salmon demonstrate how interconnected these all are and how technological arrogance can create downstream problems when we seek to outsmart the ecologies we belong to. A disruption in one part of the web of life, within a few short decades, ends up eroding the vitality of the whole system. But the good news is that ecologically guided reparation starting at one point of the web can bring vitality back to the whole. This work is becoming more critical every moment, and with every passing season, time is running out. And that ecological restoration must start with the people who were integrated into the ecology before colonialism, and who are still here working on these solutions. As Chief Caleen warns, "We believe when the salmon are gone, there will soon be no more people."

History offers some inspiration and a surprising lesson in how the circulatory system of people, goods, and money can create emergent effects across borders. Although Chinese fishing was proscribed in California,[140] Chinese workers were in high demand in salmon canneries. Their labor had been arranged through agreements between factory bosses and labor brokers. Over the course of the industry's life, cannery and longshore workers from China, Japan, and the Philippines organized.[141] At their height, they were able to challenge not only their bosses, for wages to alleviate their debts, but also the prejudices of the white working-class organizations on the waterfront.[142] It's not unreasonable, in the struggles around salmon and organized labor, to trace the origins of a multiracial labor movement in California.[143]

LIVING WAGE AND DEBT RELIEF

Militancy and demands for control over work and money are social and medical interventions for being able to manage the terms of debt. Longshore workers and stevedores have long been on the front lines of anticolonial work, using strikes to bring not just their bosses but imperial powers to the negotiating table.[144] Part of the workers' strategy: understanding that the longer a ship sat in dock waiting to be unloaded, the longer its owners would face rising interest debt, with no means to repay. Today, as household and international debt levels reach catastrophic levels, the need to return to similar tactics couldn't be greater.[145]

During the Great Recession, one US study found that among older adults, "for every wealth loss of $100,000, respondents, on average, experienced a 0.993 mg/L increase in C-reactive protein."[146] Women, the poor, and minorities experience even higher markers of inflammation. In another US study, nonpoor white men had C-reactive protein levels around 1.890 mg/dL while poor Black women had 2.976 mg/dL. For both poor and nonpoor Black women, the disparities in C-reactive protein levels peaked between the ages of forty-five and sixty-four.[147] And most US families don't have $100,000 to lose: in 2016 the median level of wealth across all households was

$97,300. The average median-age Black family's net worth that year was $17,600.[148]

At a global level, the situation is equally dire. If the silver extracted from the Americas had been invested at the historical average interest rate since 1800 (5 percent) its value now would be $165 trillion. The economist Jason Hickel calculates the value of enslaved labor to the US economy to be $97 trillion.[149] The colonial system of extraction stole this historical wealth, and this process has reproduced itself in new guises. Regimes of debt and collection use mispricing, unjust exchange rates, and the imperative of repayment to siphon billions of dollars from the Global South, in net terms, annually. Although in 2019 thirty OECD countries gave $152.8 billion in development aid, they've kept the Global South impoverished. Every year, poor countries pay rich ones nearly one trillion dollars in interest and loan repayment over a debt of $7.8 trillion.[150] The world's poorest countries continue to fund the richest ones, just as every country's poorest people keep paying for its richest. The question, then, is how to control debt and its circulation in ways that restore justice and health.

In the mid-2011, applicants for jobs at a new textile factory in the Dominican Republic didn't know that they were going to be part of a medical experiment. Workers at comparable textile factories in the country's free trade zone were paid the minimum wage, RD$5,400 per month (US$142 at the time). All workers at the new factory would be paid a living wage: RD$18,153 (US$477), 340 percent more. Fifteen months later they were given a series of tests and assessments and compared to workers on the minimum wage. Those earning the higher wages saved more but had *more* debt, but also fewer missed payments on that debt. They spent the money on things like deferred home improvements, education, and home appliances. Food habits shifted too, as they spent more money on high-sugar items and protein. Rates of overweight and obesity rose, but blood pressure fell.[151]

What does this suggest? First, higher incomes mean that people are generally healthier. Notwithstanding the dietary shift toward sugar, the stress of debt fell, and with it so did blood pressure. But harms caused by the injustices of the global circulation of capital can't be fixed by an aspirin a day to ward off heart attacks. They can't be fixed even with money. Families are choosing to incur debt from banks to invest in school fees. Government's austerity-assisted failure to provide a decent public education system drives many parents in the Global South to spend for private education.[152] That failure is a function of the reduced budgets and austerity that have been part of the Washington Consensus since the 1980s and that created low-wage export zones in the first place.[153]

Second, it's worth understanding why higher incomes lead to obesity. For the very rich, money doesn't mean weight gain. The wealthiest are able to afford the diet, gyms, nutritionists, personal trainers, and leisure time to avoid the worst elements of a food system that is overwhelmingly geared to producing obesogenic food.[154] A number of studies have found that higher income leads to worse dietary outcomes—but this is to blame the victim. When the modern diet is sold as safer, healthier, and more convenient than a traditional one, and when that diet is more likely to make consumers overweight, higher incomes are structurally certain to increase obesity. Tackling poverty through giving people higher wages won't change health outcomes if capitalism's dysfunctional toxic food and financial systems remain in place. Blaming individuals for a systemic failure is simply bad medicine.

A range of structural responses makes sense here. A debt jubilee for the poorest countries, forgiven by both public *and* private banks, would give governments room to point their economies away from sweatshops for global exports and extractive resources, which are geared only to ridding themselves of the cancer of debt, and toward the kinds of activities more compatible with a world of climate change.[155] Reparations for the historical harms caused by colonial debt are a moral requirement, as is the need to make public goods of energy, shelter, education, and health care.[156] Borrowing money to pay for medical care or education is unconscionable when the country has enough resources to support free health care and education for all.[157] The complement to universal health care and education is a system of credit controlled by public banks to help redirect economic activity.

The stress and inflammation linked to economic precarity can be healed with social commitments to good, well-paid jobs and safer ways to bank. Financial products can have the same life-altering consequences as medications. Just as we don't allow consumers to help themselves to whatever they feel like in a pharmacy, banking products need far better safeguards. Payday loans, for example, are the most toxic kind of financial product.[158] Banning them, by one estimate, would reduce the "suicide mortality rate by 2.1 percent and fatal drug poisoning rate by 8.9 percent."[159] Just as it's possible to proscribe bad banking, it's possible to invent healthier kinds. Movements like Positive Money propose to create banks that are under democratic control, to issue money and redirect resources, and to generate capital flows, according to principles of justice and ecological good sense.[160] These banks, governed wisely, will be much readier to reject the damming of rivers.

Public representation on bank boards is, of course, no guarantee of happy outcomes. Multilateral development banks like the World Bank, ostensibly public institutions, have offered to engage in only derisory debt relief, even after decades of public protest.[161]

But there is reason for genuine hope. Undamming rivers can bring biodiversity back,[162] reconnecting fish to the ocean and making their populations more resilient.[163] The number of new dams under construction is falling, and older ones are being decommissioned.[164] From the Klamath River in California to the Whanganui River in New Zealand, Indigenous people around the world are giving their rivers human rights and protections, so this kind of violence does not happen again.[165] As the world's inflamed waterways come unblocked, natural pumps are returning in surprising numbers.[166] The earth's vasculature can be restored, not through the technology of breeding and releasing fish, but by a reparative addressing of the underlying causes of inflammation.

The answer, though, is not merely to add fish and stir. Salmon are the pump, but they can't work without a thriving ecosystem to sustain them. There's a great deal of magical thinking around the conservation of individual species, with recognizing the conservation of cosmologies, ways of life, and ecosystems that surround those species. This is like trying to save a tree while surrendering the forest and its inhabitants to loggers. When it comes to the human body, new ideas about our own internal forest are susceptible to similar thinking: that with the right blend of newly drafted bacteria, we can return ourselves to health. As we'll see, nothing could be more mistaken.

3

DIGESTIVE SYSTEM

THE FOREST WITHIN

The first man who, having fenced in a piece of land, said "This is mine," and found people naïve enough to believe him . . . From how many crimes, wars, and murders, from how many horrors and misfortunes might not any one have saved mankind, by pulling up the stakes, or filling up the ditch, and crying to his fellows: Beware of listening to this impostor; you are undone if you once forget that the fruits of the earth belong to us all, and the earth itself to nobody.

—JEAN-JACQUES ROUSSEAU[1]

The Famine Irish—like the slave and the prisoner—occupy the threshold that divides human and the non-human. The Famine . . . was the price of converting the Irish into wage laborers, and to achieve that end what had to be destroyed was the *clachan* (an older Gaelic system of communal landholding and collective labor recalcitrant to capitalist modes of production).

—STEPHEN BEST AND SAIDIYA HARTMAN[2]

Joe Sanders was twenty-six years old and severely emaciated when he died in 2011. Fourteen years earlier he had been diagnosed with Crohn's disease, an illness characterized by chronic gut inflammation, with bloating and bloody bowel movements. Sanders had been a small child, but he developed stomachaches and started rapidly losing weight when he was twelve. A CT scan revealed a bowel stricture, and he was taken for surgery to remove a section of his intestines. Viewed under a microscope, the intestinal walls were found to carry the erosions that make up the signature of Crohn's.

Sanders excelled in school and enrolled at a university, planning to become either a physician or a lawyer. When hospitalized, he was an informed patient, negotiating with his healthcare team over which therapies he would or would not do. And he was in the hospital often. He had been put on various anti-inflammatory treatments—from steroids to drugs designed to target specific pathways of inflammation in the body. But nothing stopped his gut from being inflamed to the point of developing abscesses that would spontaneously burst open and ooze a mixture of pus and fetid material through the skin over his abdomen.

Food couldn't sustain him—his gut was leaking blood and nutrients. No matter how or what he ate, his digestive system couldn't nourish his body. Toward the end of his life, half of his intestines had been surgically removed. All the minerals, vitamins, amino acids, fats, and carbohydrates his body needed were given to him daily through a vein. To find some pleasure, he'd occasionally eat, only to suffer the consequences, convulsed with more bloating and more pain. Sanders was the average height for a man in the United States, around 175 cm (5 feet 9 inches). At that height, the average weight is 77 kilograms (170 pounds). When he died, Sanders weighed just 45 kilograms (100 pounds).

Sanders was a frequent visitor to the ICU as his inflammation drove his body into shock. He would be placed on broad-spectrum antibiotics and medicines to bring up his blood pressure. After several hospitalizations in short succession, he started to feel like a prisoner of his own body. Seeing no hope for improvement, he enrolled in a last-chance procedure, one that would either save or kill him: an intestinal transplant. Surgeons consider this operation only for end-stage patients, those who have exhausted every other option. But he never made it. The day of the procedure, Sanders died from a gastrointestinal bleed.

Crohn's disease is a medical diagnosis based on a number of clear symptoms. But the most telling sign of Sanders's illness was in the stool culture that was sent before his surgery. The feces of people with no inflammatory bowel disease have about 90 billion microorganisms per gram.[3] Sanders's stool had almost none.

THE ENCHANTED FOREST

Sanders's life and death are horrors that more and more people are experiencing. Inflammatory bowel disease, which includes Crohn's disease and the closely related condition ulcerative colitis, is on the rise in the United States, where 3 million people suffer from these illnesses. The rest of the planet is catching up: the global incidence of inflammatory bowel disease is 6.8 million and rising.[4] As awareness of the disease spreads, more diagnoses are likely. But rates aren't rising just because clinicians are getting better at diagnosing it. Other causes are driving this epidemic. Sanders died in 2011, just as medical knowledge about Crohn's disease and other inflammatory diseases were undergoing a revolution.

Our understanding of inflammatory bowel disease is in its infancy, not least because we are just starting to realize the consequences of Walt Whitman's truth, that humans contain multitudes. Which is ironic, because people of Whitman's era learned about the gut in ways that are still taught to this day—as a singular, almost mechanical entity.

The 2012 edition of the *Oxford Textbook of Medicine* introduces the gastrointestinal tract as "a hollow tube stretching from the oral cavity through the oesophagus, stomach, small intestine, colon, and rectum to the anal sphincter."[5] Which means the body, topologically, is a doughnut. Until relatively recently, standard medical training taught that the hole in the middle is a tube through which food passes and from which nutrients are progressively extracted: from the chewing and saliva of the mouth, to the acid fires of the stomach, to the fat-digesting bile and pancreatic enzymes of the small intestine, to the water balance in the final journey through the large intestine, each step that food takes down the digestive tract unlocks nutrients to support our vitality. When there's nothing more to wring out, we poop the residue.

But the gut isn't just a 6.5-meter-long (21 feet) tube of stomach, small intestine, and large intestine, a long sieve with progressively smaller holes. A better analogy for the digestive system would be a dense, teeming, and enchanted forest that borders two worlds within a single ecosystem, a transition zone between what we call the world and what we call our bodies. That forest encompasses human tissue, food, and a vast understory of microbial life.

Microbes—bacteria, archaea, protozoa, fungi, and viruses—are the most successful organisms on the planet. In sheer number, longevity, and adaptability, no other creature holds a candle to them. By the time mammals showed up, microbes were already over 3 billion years old. They are the unseen majority, who are critical in carbon and nitrogen cycling as well as the global food web, but they rarely get the credit they deserve for holding our planetary systems together.[6]

The human microbiota—the community of microbes who live on and inside us—comprises nearly two thousand different kinds of organisms.[7] Although Western medicine had long ignored them, these beings are the key to understanding inflammation. Like coral reefs and trees themselves, we are *holobionts*, to use the recently coined term for assemblies of plant, animal, microbial, viral, and fungal ecologies.[8]

We are host to trillions of microbes who, together with the specific niches they inhabit, make up the human microbiome.[9] To be precise, the collections of microorganisms themselves are called the microbiota. The microbiome is much more. It contains these living creatures and others for whom the description "living" is subject to debate, such as viruses, phages, and scraps of relic DNA, which are entities that cannot reproduce independently. While SARS-CoV-2 made its way to every continent in the world in 2020, by that definition, it isn't technically alive. The microbiome includes the collective genetic material and activities, as well as the conditions surrounding these organisms: in sum, their "theatres of activity."[10] Because this definition expands the microbiome beyond the microbes to include their activity and their environment, microbiome science is turning human health specialists into ecologists.

Like early European cartographers, the first scientists mapping the human genome were disappointed to discover how insignificant we are in comparison with the rest of the living world. Humans have only twenty thousand protein-encoding genes, about the same number as fruit flies.[11] Although the exact number is a subject of active debate, by some estimates, the microorganisms living within us outnumber our own cells by a factor of ten to one. All the life on or in our bodies contains at least 200 million genes, and some studies point to orders of magnitude more.[12] We are at the very beginning of learning how much of this genetic material is critical for our health. Symbiotic microbes inhabit every one of our organs, each organ having its own distinct ecosystem.[13] The gut hosts the greatest number and diversity of microbes of all our organs. The adult gut microbiome contains around 23 million unique genes, many of which matter in the busy forest of our digestive system in ways that we are only starting to understand.[14]

Our thriving internal ecosystems can withstand a certain amount of damage. But beyond a certain threshold of destruction, collapse cascades. Modern life has denuded the human microbiome, driving to extinction species we have co-evolved with since the dawn of our own. Diseases in the gut that were rare in the twentieth century, and that continue to be rare in some populations of Indigenous people, have become far more commonplace in industrialized societies. Western medicine is undergoing a seismic shift in thinking about how humans fit into a complex web of life—a web that we're beginning to understand just as we realize how much of it we've already annihilated.

Microbes aren't new to medicine. In the late seventeenth and early eighteenth century, at the zenith of the Dutch Empire, Anton van Leeuwenhoek, a draper in Delft, invented powerful glass lenses to examine the weave of his cloth. When he used them to look at pond water, he saw a world crawling with microscopic life. His observation of "animalcules" was the first known sighting of bacteria and protozoa.[15] In another sign of Western medicine's patriarchal foundations, van Leeuwenhoek became known as the Father of Microbiology.[16]

Microscopes played a supporting role in the drama of metropolitan health problems, in particular the problems of expanding European cities. Within those cities, the provenance of food that was once mediated by an exchange or two from farm to fork became a much more complicated affair. The microscope could magnify evidence of contaminations along the food supply chain. Worries about food spoilage led to the 1820 transatlantic best seller, *A Treatise on Adulterations of Food, and culinary poisons, exhibiting the fraudulent sophistications of bread, beer, wine, spirituous liquors, tea, coffee, cream, confectionery, vinegar, mustard, pepper, cheese, olive oil, pickles, and other articles employed in domestic economy and methods of detecting them*, by Friedrich Christian Accum.[17]

Microscopy also featured in the cure to anxieties about food poisoning. When the problem of food spoilage arose because of the long supply chains between the producers of wine, beer, and milk and their eventual consumers, pasteurization was the solution. Louis Pasteur's early work provided evidence for the germ theory of disease. His ideas were not, however, magnified through the microscope alone. As the philosopher Bruno Latour observes, it took an assembly of science, commercial interest, French politics, and colonial ambitions to achieve the "Pasteurization of France."[18]

Domestic and international public health were intimately linked. The field of infectious diseases was developed to support the imperial project, and its colonial roots are evident in modern-day global health programs.[19] Keeping British colonists safe from malaria during the subjugation of India, for instance, required a complex mix of science and state power. The cinchona tree was the Andean source of the antimalarial drug quinine, and the countries there guarded their exports jealously. Britain paid the modern equivalent of around $10 million a year to Bolivia, Colombia, Ecuador, and Peru for cinchona bark.[20] Through the 1860s, British agents smuggled cinchona plants and seeds to the Royal Botanic Gardens at Kew in London, whose mission was to "aid . . . the Mother Country in everything that is useful in the vegetable kingdom."[21] From there, the plants and the science fanned out to the colonies, where the medicine was given to fortify colonial troops against the malaria parasite. It was not intended to treat the people being conquered. Today colonial medicine's legacy continues as malaria remains a major cause of illness and death in the Global South.[22] As Pasteur put it, *"Le microbe n'est rien, le terrain est tout."*[23]

At the peak of colonial expansion, outbreaks of both uprisings and disease were treated with new techniques of government. The relationship between humans and microbes came to be understood as adversarial. (Think about how unusual and relatively new the term *probiotic* is.) Self and other were yet again set in opposition, in the kind of war metaphor that Darwin would've loved. Armies and police rounded up the mutineers. Doctors eradicated bacteria. In this task, the French offered a new style: hygiene. Hygienists like Stéphane Leduc cautioned that "ignoring the danger of the microbe awaiting us, we have hitherto arranged our way of life without taking any account of this unknown enemy."[24] Society needed to be defended, so medical, social, and cultural hygiene locked up, schooled, bleached, and civilized its enemies as necessary.[25] On so many levels, it was a war against life itself. For the individual, new habits of behavior made germophobia—a word first used in 1893—possible.

At a planetary level, colonialism transformed the interactions between ecologies in the web of life. Species that hadn't been in contact before were brought together by accident or design, flowing along the trade routes of Europe's empires. The pandemics of smallpox in the Western Hemisphere and cholera in the Eastern Hemisphere were consequences of this new interaction. In response, hygienists wielded tools of eradication and sterilization along lines of supremacy. Certain humans, animals, and microbes were categorized as inferior. This is why the war on microbes is inseparable from the cultural matrix that sustained it; hygiene coincided with the birth of eugenics, the heyday of Orientalism, and the expansion of European empires.

The biological consequences of an increasingly sterile planet are visible both in the world and in our bodies. At an Earth-systems level, widespread deforestation and industrial agriculture are causing the loss of rich microbial diversity in soil, a living key to carbon sequestration and water retention.[26] The lack of soil biodiversity also impacts our health in many ways. Foods that are grown in sterile soil are less nutrient dense, specifically in those molecules that counteract inflammation.[27] Microorganisms in the soil that settle on our windowsills—or lack thereof—shape our immune response.[28] The microbiota of the soil are linked to those we host in the human microbiome, and we are discovering more about those interrelationships every day.[29] We see the same trend in the gut and in the soil: microbial biodiversity in places of modern human activity is disappearing.

What's true for the forest without is true for the forest within. In 1989 the epidemiologist David Strachan studied the rising rates of hay fever in children in England and found that exposure to diverse microbial environments when young protected them against developing allergies and autoimmune disorders, like asthma and eczema.[30] What started out as a hypothesis in the field of allergy has moved into the field of immunology, as rates of chronic inflammatory diseases are similarly rising in increasingly sterile places.[31]

THE GUT MICROBIOME: A GUIDE TO THE FOREST

Your gut microbiome is as unique as your fingerprints. Even identical twins, whose host genome is 99.9 percent similar, can have gut microbiomes that are 80 to 90 percent different. This is the poetry of the web of life: what makes you unique is the multitude of beings that make your body their home. And what keeps you healthy literally depends on the relationships you maintain between yourself and others.

The gut microbiome sits at the crossroads of vital pathways that dictate how we develop and how we thrive. Its organisms digest foods that we cannot digest ourselves. Enzymes encoded by microbial genes expand our ability to extract nutrients from diverse diets.[32] If our own genes offer a Swiss Army knife of tools for digestion, microbial genes offer a whole hardware store of possibilities. Our gut microbes digest complex carbohydrates in insoluble plant fiber, for instance, creating short-chain fatty acids. These molecules have powerful anti-inflammatory properties, acting both locally in the gut and around our bodies by entering the bloodstream.[33]

Our microbes also make essential nutrients such as vitamin K, which is needed for blood to clot. There are two main forms of vitamin K. One comes from plants such as broccoli and kale. This form is absorbed by the small intestines when we eat those foods. The other—which makes up 90 percent of the vitamin K in our bodies—comes from the bacteria we host. Gut microbes possess enzymes that convert *shikimate* (pronounced shĭ′-kĭ-māt) into vitamin K.[34] Shikimate is a molecule that was first discovered in 1885 in *shikimi*, Japanese star anise.[35] Found only in plants and microorganisms, it serves as a precursor to molecules that are critical for our health, including vitamin K and the essential amino acids phenylalanine and tryptophan, which we must obtain from our diet.[36] The impact of bacteria making vitamin K is not trivial. A prolonged course of broad-spectrum antibiotics wipes out the intestinal microbes that turn *shikimate* into vitamin K, leading to decreased stored levels in the liver. Without vitamin K, blood cannot clot. This has led to life-threatening bleeding.[37]

Established communities of organisms, in addition to providing us with essential nutrients such as vitamins, also influence our resistance or susceptibility to disease. They prevent pathogens from taking hold in our intestines.[38] They can turn our own genes on and off. They shape our body's reaction to danger and are impacted by that reaction as well. They can make cancer treatments more effective.[39] Much of this work involves modulating the immune system and, with it, the inflammatory response.[40]

The microbiota in our gut are foundational to the healthy development, education, and function of our immune system (as well as our endocrine and nervous systems). Microbes are involved in training our inflammatory response, teaching us how to host—not just tolerate—them inside our bodies. In turn, we receive their many modulating benefits. In this complex web of interactions between host and microbes, inflammatory and regulatory signals are continually integrated to form the immune tone. These relationships quite literally set up how the body does or does not respond to pathogens, environmental toxicities, and even to itself.[41]

What makes a healthy microbiome is as complex a question as what makes a healthy forest. When it comes to microbes, context and relationships are everything. To a scientist trained in reductionist models of disease, these concepts can be challenging. To an ecologist trained in understanding how systems function, the

principles upon which health depends—biodiversity and balance—
are familiar.[42] An appropriately biodiverse and functional gut microbiome is our most sophisticated defense against inflammatory
disease. The less diverse our gut microbes are, the more inflamed
we seem to be.[43] A lack of gut biodiversity is associated with cardiovascular disease, asthma, allergies, obesity, diabetes, suicide, colon cancer, Alzheimer's disease, inflammatory bowel disease, and
autoimmune disease.[44] In this area of active research, early indications suggest that a microbiome that lacks diversity cannot produce
a balanced immune response.[45]

Once we lose the bacteria that temper inflammation—and they
can disappear over a single human generation—it is not clear that
we can ever get them back.[46] When mice, whose biological responses
closely approximate our own, eat a low-fiber diet, the biodiversity of
their gut microbiome drops. Resuming a higher-fiber diet alone does
not bring back the lost microbes. Once you lose a strain of microbes,
it's gone for good. You can undergo a "reprogramming of the gut,"
in which you are inoculated with the strains you lost, then tend and
nourish those strains with a high-fiber diet.[47] But this spot treatment,
as we'll learn later, is futile if the world around us, with its stresses,
food additives, and industrial pollution, constantly strips the microbial biodiversity from our bodies.

If you want microbial biodiversity, don't live in a city in the
Global North. Western urban dwellers have the least biodiverse guts
on Earth. Hunter-gatherer and rural agrarian communities in Africa,
India, and the Amazon host the most internal biological diversity.[48]
These rural and Indigenous communities have greater prevalence
of beneficial gut bacteria such as *Prevotella* and *Treponema*,[49] which
ferment fiber into short-chain fatty acids. These fatty acids push immune cells to produce molecular messengers that halt inflammatory
signals. They also directly suppress other immune cells that drive
inflammation.[50] With diets rich in fiber, non-Western civilizations
have the capacity to sustain an internal microbiome far more varied
than the flaccid modern Western diet can.[51]

Indigenous Yanomami communities in the Amazon rainforest farm, eat, and live in sophisticated ecological balance with the lives around and inside them. Their bodies are fully integrated into an ecosystem that supports a vibrant immunity, shaping how a pathogen will express itself on encounter. Virchow's hypothesis—that a bacterium doesn't create a disease, but the body's inflammatory reaction to it does—is proven in the Yanomami experience with *Chlamydia trachomatis*, a bacterium that is endemic to the Yanomami population. Outside their community, the organism is responsible for causing blindness, through repeated cycles of infection and inflammation. The Yanomami are widely infected, but they don't suffer the inflammation, and they don't go blind from it.[52] Their coevolved relationships with the microbial ecology inside and around them have trained their immunity to not react with inflammation, even in the face of infection. Instead, the greatest threat to their sight is posed by the Brazilian and Venezuelan governments, and the encroachment of their territories by the illegal gold miners that those governments allow, bringing diseases that will disrupt the ecological balance that has long supported Yanomami immunity. This example highlights how immunity is less about self and other than about balance and relationship, which when damaged leaves us vulnerable to inflammation.

Clearly the immune benefits of the Yanomami gut microbiome make it valuable as a potential inoculant: it contains a cocktail of life that most humans have lost. No doubt right now capitalists somewhere are developing a marketing plan to turn Indigenous shit into gold. But it would be a mistake to imagine that this microbiome is some sort of fossil from the past, one that can simply be transplanted and maintained.[53] It is a living reflection of people existing in a healthy relationship with the web of life that supports them. Ancient strains of microbes such as *Treponema* and *Roseburia* have been found both in fossilized feces from ancient peoples and in the guts of modern Indigenous people. These gut microbes express fewer of the enzymatic pathways prevalent in the modern-day industrial microbiome that predispose us to inflammation.[54] These ancestral strains, which abate inflammation and regulate the innate immune system, are frequently absent from US city dwellers.[55] This gives a new layer of meaning to a core value expressed among Indigenous people: we must maintain connection with our ancestors. It literally is a matter of living well or living with bodies damaged by inflammation.

We didn't just lose these ancient strains a long time ago. We're losing them still today. The Irish Travellers are genetically similar to their settled compatriots but are a distinct group who have been nomadic for several centuries.[56] Although they suffered from the usual scourges associated with poverty, Irish Travellers did not suffer the chronic illnesses of their settled counterparts, such as inflammatory bowel disease.[57] Historically, Travellers moved in caravans, living in tight quarters in large family groups and often in close proximity to their horses. In 2002 the Irish government forced their settlement into single-family homes, in an act of ongoing demonization of this minoritized group. Before settling, their guts contained hallmarks of an ancient or nonindustrialized microbiome that is believed to be the cause of their protection against modern diseases.[58] In the twenty years since settlement, their microbiota have become less diverse, now mirroring an industrialized microbiome—even though their diet has stayed the same.[59] Researchers are currently investigating the consequences that this loss of ancestral strains and biodiversity has had on their health, looking specifically at the prevalence of chronic inflammatory diseases.

The presence of certain species of bacteria alone does not make for a healthy microbiome: the balance of bacteria matters as well. Disruption of this balance in the gastrointestinal tract, called gut dysbiosis, is associated with a wide range of inflammatory diseases. The community of bacteria living in the large intestines determine—through direct contact or through their metabolic products—whether host cells maintain homeostasis or trigger an inflammatory response. Some species and some metabolic pathways appear to confer protection against inflammatory diseases, while others seem to promote inflammation, with relative consistency across populations.[60] For example, an unfavorable balance between *Bacteroidetes* and *Firmicutes* is associated with obesity and its accompanying chronic inflammation.[61]

The guts of people experiencing obesity tend to have a higher ratio of *Firmicutes* to *Bacteroides*, while those of people without obesity have the reverse pattern. This microbial imbalance results in the extraction of more energy from food, which leads to its storage as fat.[62] Conversely, for individuals who experience obesity, losing weight is more strongly a function of rebalancing their gut microbiome than of changing calorie content over time.[63] While food choices matter in weight loss, microbes are a critical part of our own energy balance. If farming practices, food additives, and the stresses of modern society destroy healthy microbial ecologies, obesity must be reframed as a condition caused by a damaging exposome rather than solely as a problem of individual indiscretion.

Dysbiosis can result from disease, antibiotic use, or repeated exposure to stress and pollutants.[64] People exposed to multiple rounds of antibiotics in childhood have an increased risk of developing inflammatory bowel disease.[65] This may seem odd—antibiotics are routinely prescribed to treat harmful bacteria. But antibiotics kill indiscriminately. Taking them has the effect of clear-cutting an old-growth forest. A secondary forest may return, but without care, it's not likely to be as robust or diverse as its antecedent.[66] *Clostridium difficile* lives in the soil and in our intestines. When it's held in balance, it's benign. A round of antibiotics, however, can clear the way for *Clostridium difficile* to take over, causing diarrhea and life-threatening infection.[67]

Scientists are still teasing apart what the relationship between various diseases and dysbiosis signifies, being careful not to infer causality when an association is found. But the associations alone are providing stunning insights, expanding our limits of understanding what determines sickness or health. In complex diseases that are the outcome of interacting environmental and genetic forces, such as colorectal cancer and schizophrenia, the genome of one's gut microbiome predicts the presence or absence of disease better than does the human genome alone.[68] Such associations point to the need for deeper investigation to establish causality. Mapping the effects of dysbiosis and the biological by-products of various microbiota is an important first step in understanding what part microbes play in human wellness and disease.

SEEDING THE FOREST

Cultivating a rich forest of microbes requires a lifetime of engagement. It involves more than following a particular diet or taking a slurry of probiotics. The seeds of your microbiome were first planted when you were still inside your mother: humans can be exposed to microbes in the womb. Meconium, a baby's first, tarlike bowel movement, is already rich with biological life. As early as fourteen weeks of gestational age, clusters of bacteria in fetal intestines begin to educate the developing fetal immune system, which in turn decides which microbes the body will become home to.[69] This two-way dialogue between developing immune cells and microbes sets the tone for how a person's immune system will function later in life.[70] A lower risk of childhood chronic inflammatory diseases such as asthma is associated with reduced maternal stress and prenatal antibiotic exposures and increased exposure to different microbially rich environments during pregnancy, suggesting the mother's microbiome is also involved.[71] The exposome of your own life starts in the womb, shaped by your mother's.

The first large microbiome inoculation happens during birth itself. Babies born through the vagina tend to develop a gut microbiome that closely mirrors their mother's. Babies born via C-section are less likely to receive their mother's microbes and are more likely to pick up bacteria from their surroundings, usually a hospital,[72] predisposing them to higher risks of developing several inflammatory diseases, including inflammatory bowel disease, leukemia, asthma, and type 1 diabetes.[73] In addition to vaginal birth, breastfeeding and skin-to-skin contact are primary ways that microbes spread from mothers to children.[74] This transfer represents a previously unconsidered component of genetic inheritance, because when microbes move, their genetic toolkit goes with them. Over the first two years of life, microbiomes rapidly develop across the human body. In the gut, the accumulation of microbes relates to early-life encounters including the baby's diet, antimicrobial administration, and other environmental exposures.

After birth and throughout our lives, our gut microbiome develops in response to exposures. What we eat selects which organisms will thrive in our gut. Breast milk selects for specific microbes to establish themselves in an infant's digestive system. Formula selects a different set, with a predominance of fungi. These fungi extract energy from formula at much higher rates than organisms in breastfed babies. This intensified energy extraction from food may be one reason why formula-fed babies have higher rates of childhood obesity by age two. The microbiome profile of formula-fed babies is also associated with higher rates of asthma, eczema, and pro-inflammatory markers.[75] How the early gut microbiome is shaped has consequences throughout life. Early exposure to antibiotics before the age of five is associated with developing Crohn's disease later in life. Disruption of the early-life gut microbiome, which trains immunity and shapes host cell physiology, is a proposed mechanism of causation.[76]

One microbe that is more common in exclusively breastfed babies is *Bifidobacterium infantis*, which feeds on the oligosaccharides in breast milk, creating the beneficial anti-inflammatory short-chain fatty acid acetate as a by-product.[77] Breast milk oligosaccharides provide no direct nutritional benefit to the infant, but they do serve as the perfect food for *Bifidobacterium infantis*, which evolved the enzymes necessary to digest these sugars—a perfect example of microbial-human coevolution. This microbe optimizes the infant's internal ecosystem by tightening the intestinal barrier and by training the baby's immune system prior to weaning.[78] It teaches a newborn's gut to tolerate its developing microbiota by inducing regulatory T cells that then shape autoimmune and inflammatory responses.[79] Reduced presence of this educating organism in infancy has been associated with lifelong problems such as asthma, obesity, and autoimmune disease.[80]

Recently probiotics containing *Bifidobacterium infantis* have also been used therapeutically on adults. A randomized controlled study looking at three separate inflammatory conditions in adults—ulcerative colitis, chronic fatigue syndrome, and psoriasis—found that taking *Bifidobacterium infantis* for eight weeks significantly decreased systemic inflammatory markers, including C-reactive protein, IL-6, and TNF-α. This central impact was attributed to the organism's ability to increase the number of regulatory T cells, which in turn decrease inflammatory activity.[81]

The microbes in infant feces have anti-inflammatory qualities that were observed in sixteenth-century China, where baby poop was used to make medicine. This concoction, called yellow soup, was prescribed for abdominal pain and diarrhea. Even earlier than that, during the fourth century Dong-jin dynasty, traditional Chinese medicine doctors used oral suspensions of human feces to treat food poisoning. This practice is documented in the first Chinese handbook of emergency medicine, *Zhou Hou Bei Ji Fang*, "Handy Therapy for Emergencies," which dates to the same era.[82] These were the first recorded fecal transplants, which have come back into vogue seventeen hundred years later.

Fecal transplants have induced remission in some cases of inflammatory bowel disease and have proven highly effective against recurrent *Clostridium difficile* gastrointestinal infections, which have become increasingly tricky to treat.[83] The organism has evolved multiple pathways of drug resistance, and more patients are suffering relapses, as the infection reestablishes itself as soon as antibiotics are stopped.[84] A surprising number of patients who suffer from recurrent *Clostridium difficile* infections say they prefer the fecal transplant to antibiotics.[85] If you're one of the 40 percent of melanoma patients who don't respond to new immunotherapy drugs, there's hope. Fecal transplants can overcome resistance to these therapies, making the drugs more effective in eliminating cancer.[86] As far as guests go, that's a remarkable "thank you for hosting me" gift.

One unexpected side effect of receiving a fecal transplant is improvement of another disease associated with poor gut biodiversity: depression. In a small study, 38 percent of people who received a fecal transplant for the treatment of *Clostridium difficile* reported improved mental health after the procedure, compared with 8.9 percent of those who received antibiotics, which is the current standard of care treatment for the infection.[87] Fecal transplantation is currently being studied in the treatment of diabetes and obesity, and early results are worthy of tempered enthusiasm.[88]

TENDING THE FOREST

Our microbiome settles into an adult pattern by the age of three, but it never remains static. It changes constantly, in response to how we live and what makes up our exposome. It is a living reflection of our historical and contemporary exposures.

In a little under a week, for example, you can alter which organisms flourish in your gut by altering what you eat.[89] Microbes are one of the main reasons for the success of the Mediterranean diet.[90] Its high-fiber content nourishes those organisms, like *Prevotella*, who produce the beneficial short-chain fatty acids that cool inflammation. Likewise, vegan and vegetarian diets promote greater gut biodiversity, which also has a beneficial effect on systemic inflammation.[91]

By the same token, a diet rich in the industrial chemicals that currently flood our food system is far more likely to harm our microbiome.[92] Dietary emulsifiers that are used to make ice cream smoother hamper microbes' ability to mitigate inflammation, and synthetic sugars have totally altered the composition of the Western gut microbiome.[93] Not to mention the world's most widely used herbicide: glyphosate. As we saw in Chapter 1, this active ingredient in Roundup likely killed Lorenzo Hidalgo.[94]

Since the early 2000s, an off-brand use has been driving Roundup sales: farmers will wait for a few days of dry weather in late summer, then spray their nonresistant cereal crops with glyphosate to kill them. The dead crops shrivel in the sun, which means they're ready to be mechanically harvested a couple of days later. Using glyphosate as a desiccant allows farmers to synchronize their harvest to a window of time that matches the weather, the availability of a combine harvester, and the needs of the market.[95] But it also ensures much more direct contact between humans' guts and the pesticide. We have much more chance of eating glyphosate if it was used to kill the crop days before the crop was turned into flour than if it was used to kill weeds weeks before harvest.

Its manufacturers insist that glyphosate has no biological impact on health, because it inhibits an enzyme pathway present in plants, fungi, and bacteria but not in animals—the *shikimate* pathway. But this is the same pathway that makes vitamin K and several essential amino acids. Without it, many microbes die, and other beneficial microbes appear to be disproportionately impacted.[96] Even at levels deemed to be safe for health, glyphosate has been shown to disrupt the rat gut microbiome.[97] It does the same to the honeybee gut microbiome,[98] to poultry gut microbes,[99] and to the microbes in the soil, because it inhibits this metabolic pathway common to all microbes. Not only does glyphosate disrupt microbial communities, it creates the conditions where pathogens can thrive. *Clostridium* species, including *Clostridium difficile*, and *Salmonella* species—both significant human pathogens—are resistant to glyphosate's impact on this pathway.[100] These pathogens are left to multiply, in the gut and in the soil, after glyphosate's assault on microbial biodiversity. In addition to the overuse of antibiotics in animal feedlots, glyphosate may be implicated in the increased presence of community-based *Clostridium difficile* infections seen in people living close to industrial farms.[101]

As we observed in Chapter 1, glyphosate is everywhere, from cereals to baby formula to beer and wine.[102] For researchers looking to see how it causes gut dysbiosis in humans, that ubiquity is a problem because it's next to impossible to find a control group that hasn't been exposed. It's hard to truly farm organically when the groundwater from below has been tainted by synthetic pesticides in agricultural communities around the world.[103] As with public tobacco use, the only way to understand the impact pesticides are having on the gut microbiome and on human health may be to eliminate them altogether and watch what happens.

Beyond the foods we eat, other aspects of the exposome dramatically shape the composition of the gut microbiome. Stress is one of the most damaging, illuminating a bidirectional communication between the gut and the brain—what is called the gut-brain-microbiota axis. This communication is regulated through the immune, endocrine, and nervous systems, all of which are under the influence of the creatures that make their home in the folds of our intestines.[104]

One of the most important functions that gut microbes play throughout human life is the development and maintenance of the intestinal barrier, the space that separates the hollow inside of the intestine—called the lumen—from the blood and hence from the rest of the body. The intestinal barrier absorbs nutrients, water, and electrolytes and blocks the entry of pathogens and toxic substances.[105] Microbes live at this edge, and if you don't have enough of them when you're an infant, you might have an exacerbated stress response when you're grown up.[106] It turns out that in those early months, gut microbes program the HPA stress response axis (see Chapter 2).[107] As an extension of the hygiene hypothesis, which asserts that our sterilized world has created an increase in allergic disease, the lack of a robust gut microbiome in early life may contribute to the rise of stress-related disorders such as depression.[108]

While gut microbes program our stress response from an early age, stress in turn also impacts the microbiome.[109] Stress changes the composition of microbes and their metabolic products, making for a more inflammatory milieu.[110] This may explain how stress can lead to a flare of inflammatory bowel disease. Stress also compromises the integrity of the intestinal barrier, making the gut leaky. Molecules and microbes that usually sit in the hollow lumen can then seep into the blood circulation, setting off an inflammatory response when they do.[111] What is incredible about these changes is that they respond to probiotic intervention. Strains of *Lactobacillus* can suppress stress-induced changes in gut permeability and improve the mucus barrier.[112] As with microbes programming the HPA axis, early-life stress also impacts the integrity of this intestinal barrier later in life.[113] In rats, neonatal separation from a mother predisposes the baby to intestinal barrier dysfunction in the face of stress when it grows up.[114] This may be another mechanism by which early childhood trauma leads to adult inflammatory diseases.

Perhaps one of the most pernicious reasons for changes in the gut microbiome are adverse childhood experiences (ACEs, if you're looking in the literature). A landmark study found that the more a person reportedly experienced physical and sexual abuse or neglect as a child, the more they were likely to develop diseases of the heart, lung, and liver, skeletal fractures, and cancer in adulthood.[115] Childhood traumas are stressors that lead to an imbalance of microbial life in the gut. This creates an exacerbated stress response throughout life and, as a consequence, chronic inflammation.[116]

One small study showed how ACEs can alter the gut microbial composition in a way that affects future generations. The more adverse events a pregnant woman experienced when she was a child, the more likely she is to have microbes that promote inflammation in her gut, which in turn affect the microbiome of her fetus.[117] Genetic transmission of trauma happens through microbes in addition to epigenetics, as we saw in Chapters 1 and 2. Not only does stress erode telomeres, it yields microbes that may compound the impact, further connecting ACEs to adult chronic inflammatory diseases, such as heart disease and diabetes.[118] This just goes to show that when one relationship falls out of sync, it affects all the others that are interconnected.

Thanks to colonialism's dissection of the web of life, humans must now contend with its legacy in today's toxic world. The air we breathe, including its pollution, impacts our gut microbes.[119] Environmental contaminants such as the perfluorinated compounds PFOS and

PFOA disrupt the gut microbiome.[120] These compounds have been used for over fifty years in everything from nonstick frying pans to pesticides. North Americans and Europeans are likely to experience long-term and ubiquitous exposure to these "forever" chemicals in contaminated food supplies and drinking water.[121] (Recall the case of Shelia McCarley.)

It shouldn't be surprising, then, that in ecosystems that have resisted the call for industrial chemistry, on farms where the land is managed through agroecology, microbes seem to confer the most anti-inflammatory benefits.[122] Spending time in a forest can have similar results, according to Japanese scholars who have described the health benefits of *shinrin-yoku*, "forest bathing."[123] The German equivalent is *Heubad*, or "hay bathing," which Alpine farmers have promoted for centuries to help with aches and pains, bringing about a sense of wellness.[124] We have identified one soil microbe, *Mycobacterium vaccae*, that has anti-inflammatory properties that make our bodies more resilient in the face of chemical and emotional stress.[125] There are likely countless more where that came from: each organism creates its own sound that, together with all others, forms a complex chord of immunomodulating action when we lie down on the Earth's floor. While the molecular mechanism of how *Mycobacterium vaccae* mitigates inflammation is still being investigated, it and others offer insight into why these bathing practices have such an impact on mental and physical health.[126] As urbanization and industrialization expose us to more environmental pollutants and reduce our opportunities to interact with vibrant, rich soil, our internal worlds are becoming more and more depleted.[127]

Our microbes adapt to what we eat and where we live, what we are surrounded by and how we feel.[128] Their genes offer us tools to digest foods we otherwise can't, giving us more metabolic possibilities. Bacteria are also highly promiscuous. They swap their genetic material across species, so a pathway for digestion can leap from a species found in the soil to one found in the gut. This can be a benefit but also a liability. A genetic pathway to digest seaweed, for example, is found in marine microbes but also only in the guts of Japanese people for whom seaweed is a staple. The genes encoding this pathway don't exist in any other human microbes. They jumped from a marine organism to a gut microbe and stayed there, helping Japanese people unlock the nutrients in seaweed.[129] Genes that encode metabolic pathways move from one organism to another, offering new tools for survival.[130] But this can pose a problem when the surrounding environment is toxic.

Just as on farms, not everything in the sea is benign or natural. By 2050, there will be more plastic in the sea than fish.[131] Bacteria adapt. *Ideonella sakaiensis*, first identified near a Japanese recycling plant, uses enzymes to digest polyethylene terephthalate, a widespread plastic, as its sole energy source. Its enzymes break plastic down into by-products that induce cancer and cause localized inflammation in humans.[132] Since we first put plastics into the world, we have been accumulating them in our bodies. People consume up to 52,000 microplastic particles a year. If you add what we are breathing, that brings the total to 121,000 particles a year.[133] Even the unborn are exposed.[134] If the genetic code for the enzymes digesting plastic ends up in the human microbiome through bacterial gene swapping, our microbes will digest them, and those by-products will create more inflammation and more cancer. Environmental pollutants such as these have been associated with the development of type 2 diabetes, obesity, cancer, and immune and reproductive dysregulation. Our gut microbes are feasting on these chemicals, and their biological excreta are poisoning us.[135]

The adaptability of gut microbes was helpful when early humans had to follow different food sources or move away from unwelcoming climates. But in a world where industrial contamination is now ubiquitous, this adaptability has become a liability. Gut microbes harmonize our bodies with the ecology around us. When our surrounding exposures are harmful, the result is inflammation.[136]

The microbiome illustrates how virtually everything around us affects our health, especially our social structures: our industries, farming practices, communities, and homes. Systemic injustice, then, maps itself directly onto our bodies. Indigenous people have known for thousands of years what modern science is just beginning to understand:[137] that good health is all about relationships and living with others in harmony. Instead of domination (of germs, of people, of life), good health is about hospitality, reciprocity, and care. By disturbing our traditional relationships with the land and with one another, colonialism has disturbed our internal ecologies as well.[138]

WEB OF LIFE AND OF DEATH

Homo sapiens sapiens (as distinct from *Homo sapiens neanderthalensis*) emerged ninety thousand years ago. If the history of humanity lasted a single day, starting at midnight, then for most of the night and day, we were hunters, foragers, and gatherers. Around eight-thirty in the evening, humans domesticated our first species: dogs.[139] Almost immediately, we changed their bodies, selecting not just for a lack of aggression but also for the ability to eat a human Paleolithic diet. Dogs developed guts that were ready to manage the high-starch diet of their hominid companions.[140]

Just past nine, in what is now Iraq, humans domesticated sheep.[141] And sheep appear to have domesticated humans in turn, because around that time our ancestors stopped being nomads and finally settled down—the first continuous human settlement emerged in the Fertile Crescent.[142] About half an hour later, the retreat of ice sheets spurred the near-simultaneous domestication of plants in half a dozen regions of the world.[143]

Humans' seasonal migrations for food took them from settlement to settlement. Meanwhile certain plants thrived in the disturbed soil of human habitation. Although we may imagine humans scouring the world looking for the right kind of plant to turn into daily bread, the plant breeder Stan Cox notes that "many crop ancestors were just as responsible for seeking out humans and human-made environments as were people for tracking down the plants."[144] What ensued was a delicate, reciprocal relationship between humans and plants called *commensal symbiosis*.

A species of plant advertised itself to humans, who in turn elected to cultivate it once they found they did better by eating, drinking, or healing with it. The plant also did better because humans began experimenting with the surrounding ecology to encourage its growth. The origins of agriculture, then, lay in a mutually beneficial symbiosis between humans and plants. Note that this is a relationship, not a hierarchy.

Humans domesticated plants, but their ambitions weren't modern ones. It's an anachronism to imagine that in the late evening of human evolution, our ancestors domesticated plants according to which ones were most productive or nutritious or had the highest yield. Neolithics were not neoliberals. Early humans wanted more than just a return on investment. Archaeological evidence suggests that they sought fermentability, snackability, and sweetness.[145] In other words, party food. Pleasure and joy, as we'll see again and again, can be vital forces.

Over generations of experiments, humans developed subtle and increasingly sophisticated knowledge about plants and animals,[146] as well as rich and varied relationships with them. The Haida people of the Pacific Northwest have a story, retold by the ethnobotanist Nancy Turner, about what in English we call the highbush cranberry:

> Yaał (Massett dialect) [Raven] was visiting the Beaver People. Two days consecutively, he was served salmon, highbush cranberries [łaayi] and the inside parts of the mountain goat. On the second morning, yaał was taken behind a screen where there was a fishtrap in a creek filled with salmon, and several points on a lake which were red with cranberries. After the beavers had gone for the day, yaał ate the usual meal. Then he stole the salmon-filled lake and the house, rolling it up and hiding it under his arm, and climbed a tree with it. When the beavers returned, they tried to catch him

by chewing down the tree, but yaał simply flew to another. Finally they gave up, and yaał flew inland and unrolled the lake there and kept the fishtrap and house to teach the people of Haida Gwaii and the Mainland how to live. Since then, there have been many highbush cranberries in Haida Gwaii.[147]

The peoples of the Pacific Northwest know the highbush cranberry by different names depending on whether they speak Tsilhqot'in, Nuxalk, Comox, Sechelt, Lushootseed, Twana, Stl'atl'imx/St'át'imc, Secwepemc, Haisla, Heiltsuk, Oowekyala, or Kwak'wala.[148] The stinging nettle has twenty-two distinct names in this region, each telling a story of its relationship to everything around it—in this case, how Raven brought łaayi to the region.[149] In contrast, the Linnaean system has just one name for the highbush cranberry: *Viburnum edule*, a term that is derived from a hierarchy of plants, classes, orders, families, and genera. This demonstrates two different ways of thinking about the world. The Indigenous cosmology celebrates multitudes and the complexity of the various relationships comprising the web of life, whereas the colonial cosmology merely seeks to categorize, to civilize, and to impose social order.

When colonial powers civilized Indigenous people, they used the Linnaean genetic theory to identify each resource they would plunder. Not only that, but the civilizing campaign included the optimization of planting and grazing on the land those colonial powers seized. Ranches replaced wild bison ranges.[150] Plantations replaced camas fields, made through centuries of careful burning.[151] Early white Australian settlers beheld the landscapes that had been tended by millennia of Aboriginal work, and saw the sophistication of Aboriginal agriculture, aquaculture, and pyrogeography, but failed to recognize it as such due to the a priori notion that Aboriginal people were uncivilized and thereby incapable of such cultivation.[152] Instead, they concluded that Australia was naturally beautiful—God's Own Country.[153]

Colonialism erased many traces of this Aboriginal agriculture and the cosmology of relationships that attended it.[154] Linnaean nomenclature describes this erasure: the standardization of names meant that one European-approved term overwrote the multitude of Indigenous words that reflect local lifeways. Doing so flattened living things—plants, animals, even people—into assets to be managed from afar in the service of an economy.

Perhaps the most important contrast with plants that have dozens of names is a plant product which has only one: sugar. Sugar was the world's first factory food. The name of sugar is almost universal: from its origins in what is now Papua New Guinea,[155] sugarcane and its products spread from the Chinese *sha-che* to the Sanskrit *sakkar*, the Arabic *al-shakker* and the twelfth-century French *sucre*, and thence to fourteenth-century English, where the *Oxford English Dictionary* first registers the word.[156]

With its beginnings in the Middle East and Spain, mass-produced sugar was at the very spear tip of modern colonialism. It was the crop that transformed Madeira, a colony in the northeastern Atlantic that Portugal claimed in 1415.[157] Initially, the *ihla da madeira*—"island of wood"—was densely forested. The trees were used for lumber, particularly for shipbuilding. But sugar was rare and demand for it in European courts was high. (The king of England wanted 1 kilogram [2 pounds], "if so much could be had at one time.")[158] To meet that demand, colonists transformed Madeira. Hydrological engineers channeled rain to the low plains, where sugar grass could grow. Slavers brought Indigenous people from what are now called the Canary Islands to work the land, and when they perished, Africans from other colonies took their place. Trees became fuel, and within seventy-five years the sugar trade burned through the island. By the 1530s, Madeira was an island of clear-cut stumps, a way-point for slavers and colonists seeking greater returns in the cane fields of Brazil.[159]

Slaves, markets in the metropolis, and speculative finance made gambles on acquiring territory for the purpose of sugar production increasingly lucrative. Colonialism also drove innovations in production, weaponry, marketing, distribution, and consumption. As the price of sugar fell, its base of consumption widened. Today, the world produces 188 million tons of sugar per year, and we eat far more than we should, from far too early an age. In the Global North, free sugars range from 20 to 40 percent of total energy intake among children under four.[160] Although the numbers in the Global South are generally a little lower, it is not by much. The World Health Organization strongly recommends limiting free sugars to 10 percent of total energy intake, although data suggest that figure should be closer to 5 percent. Added sugar is a cause of diabetes and is linked to heart and liver disease, dementia, cancer, and an expanding range of other metabolic ills.[161] Early research suggests that sugar's impact on the gut microbiome is not beneficial.[162]

Although sugar was the first, and perhaps the most pernicious, global crop, the markets for other plants have also driven Earth's destruction. The forces that compelled Madeira, Brazil, the Caribbean, and a belt of the tropics to plant sugarcane also broadened appetites for tea, cotton, and tobacco. Moreover, colonists hungered for the types of crops that were grown back in Europe, especially if they could be bought more cheaply under colonial duress. Thus, through the processes we noted in our discussion of *immunes* in Chapter 1, Ireland became an exporter of potatoes and India of wheat under British colonial rule, and both were forced to continue along this path while their own populations suffered catastrophic famines—in 1845–49 in Ireland and throughout the nineteenth century in India.[163] Modern states have internalized such colonial discipline, pursuing policies of exploitation with abandon. Today 1.3 billion hectares are reserved for just fifty-two crops,[164] and 5.3 billion for livestock.[165] Humans and our cattle, sheep, goats, chicken, and pigs account for 96 percent of all vertebrate biomass on Earth.[166] We've left other mammals, and much of the rest of the web of life, no quarry.[167]

Central to tilting the scales of life on Earth has been the refinement of industrial agriculture. Although first practiced in the fields of Madeira, industrial agriculture has since sharpened its tools of life and death. By 1962, when Rachel Carson published *Silent Spring,* the United States was using around 200 million pounds of pesticides annually, a number that tripled over the next twenty years.[168] Globally, over 4 million tonnes (9 billion pounds) of pesticides were used in 2018.[169] Herbicides and fungicides were used routinely to mimic in miniature the clear-cutting of forests. No species other than those favored by human consumerism would be tolerated in the soil. Modern industrial agricultural techniques were developed in sterilized laboratories. When the real world proved more complex, the solution was to render it more tractable by administering chemistry that would kill and clean and simplify the fields, in a continuation of colonialism's long war of sanitation—a war against life in all its complexity. This process of simplification has brought the loss of biodiversity and knowledge, particularly women's traditional knowledge of seeds, life, health, and the multitude of interactions within the web of life.[170]

The consequences of this seasonal annihilation can be seen in California's Salinas Valley, whose boosters call it "The Salad Bowl of the World." The lettuce here comes from dead earth, soil in which there is a paucity of microbes.[171] The community of bacteria in abused soil bears striking resemblance to the community of bacteria from an inflamed gut. Whereas taking a course of antibiotics can disrupt the gut microbiome, potentially leading to diarrhea, disrupting the soil microbiome through chemical fertilizers, pesticides, and industrial monoculture has far more devastating, long-lasting consequences for human health and the health of the whole ecosystem.

In the early 2000s, physicians in the United States puzzled over rising rates of community-acquired *Clostridium difficile* in people with no prior antibiotic exposure.[172] They found that living near a farm and living near livestock were risk factors for developing community-acquired *Clostridium difficile.*[173] Perhaps this killer was being cultivated and concentrated in the soil where our food is grown, or in the animals who were being treated with antibiotics in massive feedlots. Communication between the human gut microbiome and the soil microbiome—these two superorganisms—may be a critical link. From the field and the factory farm, these bacteria end up on our food, and from our food they move through our intestines. The consequences can be fatal, as is often the case when our microbial community gets knocked out of balance.[174]

HOW TO COLONIZE A BLUE ZONE

There is a simple way to improve soil biodiversity: don't kill the things that live in it. Agroecological soil management can reduce glyphosate concentrations and rebuild complex biomes within soil.[175] But the twin habits of domination and extermination are hard to kick. They are as ingrained in conventional practices in farming as they are in the practice of medicine. Both fields are characterized by a deep lack of understanding of the web of life. And often the ignorance is willful, mandated by the profit motive.

So instead of humility, colonial capitalism cultivates a tendency toward extermination. Farming deals with weeds and pests through the purchase of chemistry and machines; medicine, through surgery and pharmaceuticals. These quick fixes are more lucrative than supporting the capacity of surrounding systems to address the problem at hand—in farming the soil-food biome, in medicine the microbiome and immune system. Under capitalism, deficiencies are spot-treated with inputs that are essentially commodities; in farming, you buy phosphorus and nitrogen, for example, and in medicine, thiamine and vitamin D. The result is a metabolic rift, the consequence of isolating a single component from the systems that bring them vitality.[176] By contrast, deep medicine seeks to enter reciprocal relationships with the entities that attend to those deficiencies by way of their biological intelligence—soil and plant microbes in farming, and gut microbes and sunshine in medicine.

As we begin to grasp the mutualism between humans and the web of life, the beneficial consequences of symbiosis and the holobiont, the search has begun for those places, communities, and cultures that have managed to maintain better dynamics between themselves and the world around them.[177] One of the earliest ways Western medicine came to understand the link between the microbiome and health was by looking at longevity. When Élie Metchnikoff was a researcher at the Pasteur Institute in France, he'd heard that Bulgarian peasants were living unusually long lives, possibly because they ate unpasteurized dairy. His discovery of *Lactobacillus bulgaricus* and its effects on human lifespans later made him a darling of the human biohacking community.[178]

Okinawa, the largest of 150 islands halfway between Taiwan and the Japanese mainland, has one of the world's highest concentrations of people who live to be one hundred years old. Such areas of extreme longevity have come to be known as Blue Zones.[179] Okinawa has more centenarians than anywhere else: 68 people per 100,000 live to be one hundred years, compared to 48 in Japan, 22 in the United States, and 2 in India.[180] Okinawans' long lives are the result of a combination of good medical care, good sleep habits, more years of education, networks of friends, good genetics,[181] and even spiritual life.[182] Some researchers suggest the lack of harsh winters compared to the Japanese mainland helps.[183] Perhaps most famously, the food is rich in the kinds of things that keep people living long—antioxidants, fiber, complex carbohydrates—and is low in salt, fat, and sugar.[184] Food culture is also important. Okinawa is the home of *hara hachi bu*—the art of eating until you're 80 percent full. The Okinawan diet is a poster child for what to eat for a healthy microbiome. So why is life expectancy there now beginning to fall?[185]

Researchers generally agree on the cause: colonialism. Okinawans used to have a food system that was bound to their soil and sea. The Ryuku religious traditions emphasized the connections of humans to the web of life around them; women spiritual practitioners acted as guardians of sacred *utaki* groves.[186] Colonial incursions by the Japanese and then by Americans destroyed many of those sites; those that remain are tourist attractions, for those who want to see pockets of the biodiversity that was once widespread across the islands.

When the Allies arrived in 1945 after the Battle of Okinawa, at the end of World War II, the islanders received the Americans ecstatically. Okinawans had suffered mightily under Japanese rule—most intensely at its very end. In the eighty-two days of fighting before the Americans declared victory, over one hundred thousand Japanese and US soldiers died in the battle. Civilians fared worse: between one-tenth and one-third of Okinawa's population died either from starvation or as "collateral damage" in battle or were forced to commit suicide by the Japanese.[187] Okinawa's current centenarians are all lucky—or not, depending on how you look at it. They survived, and still recall, their population's decimation.

After World War II, occupation brought the American way of living, working, and eating to a starving Japanese population. Milk and white bread were eaten in schools—an edible education in the ways of North American civilization. With China mere hours away, prominent US politicians, industrialists, and philanthropists worried that hungry Japanese would see their future not under the umbrella of American capitalism but under that of communism. So they shipped American cereals to quiet the rumble of stomachs and of discontent. The red scare was the reason white food made its way to Okinawa.

Hidemi Todoriki, who teaches in the department of environmental and preventive medicine at the University of the Ryukyus, is a leading researcher on Okinawa's generational shifts. In the 1960s, he notes, the Okinawan diet had around 10 percent fat. The level is now around 30 percent. The fat found its way into the diet far faster in Okinawa than in mainland Japan because of the US occupation. (Okinawa was handed back to Japan only in 1972.) The proliferation of Western eateries, and food culture, centered on the US airbase are to blame.

Okinawa's shifting fortunes have resulted in one of the saddest demographic curves in the world, one that shows relatively high mortality rates among the young and low rates among the old.[188]

The series of data points describe a time and place in which adult children are today more likely to be buried by their parents than anywhere else on Earth. The effects have whipped down the demographic pyramid, as the prefecture has become home simultaneously to the longest-lived and most overweight Japanese.[189]

How, then, might Okinawa respond? At the heart of traditional Okinawan cuisine is the purple sweet potato. Consume lots of it, together with the vegetables that surround it on an Okinawan plate, and you'll be healthier.[190] Okinawa's nearly vegan, fermentation-rich diet will reduce your blood pressure as well as your risk of diabetes, stroke, heart disease, and cancer. The Okinawan diet works, and it works well.

The problem is that there's no longer a traditional Okinawa in which to eat like a traditional Okinawan. Diets are products of society. To demand that people individually take responsibility for changing their diet is not only to consign many to failure but also to ascribe the fault of all who fail exclusively to a deficit of will on their part. Food and health are part of our social world. Modern medicine, ignoring the web of life, offers a sophisticated solution: probiotic pills based on the kind of intestinal fauna that the Okinawan diet helps breed.

Dietary supplements are an individualized solution, a philosophy that finds its apotheosis in microbiome companies that can map your internal ecology and identify the deficits. But as we've already seen, this "add biota and stir" approach doesn't address the underlying causes of dysbiosis. There's merit in promoting anti-inflammatory foods,[191] and the modern Paleo diet certainly changes our microbiome,[192] but these diets are reserved for the 1 percent. Although vegetables may be cheaper than meat, a balanced diet requires a range of plants, many of which are expensive. In the Global North, empty calories are far cheaper than nutritious ones; one UK study found that a healthy diet is double the price of an unhealthy one.[193] Even the Mediterranean diet works only for the rich who can afford the best foods from that cuisine.[194] As the world becomes yet more inflamed, both inside our guts and out, and as high-end food becomes scarcer under climate change, we need a diet that everyone can eat.[195] Okinawan longevity emerged in symbiosis with the land and sea. You can't get that back just through a menu or a fecal transplant.[196]

Some Okinawans have been pushing for deep systemic changes for a while. Shoko Ahagon, a man some call "Japan's Gandhi,"[197] lived through the destruction of the Allied bombing campaigns of World War II. After the war, he returned to his ancestral fields to discover that they, together with 63 percent of his home island of Iejima, a spit of land northwest of the Okinawan mainland, had been occupied by US Marines.

He asked for access to land for his family and community to farm once again. The US Air Force wanted to use his community's part of the island as a munitions range and evicted them. He organized and led a "Beggar's March" around the prefecture. United States soldiers burned down his house while he was out protesting in front of the government buildings. But Ahagon inspired other farmers, on Iejima and on Okinawa Island. They started to encroach on military land, to farm again on land that had once been theirs. The military decided it was easier to tolerate this than to routinely burn these farms down. Soon hundreds of farmers were slipping onto bases on the Ryukyu Islands, growing food under the flight paths of B-29s.[198]

Ahagon's ultimate goal was to return some autonomy to Okinawa. He died in 2002 (at around eighty-nine)[199] without seeing that happen. One of his most loyal students, Etsuko Jahana, first met Ahagon after the war.[200] Although she uses a wheelchair when she gets tired, she's still able to garden a little and teach a lot. She explained why Okinawa's food crisis is happening, and why out of Japan's forty-seven prefectures, Okinawans had fallen from the longest lived to being ranked twenty-sixth in the country: "74 percent of all bases in Japan are in Okinawa, which is only 0.6 percent of all the land in this country. The reason why Japan's longest-lived Okinawans are reduced to the 26th is clearly because of the bases."

DECOLONIZING OUR GUTS

For the Okinawan diet to be effective, eaters must be able to connect to the soil and sea from which food comes. Otherwise they become spectators to the land, separated from it by barbed wire and barbecue joints. And there's no possibility of symbiosis when the land on which plants grow is occupied by airstrips and warplanes.

Even if the land is reclaimed from occupiers, there's no guarantee that it'll be safe. After the Canadian government allowed tar sand extraction on Mikisew Cree First Nation and Athabasca Chipewyan First Nation land in Northern Alberta, it was reopened for recreation, and Indigenous food rights—which had been violated until that point—were restored. But now the land was contaminated with heavy metals, such as mercury and arsenic, and the detritus of oil sand extraction.[201] Local doctors in Fort Chipewyan were alarmed by elevated cancer rates among Indigenous people in the region.[202] Tragically, harvesting traditional foods in modern times can make Indigenous people sick.

Heavy metals will endure for generations, entering our children through things as innocuous as commercially available baby food,[203] but we can start to decontaminate the cosmology that polluted the planet right away. Part of the process of decolonization is identifying and correcting the way colonialism makes us see the world. For that, you need a school, like the Muckleshoot Tribal School in Enumclaw, Washington. A light-filled modern building, it looks at first glance like any other campus. Alphabet posters feature images of trains entering tunnels: L is for lilud (pronounced layload, meaning "railroad"). Other posters are more surprising: S is for sčədadxʷ (schedad, salmon). A is for ʔaciłtalbixʷ (atsichtalbiw, human being), and ƛ̓ is for ƛ̓əlay? (chuhlay, shovel-nosed canoe). The language is Xʷəlšuʔcid (Twhoolshootseed), the Muckleshoot language, the last native speaker of which died in 2016.[204]

In the main hall, thirty-three-year-old Native food nutrition educator Valerie Segrest shares some homemade food, helping a class of sixth graders understand how food fits patterns of ill-health that will afflict them directly: Native Americans and Alaska Natives have the highest rates of diabetes of any group in the United States. Segrest is a leader of the Muckleshoot Food Sovereignty Project. When she teaches about a decolonized food system, her first task is reversing colonial thinking about the web of life. Rather than see "nature" as separate from "society," she encourages her students to read the landscape so that they might unlearn the idea that wild spaces are "untouched and unmanaged."

When she teaches her fellow Muckleshoot educators about the process of decolonization, she takes them on five-mile treks up mountainsides. "I schlep them up to look at a huckleberry meadow that they could have seen two miles down, from out the door of the car," she says. "But that huckleberry meadow is an archaeological site that has six-thousand-year-old smoldered logs that show we had been drying berries and burning up there and maintaining those wild ecosystems for four, five, to seven thousand years, depending on where you're at in the Cascades. At that time, Pompeii and Rome and Athens and all these historical amazing civilizations weren't even a dream."

The trek is a physical and metaphorical journey away from the hubs of colonial control and into domains that have been tended by Indigenous people for centuries. Medical students complain that their degrees put them into the workforce only in their thirties, and that specializations take even longer because of the number of classes and rotations needed to achieve mastery over a particular organ or system. In the Pacific Northwest, however, a relationship with a single species takes even longer. Segrest explains, "You wouldn't dare study more than one plant in a given year. You would be focused on one plant at most. And that study may go on for the rest of your life."

Segrest is well aware of the forces that seek to school her students differently. Outside the reservation, there's a great deal of talk of resource exploitation, of taking quotas of salmon, of "developing" land. In Twhoolshootseed, the closest idea to exploitation is *tiχdx*, which might be translated as "cultivation."[205] Exploitation allows the sundering of connection between people and the world. Much of Segrest's work is directed toward treating the consequences of this disconnection and the miseducation of Muckleshoot youth, who like most Native Americans have disproportionate rates of type 2 diabetes.[206] She urges upon the young people she counsels a diet free of sugar-sweetened beverages and rich in the teas and fresh water of Muckleshoot medicine. It's a hard sell. She's pitching to kids who are the targets of multimillion-dollar marketing campaigns to drink soda. And she's living in the middle of a settler state with a cosmology dedicated to turning *tiχdx* into profit.

Despite colonial forces seeking to exterminate the web of life, abundant knowledge about it remains. Segrest has ideas about healing these disconnections, but she cautions, "Don't come to Indian country with your pity—come to us because we have answers and the ability to make normal look different." Segrest advocates a deep and difficult medicine: decolonizing our views of the forest. It's difficult because it requires not just reappraising what counts as nature but unpacking the impulse to defend "society." To recognize that "society" was formed in opposition to wilderness depends on understanding what Solomon Reese, a Tsimshian Saulteaux man living in the Pacific Northwest, believes: "When we say we are the land, we are not being poetic. The land is made of our ancestors' bodies reentering the life cycle, and our bodies are derived from that very land where our ancestors have been."

How we treat the soil reflects what will eventually happen in our own gut. Those who tend the soil—our farmers—are critical stewards of our health, because our health starts in the ground under our feet. Just as the body keeps the memory of trauma alive in our cells, the soil also remembers. Microbes are a part of that living memory, ancestral beings that travel, in whole or in part, through the spaces around and inside us, circulating life from the soil to the body and back again. We have to understand how the forces of history have now made our insides less hospitable to these passengers who act as our own internal healers, offering up their medicines in reciprocal exchange for our accommodations. We feel their absence and presence in how we suffer or how we thrive. Although the microbes that share our lives are not human, they make up so much of who we are that it raises the question of what it means to be human in the first place.

4

RESPIRATORY SYSTEM

THE LAST THING YOU SMELL IS A FOREST FIRE

Can't talk because I choke and can't breathe.

—KIOUS KELLEY, RN[1]

I will tell you something about stories, [he said.] They aren't just entertainment. Don't be fooled. They are all we have, you see, all we have to fight off illness and death. You don't have anything if you don't have the stories. Their evil is mighty but it can't stand up to our stories. So they try to destroy the stories, let the stories be confused or forgotten. They would like that. They would be happy. Because we would be defenseless then. He rubbed his belly. I keep them here.

—LESLIE MARMON SILKO, *CEREMONY*[2]

A people are as healthy and confident as the stories they tell themselves. Sick storytellers can make their nations sick. And sick nations make for sick storytellers.

—BEN OKRI[3]

Dr. Coleen Kivlahan was sixty-seven years old, with no underlying illness except occasional asthma. She took no regular medications and was in great physical shape before she got sick. On March 3, 2020, at the University of California, San Francisco hospital, she was seeing patients who came into the urgent care clinic with the same symptoms: fever and a dry hacking cough. She was wearing a surgical mask, and her patients were too. She believes she knows who gave her Covid: "He was seventy years old, receiving hospice care, and came in because of a harsh, dry cough and low-grade fever. I had a surgical mask. He had a mask. But I spent forty-five minutes in his room. I did a full head-to-toe exam on him because I felt, 'What am I missing?' His chest X-ray was negative, but at that time we had no Covid tests available. He was never tested."

Three days later, on March 6, Kivlahan attended the first in-person strategic meeting for one hundred leaders in the UCSF health system to address the pandemic, where she learned that the chief symptoms to look out for were fever and cough. The meeting lasted most of the day, and by the afternoon she was experiencing rigors—intense shaking chills with no fever. She stayed until the end, though, and when she got home, the chest tightness and cough started.

On March 9, Kivlahan went to a newly created Covid clinic and got tested for Covid and influenza. Both tests came back negative. She rested at home and began to keep a journal documenting her heart rate and oxygen level whenever she felt symptoms. She was a physician known for maintaining her cool under pressure. In addition to overseeing 350 doctors as the director of the primary care clinics of a major university health system, she had worked in Syria during its civil war and in the Democratic Republic of the Congo in the midst of the Ebola outbreak.

On March 15, as her symptoms persisted, Kivlahan was tested a third time. Negative again. But she tested positive for the respiratory virus human metapneumovirus (HMPV), which can cause bronchitis in young, old, and immunosuppressed people. Then on March 25, almost three weeks after her first strange cough, she developed violent coughing spells, chills with fever, and drenching night sweats so intense, she had to change her sheets twice. The next morning she went back to the Covid clinic and got tested a fourth time. This time the test came back positive. "I felt relief, actually," she remembers—"I knew it had been hiding away, under the banner of HMPV, and waiting to take hold of me. I was full of fear about when the worst days of Covid might make me surrender to hospital care and ventilators, and I felt tremendous pressure to finish my will, my trust, and to find two people to witness my advance directive edits."

Shortly afterward she lost her senses of smell and taste. Instead of the hot chocolate she made in the morning, for instance, she smelled something else, spawned by the disease. It was the smell of a forest fire.

Over the next two weeks, the worst of the virus set in. Kivlahan's blood pressure plummeted from her normal of 100 to a systolic of 60, with no reading in the lower number. Her heart raced into the 150s. Her oxygenation saturation dropped to 91 percent. She knew these were dangerous indications to go to the hospital, but didn't want to end up on a ventilator, so she did everything she could to stay home. "From March 27 through 31," she recalls, "I experienced nightly terrors: the relentless cough lasted all day, as did the chest pain. Then, as evenings fell, I was convinced that I smelled smoke, like during the Camp Fire. I could not take a full breath; the pressure in my chest was so intense I had to lie very still in bed to avoid breathing deeply."

In 2018 the Camp Fire became the deadliest wildfire in California's recorded history, after record-high temperatures in preceding years turned the state's forests into a parched tinderbox. The Camp Fire burned more than 60,000 hectares (150,000 acres) and killed eighty-five people, who were engulfed either in their homes or in their cars trying to escape. Driven by winds of up to 80 kilometers (50 miles) per hour, the blaze consumed an area the size of eighty football fields every minute. The fire ultimately burned an area three-quarters the size of New York City.[4] Smoke from the blaze, which was 240 kilometers (150 miles) away, choked the entire San Francisco Bay Area for two long weeks. The air quality registered as "hazardous for human health," and the smell from that time is seared into the memory of all Bay Area residents.[5] For years before this blaze, the electrical utility PG&E, whose equipment had sparked the inferno, gave executives bonuses instead of updating its infrastructure.[6] For Kivlahan, it was this smell that accompanied her Covid symptoms.

Her illness was more manageable in the daytime, so much so that she felt she was getting better each morning. But then each night the monster returned: the fever with shaking chills, cough, and chest tightness became more pronounced. These symptoms were always accompanied by phantosmia, smelling something that isn't there. Worse yet, the forest fire scent would linger for most of the day, recede at dusk, then strike again at night, when the coughing fits convulsed her once more.

Four months later Kivlahan was doing much better. She climbed fifty stairs at a time twenty times per day to build her endurance, and her heart rate was back in the normal range. But she could still neither taste nor smell the world around her. Every two to three days, a wave that she described as an inflammatory phenomenon hit her: "I am confident that the inflammation surrounds the olfactory nerve. It is not posterior pharyngeal. I don't feel inflamed in the back of my throat. It must be deep in the nerve." The smell of the fires kept returning.

HOW FORESTS BURN

Covid settles disproportionately into the lungs of those who have been exposed to air pollution. We have yet to understand how the long-term symptoms of the virus compare to the effects of toxic air, from chronic obstructive pulmonary disease to diabetes. Each year millions of people die, inflamed, by the consequences of fire.

Humans burn forests and fields and harness fossil fuels in stoves and internal combustion engines. As a result, air pollution is the fourth-leading risk factor behind premature death.[7] Worse, the effects of climate change are such that we will be living with the consequences of the past five hundred years of fire for centuries to come. Air pollution causes climate change, which in turn increases pollution. The heat trapped in the atmosphere alters weather patterns, drying forests, increasing the chance of lightning strikes, and suspending more sand and dust in the air.[8] As a result, climate change itself raised particulate air pollution by 5 percent over the period 1860–2000.[9] Even if we begin now to address the climate emergency, it will take generations to clear the effects from our lungs. Until then, it is in the respiratory systems of those least responsible for causing the catastrophe that the residue of this history will settle.

Let's practice the art of diagnosis by examining a death by fire. Hina Pandey[10] was one of the 1.67 million people who died of air pollution in India in 2019.[11] She felt the filth in the air build in her lungs over her lifetime of work, picking and sorting trash on a municipal dump. If she had lived in a richer country, or if she had had resources, she might have been diagnosed with COPD, an inflammatory disease of the lungs, and given a portable oxygen machine. But waste pickers, particularly women waste pickers, don't have access to that kind of money.[12]

By day Pandey breathed in the fetid air of the Bhalswa dump in northern Delhi, a teetering municipal landfill that routinely crushes the waste pickers working on it, because of the decomposition of material within it. She would often complain about the smell of rot mixed with a burnt chemical odor. The dump frequently caught fire: in 2016 alone, there were 117 separate blazes.[13] By night, she cooked dinner over an open flame for her family. Every exposure sent small particles through her respiratory system into her body. The heart attack that killed her in her sleep in her early forties was precipitated by these particles that brought fire down the tree of her lungs and into her blood vessels, singeing the delicate tissues as they traveled.

The Punjab region of South Asia, before the colonists invaded, was once home to large forests. Over thousands of years, Macedonians, Mauryans, Shakas, Mughals, and British all made their mark in this part of northern India and southern Pakistan, named for the five rivers fed by the Himalayas (*panj* = five; *āb* = waters) that nurture the rich soil.[14] As each colonial empire expanded its borders and the footprint of settled agriculture, it further encroached on the forest.[15] Cities grew and occasionally shrank. Trade networks became more intricate and sometimes collapsed. Pastoralists and nomads were conquered and conscripted and settled. In one wave of colonization, two thousand years ago, the jungle in Punjab, around Patiala, burned. The *Mahabharata* tells of the systematic destruction of the forest together with the Adivasi (India's Indigenous people) who lived there, all in the name of advancing civilization.[16]

Many centuries later the British did worse, because the British weren't just colonists but capitalists, too.[17] Under feudalism in Europe, forests had been commons on which the poorest depended.[18] After the Black Death, and after Europe began its transition to capitalism, those forests became less a refuge and source of sustenance than a resource to be exploited by the rich.[19] Laws of enclosure, beginning in thirteenth-century England, brought public lands under private control, rerouting and concentrating the circulation of wealth and power. The poor fought to preserve their rights to the forests but were ultimately defeated in a series of early modern peasant wars.[20]

Arguably, capitalism's original sin was to transform the forest: from a space in which humans might find the fuel, food, building material, medicine, and sanctuary necessary for life to a thing that could be privately held and exploited. As Europe's forests dwindled, its appetite for resources and workers to convert into wealth compelled them to invade other lands and to expand out across the rest of the planet.[21] This imperative drove the British East India Company and its colonial ambitions.[22] In Ireland, British clear-cut forests for shipbuilding. In India, the forest became a resource for the next generation of technological capitalist advancement: the train. Across the empire, a new, displaced class of people were sundered from the forest as they came to be embedded in new international flows of extraction and trade, with nothing to save them from hunger but the sale of their labor.

India's forests were central to the British imperial economy. Early modern travelers' accounts and court documents tell of rhinos and elephants featuring in court rituals and hunts. After the British arrived in the seventeenth century, the forests were cleared of megafauna.[23] Many of those forests are gone now, as are the *junglees*—the pejorative term used by settled agricultural civilizations to refer to nomadic and pastoral people. The best translation: savages.[24] In the colonial cosmology, this was a holy war of society against nature. British officials reported that "previous oriental governments"[25] in India had allowed forests to remain untouched, and that the untapped resources, "the waste and forest lands never . . . attracted the[ir] attention."[26] In order to create one of the largest railway networks on Earth, railway builders turned the trees into sleeping cars, and large parts of the forest were "felled in even to desolation." The lumber became the infrastructure beneath, then the fuel inside, British locomotives.[27]

British trains moved vast quantities of grain, along with other goods and workers and colonial administrators, and connected the interior of the subcontinent to ocean trade networks. Under the well-worn technologies of imperial taxation, the British made it harder for poorer peasants to stay on the land and easier for richer ones to pay their debts by growing commodities for the UK.[28] Just as in the first British colony, Ireland—where food exports continued through the Great Potato Famine[29]—grain exports from India were maintained even when pandemic hunger struck. In 1901 *The Lancet* estimated that between 1890 and 1900 alone, famine and hunger-related disease caused 19 million deaths in India.[30]

Many in India's first government, following independence from the British in 1947, had suffered the devastation of famine directly. The traumatic memory of the 1943 Bengal Famine, which killed between 2 million and 3 million people, informed the post-Independence Public Distribution System, a network of government-run food outlets. The drive to provide cheap food to the cities took a particular turn in the late 1960s, when the Green Revolution hit India.[31] Sponsored enthusiastically by the United States and embraced at first reluctantly and then wholeheartedly by the Indian government, the program supplied seeds, fertilizers, pesticides, herbicides, and subsidies, provided funding for irrigation projects, and put in place policies to shore up the landholdings of richer peasants.

The "Green" in Green Revolution was a political color. William Gaud, the administrator of the US Agency for International Development, coined the term and made clear that it wasn't like the "Red Revolution . . . of the Soviets, nor is it a White Revolution like that of the Shah of Iran."[32] The intervention was designed to stop restive workers in South Asia from becoming communists by appealing to their bellies with cheap food. If feeding urban proletarians meant that small farmers and landless workers were rendered irrelevant, and if the program demanded the planting of two crops to the exclusion of all else, so be it. The result was that India's crop diversity fell, and levels of rural hunger remain apocalyptic even today.[33] From a polyglot diversity of life on the land, Punjabi soil has been reduced to a stuttering bilingualism: rice in the monsoon *kharif* season, wheat in the winter *rabi* season.[34]

For India's so-called agricultural miracle to work, massive amounts of water had to be pumped from the ground. In 1950, 28 percent of India's agriculture was irrigated. By 2010, 61 percent was. Today, as a consequence, 91 percent of people in South Asia experience water shortages.[35] Facing steadily declining groundwater levels, farmers dug wells so deep that they needed powerful electrical pumps to bring the water up. In Punjab, the heart of the Green Revolution, the state government provided free electricity—generated by burning fossil fuels—to farmers so they could power their irrigation systems.[36] Currently, 70 percent more Punjabi groundwater is pumped out of the ground than the monsoon and Himalayan snowmelt recharges every year. The water evaporates or is taken up by plant roots, leaving behind dissolved salts from agrochemical inputs that contaminate water and soil.[37] At the beginning of the twenty-first century, the government of Punjab found itself suffering an ecological catastrophe, with rising rates of farmer distress and suicide and few options.[38]

It was politically impossible to rescind the grant of free electricity to pump water. So instead, the Punjabi state government changed the seasons. One of the most water-intensive parts of rice cultivation involves the transplanting of seedlings. A 2009 law was introduced to prevent transplanting before June 10. Farmers could then water their transplants with July's monsoon rain rather than with pumped groundwater. But a late transplanting means a late harvest: June-planted rice can be gathered only in October. Winter wheat must be in the ground in November. Farmers need to clear fields in a hurry. So every year during the final weeks of October, across 10 million hectares (25 million acres) in northern India, an area the size of Kentucky, thousands of fires are set to burn off the rice stubble.[39] This is when Delhi's air pollution, already bad because of seasonal dust, industrial pollution, and vehicle emissions, becomes cataclysmic.[40]

SIZE MATTERS

Fire never burns completely. The "fire triangle" of fuel, oxygen, and an ignition source is the basic physics of fire that most of us remember from school. If our memories are even more forgiving, we can recall that when fuel burns, hydrocarbons react with oxygen to make carbon dioxide and water. But field fires are never hot enough to reduce *everything* to water and gas—so burning rice stubble produces a great deal of fine-particulate matter.[41]

Our diagnosis must follow the circulation. Winds in the lower atmosphere carry such particles from Punjabi fires hundreds of kilometers to the southeast, over the Delhi region. There they mingle with factory and tailpipe emissions, the smoke from burning fossil fuels and funeral pyres. The end of the *kharif* season, in October and November, brings cold but little wind to northern India. India's poorest keep warm with indoor fires, and low-income Delhiites tend to use smokier solid fuel stoves.[42] During the Hindu Festival of Lights, Diwali, firework smoke raises the atmospheric pollutant levels of aluminum, potassium, and magnesium above those of some industrial sites.[43]

In India, the response to pollution has been the same as the response to the water crisis: displacement, division, and diversion. For one two-week period, the Delhi municipal government split the days that cars could drive on the roads: vehicles with odd-numbered license plates alternated with those with even-numbered ones.[44] Tailpipe emissions account for around 40 percent of Delhi's pollution, so one might have expected to see a dip.[45] There wasn't one.[46] There was no wind, and there was no rain. The toxic pollution hung in the air.

In global rankings of air pollution, Delhi and the neighboring city of Ghaziabad are typically in the top five, and fourteen out of the fifteen worst polluted cities on Earth are in India.[47] Three-quarters of Indians are exposed to pollution levels four times the limit set by the World Health Organization.[48] Children in Delhi suffer from high rates of asthma and lung infection. One in three have reduced lung function.[49]

Air pollution is a cocktail of dangerous gases and particulate matter. The smaller the particle, the farther it can get into the tiny branches of the lungs. Inhalable particles, with diameters of 10 microns or less (designated PM_{10}), have a terrible impact on human health. By comparison, a human hair is 50 microns across; human eyes can't see anything less than 40 microns wide, and the coronavirus has a diameter of 0.06 to 0.12 microns. Fine-particulate matter, which comprises particles that are 2.5 microns in diameter or less ($PM_{2.5}$), wreaks the most havoc. Such particles are small enough to travel deep into the lungs and have a large enough surface area to carry hitchhiking molecules of toxic stuff along with them.[50]

Fine-particulate pollution is primarily derived from the burning of fossil fuels for transportation, manufacturing, and power plant operation. It tends to include soot, acids, and sulfate and nitrate particles.[51] It can also potentially carry the SARS-CoV-2 virus, which may explain, above and beyond population density, why the pandemic has spread so rapidly in places with high levels of air pollution.[52] Whether those particles are infectious or not is an area of active study. Likewise, the presence of influenza on PM_{10} may be participating in its annual global spread.[53]

The more fine-particulate pollution you are exposed to, the more likely you are to die from cardiopulmonary disease or lung cancer.[54] The impact is dose-dependent: for every $PM_{2.5}$ increase of 10 micrograms per cubic meter of air, the risks of all-cause, cardiopulmonary, and lung cancer mortality rise by 4 percent, 6 percent, and 8 percent, respectively.[55] The good news is that this effect is reversible: the more a city cleans up its air pollution, the longer the life expectancy of its inhabitants becomes.[56] The bad news is that air pollution has been shown to impact every organ system in the body. Super tiny particles enter the bloodstream and gain direct access to our organs, setting off a localized and systemic inflammatory response, creating cascading health problems.[57]

Chronic exposure to air pollution leads to worsening lung function, wheezing, asthma attacks, and COPD.[58] Acute exposure causes morbid heart arrhythmias and heart attacks.[59] Although we don't know definitively whether SARS-CoV-2 can hitch a ride into our bodies through particulate matter as influenza can,[60] long-term exposure to air pollution is clearly connected to increased risk of death from Covid.[61]

While most people with Covid experience mild flu-like symptoms, a moderate number have symptoms severe enough to require hospitalization, and of those, a sizable number die.[62] Those deadly cases progress through overwhelming inflammation of the lungs known as acute respiratory distress syndrome, or ARDS. Another hallmark of ARDS is profound systemic inflammation, with elevated levels of pro-inflammatory cytokines including IL-1β and IL-6.[63] Serial chest X-rays show ARDS rapidly whiting out the air spaces in the lungs, which normally in well-aerated lungs appear black. The fluffy white cotton-ball-like areas represent fluid that builds up as inflammation runs amok and makes impossible the gas exchange that circulates life-sustaining oxygen throughout the body.[64] People are literally drowning in their own fluids, a gruesome death made worse—and more widespread—by the very air they are fighting to breathe.

An increase of only 1 microgram of $PM_{2.5}$ per cubic meter of air is associated with an 8 percent increase in the Covid death rate.[65] This correlation is echoed in the findings of two studies of chronic exposure to air pollution. One involving over sixty thousand people in Japan found that pollution is associated with a higher incidence of pneumonia. Another found that pollution increases mortality from influenza.[66] During the 1918 flu pandemic, cities that burned more coal had tens of thousands more deaths than cities that burned less.[67] Similarly, another study found a linear relationship between the Chinese air pollution index and mortality rates from the deadly SARS outbreak in 2002: the more polluted the air, the deadlier the virus.[68] In India, the cause of over 10 percent of the years of life lost to premature mortality was air pollution exposure inside and outside the home.[69]

Exposure is always a function of wealth and power. The first nurse in New York who we know to have died from Covid was Kious Kelley.[70] Had sufficient personal protective equipment (PPE) been available for frontline providers, he might be alive today.[71] In the hierarchies of the health care system at the beginning of the Covid pandemic, plastic masks and gowns were more valuable than nursing staff, and so it was they who were discarded like trash. While the pandemic covered every continent under the sky, people living in specific exposomes experienced it differently. Where the air was more polluted, the virus spread more intensely.[72] The pandemic revealed in stark terms the reality of how environmental and social injustice affects health, and also the deeper truth that under a colonial cosmology, many humans have been made disposable.

THE FANTASTIC VOYAGE OF PM$_{2.5}$

In Delhi, to be a waste picker, scavenging for plastic to recycle, is to be part of a fix. It's to be responsible for cleaning up the mess that others have made, recovering resources from the detritus that modern life generates. Yet it is also to suffer daily contempt, legal prejudice, and persistent economic inequality. In Delhi, waste dumps have been moved out of the city's center and toward its edges, clearing the air of stench for the middle class and displacing those who work on these sites.[73] Tethered through long histories of colonialism, capitalism, class and caste prejudice, patriarchy, and environmental chauvinism, dumps and bodies are moveable sites of environmental damage.[74] As workers scour through Delhi's detritus, they face dangers of highly polluted air, laceration, and infection.[75] Hina Pandey, who died an early death by heart attack, was one of legions of women and men who clean up after the city, part of an underclass unseen by the city's patricians: one of its *immunes*.

Fine particles—from dust in the waste dump, local industrial facilities, Punjabi fires, and cooking stoves—enter a human body through the nose or mouth.[76] A particle from the fires heads down the windpipe to the point where the trachea splits into two bronchi, then farther as they branch many times into the smallest airways, the bronchioles, which are a half a millimeter in diameter. The system as a whole resembles an upside-down tree, with the base of the trunk at the mouth and the tiniest twigs deep in the chest. Each bronchiole

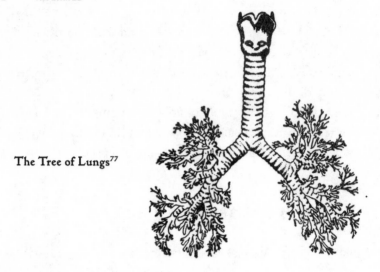

The Tree of Lungs[77]

terminates in thousands of air sacs called alveoli, which expand and collapse like tiny balloons with each breath. Here, at the tips of the respiratory branches, is where gas exchange happens. The average human lung has between 274 million and 790 million alveoli, depending on the size of the person and their lungs.[78] Each individual air sac measures about 200 microns in diameter, and together the millions of them in a human lung have a surface area of around 100 square meters (about 1,000 square feet).[79] But even though the lungs feel deeply tucked away and safe in our chests, this surface area is completely exposed to every inhalable fine particle in our air.

The wall of an alveolus is one single cell thick. This flat membrane with the capillary membrane against which it is sandwiched constitutes the 0.2-micron distance that molecules of gas must cross:[80] capillaries deposit the carbon dioxide created through cellular respiration into the alveoli to be breathed out, and fresh oxygen is loaded into the long line of red blood cells that the heart's right ventricle pushes single file through the capillaries that line the alveoli.[81]

Once a fine particle of air pollution arrives in an alveolus, carried deep into the lungs on the current of the breath, it sets off a cascade of inflammation, both locally and systemically. In the lung, $PM_{2.5}$

causes damage through several mechanisms. For one thing, the substances it brings in can generate an excess of free radicals in the tissue, such as reactive oxygen species (ROS) and reactive nitrogen species (RNS), which the body also creates during normal cellular respiration. A free radical is an unstable molecule with an unpaired electron that will scavenge an electron from another molecule. Antioxidants, such as vitamins C and D, easily donate electrons to free radicals, neutralizing their damaging impact.

If a microenvironment has an overabundance of free radicals, they will use up all the antioxidants and start snatching electrons from other molecules, such as DNA, proteins, and fat. The damage that ensues is called oxidative stress, which is one of the main tissue injuries responsible for the aging process. When it occurs at a fast enough rate, it can generate damage to DNA that cannot be corrected,[82] a first step in the development of lung cancer.[83] Free radicals also directly set off the inflammatory response, causing cells that line the entire respiratory system to start making inflammatory cytokines.[84] Moreover, the presence of $PM_{2.5}$ itself causes white blood cells to elaborate pro-inflammatory cytokines and to suppress those cells that express anti-inflammatory cytokines. This leads to the recruitment of more inflammatory cells. Inflammation in the lung tissue is implicated in the prevalent forms of lung disease, such as COPD, emphysema, asthma, fibrosis, and lung cancer.[85]

$PM_{2.5}$ hampers the respiratory system's capacities for self-defense. Both the upper and lower respiratory tracts are lined with several kinds of cells that constitute the first line of protection against infection. Some produce mucus, which can trap dirt and infectious organisms. Others have many finger-like projections, called cilia, that under the microscope look like a carpet of sea anemones. The cilia beat rhythmically upward together, to move that mucus and anything it has trapped up the airway, whence it's either coughed up or swallowed down.[86] Inhaled particles of air pollution, as well as tobacco smoking, shorten these cilia and render their motion dysfunctional, unable to clear particles that then make their way deep into the lungs. This leaves the lungs vulnerable to infection.[87]

It's intuitive that if you inhale toxic material, it will damage lung tissue. What's less intuitive is that the harm from $PM_{2.5}$ doesn't stop there. Studies of the systemic effects of air pollution are startling in their range. In healthy young individuals with very low cardiovascular disease risk, episodic exposure to air pollution is associated with the apoptosis—programmed death—of endothelial cells that line the blood vessels.[88] This is one mechanism by which $PM_{2.5}$ initiates the development of atherosclerosis and hypertension, contributing to premature death worldwide.[89]

Long-term $PM_{2.5}$ exposure puts people at risk for developing type 2 diabetes, especially the elderly.[90] Even among counties with an amount of $PM_{2.5}$ pollution deemed acceptable by the Environmental Protection Agency, those with the highest level had over 20 percent more cases of diabetes than those with the lowest level. This association held even after controlling for diabetes risk factors, such as obesity.[91] Experimental models demonstrate that inflammatory pathways mediate the connection: particles of air pollution recruit inflammatory cells to insulin-sensitive tissues, where they generate inflammation that appears to promote the development of insulin resistance, a characteristic of type 2 diabetes.[92] The air we breathe directly impacts how our endocrine organs function.

Poisoned air is also causing inflammation in our brains.[93] Inflammatory markers and buildup of a protein called β-amyloid were found in the brains of people exposed to high levels of air pollution.[94] This protein is associated with the development and acceleration of Alzheimer's-like illness and cognitive dysfunction, as we will see in more detail in Chapter 8.[95] Alzheimer's in the elderly has been tied to elevated exposure to $PM_{2.5}$.[96] And increasingly, Alzheimer's signature has been found in the brains of children.[97] In Mexico City, one study has tracked how air pollution has led to systemic inflammation and structural brain changes, which in turn causes cognitive dysfunction.[98] Some of the effects can be reversed: just adding an air filter to an inner-city classroom in Los Angeles improved test scores as much as cutting class size by one-third.[99] But for some children, the damage is permanent.

Exposure to traffic-related air pollution, nitrogen dioxide, $PM_{2.5}$, and PM_{10} during gestation and the first year of life is significantly associated with autism.[100] Tailpipe exhaust fumes have been linked to a higher prevalence of brain cancer, so much so that the elevated exposure that would occur if you moved from a quiet street to a busy street, and stayed there for a year breathing the air, would increase your risk of developing the disease by 10 percent.[101] Magnetite nanoparticles, which are created through car exhaust, are especially dangerous. At 0.2 microns (or 200 nanometers) and smaller, they can enter the brain directly through the nose, carried up along the olfactory bulb.[102] When your parents told you not to stick a pencil up your nose because it could end up in your brain, that's the pathway the nanoparticles take, right up through the delicate plate that separates the nasal passages from the brain. Once in the brain, they set off dangerous inflammation implicated in Alzheimer's and contribute to the increased risk of brain cancer.[103]

The average city dweller breathes in 10,000 liters (2,600 gallons) of air a day, air tainted with tobacco smoke, automobile exhaust, diesel soot, ozone, sulfur dioxide, nitrogen dioxide, and a smattering of other pollutants.[104] Ten years of exposure to air pollution in US cities impacts the lungs as much as smoking a pack of cigarettes per day for twenty-nine years, leading to end-stage COPD or emphysema.[105] Again, the effects are dose-dependent: in parts of China, inhaling air pollution is equivalent to smoking up to three packs per day.[106] In India, pollution reaches levels beyond what machines are calibrated to measure. "Everyone is a smoker in Delhi" is how one doctor puts it.[107] If you are a waste picker, disproportionately exposed to environmental harm, you're much more likely to inhale more than the average level of pollutants, which at one point in 2019 was the equivalent of smoking fifty cigarettes per day.[108] The fires on the Bhalswa dump can rage for days, deep within the piles of trash, emitting smoke filled with dioxins.

Not everyone smokes equally, and the calculus of exposure is complex. In Delhi and Rio de Janeiro, being wealthy reduces the symptoms of lung disease,[109] but in Rome the rich live on downtown streets with higher levels of traffic.[110] Rome is an outlier, though.[111] Most air-pollution-related deaths happen in low- and middle-income countries, and, as the *Lancet* Commission on Pollution and Health noted in 2018, "in countries at every level of income, the health effects of pollution are most frequent and severe among the poor and the marginalized."[112] Working-class people are more likely to be exposed to higher levels of pollution and are more likely to have diseases driven by inflammation that makes that exposure more lethal.

No one imagines this situation is going to get better. Trying to solve air pollution by creating more rich-only spaces with air conditioning and filtration just makes it worse for everyone, as the machines spew out heat and demand energy to generate electricity, burning more fossil fuels in order to protect the wealthy from the effects of the fires.[113]

INVESTMENT CLIMATE CHANGE

Hina Pandey's death by air pollution can't be explained simply by tracing the particles that precipitated her heart attack. Her death also demands an accounting of the caste and class prejudice that create an exposome for India's Adivasi population of horrific oppression, which put her in harm's way and put health care out of reach. Pandey's lungs were also the location that connected eons of coal formation, millennia of forest destruction, and centuries of persecution of Indigenous people, through successive waves of colonial restructuring that persists in India today. Certainly, twentieth-century geopolitics and the Green Revolution play a part in the Punjab fires that send smoke to Delhi. But the electricity for Punjabi farmers' pumps comes with its own costs, ones that are continuous with an older colonial history. The vast majority of India's energy, 72 percent,[114] comes from coal, and India's largest coal mine, Jharia, is in Jharkhand—literally "the land of forest."[115] It's also the site of one of India's longest-burning fires, a subterranean blaze that began on a coal face in 1916 and will fester for centuries to come.[116]

A key player in Jharkhand's coal industry is Panem, a public-private joint venture between a mining company and the Punjab State Electricity Board. In the forests of Jharkhand, which is geographically located on the opposite side of India from Punjab, Panem has persecuted Indigenous people and has been implicated in killings of locals, including clergy, who have stood in their way.[117] In colonial fashion, the price for Punjabi farmers' free water-pump electricity is paid in blood in Jharkhand.[118]

The lands of Indigenous people offer an "internal frontier" for extraction under the flag of national economic development. The national debt and international development funds that the Indian government has borrowed have to be repaid, and the World Bank advises that investors might be courted by "improving the business climate."[119] When Indigenous groups have organized to resist those imperatives, the government responds with violence.[120] The anthropologist Alpa Shah writes of an attempt to extinguish such a rebellion in Jharkhand in 2005. In what the local politician who led it called "the Purification Hunt," "entire villages were plundered and burned down, children thrown into fires and pregnant women killed; hundreds of women were raped, others mutilated and murdered, and more than 350,000 people were forced to leave their homes. . . . It was reminiscent of the brutality of British counterinsurgency tactics used to kill the support of the National Liberation Army of the Malayan Communist Party more than sixty years before."[121]

In the twenty-first century, the Indian government's logic is a continuation of British strategies in the nineteenth century. With anthropological sophistication, the early British colonists dissected Indian society and produced official categories like "criminal tribes" to refer to those groups who most stubbornly resisted colonialism and modernization.[122] When India's prime minister Manmohan Singh in 2009 called the insurgencies "the greatest internal security threat to our country," he was merely putting a contemporary spin on an old colonial worry.[123] He offered the following economic prognosis: "if Left Wing extremism continues to flourish in important parts of our country which have tremendous natural resources of minerals and other precious things, that will certainly affect the climate for investment."[124] In order to create an investment climate untroubled by displaced people's rebellion, the Indian home minister, P. Chidambaram, a former nonexecutive director of the mining giant Vedanta,[125] authorized Operation Green Hunt. In 2009 forty thousand paramilitary troops were deployed across the country in a genocidal campaign against Adivasi communities.[126] The Operation has yet to end.[127]

Jharkhand's fires are part of a global problem: fire is profitable. Coal shows up as a positive in the national accounts. Because of its dependence on coal, by 2025 India is scheduled to emit more CO_2 than the United States.[128] Although there's support for electric vehicles and rural solar power, the coal industry is deeply entrenched in India, and it has deep connections to the global economic system.[129] To achieve a higher GDP, India is ready to sacrifice the lungs of its workers, the homes of its Indigenous people, and through fossil-fueled growth, the planet.

Reasonably, the Indian government could point to the carbon-driven growth trajectories of the Global North, and even China, and say, "If you can do it, why can't we?" While countries in the Global North shirk their climate debts, Indians have every right to feel the burn of injustice.[130] But it's important to get clear about who the "we" is. The creation and recreation of nationhood involves the policing of borders and the tacit anatomizing of whose bodies count in the collective identity. Consider how, for instance, the bodies of women in India will be affected by the changing climate. Indoor air pollution is responsible for 2.9 million annual deaths worldwide.[131] The area around the kitchen stove, especially if its fuel source is wood, dung, or coal,[132] has more air pollution than the outdoors, disproportionately exposing women and children through the gendered expectations of women's care work.[133]

A changing climate also means more extreme weather. In a drought, women have to walk farther to perform their expected work of fetching water, risking higher rates of heat stroke. In floods, women's domestic work puts them closer to standing water, which raises their exposure to mosquito-borne disease. In a climate disaster, as in any disaster, women are disproportionately vulnerable to domestic, physical, and sexual abuse.[134] And extreme heat raises the risk of adverse reproductive outcomes.[135] The consequences of the planet's inflamed atmosphere will not be borne equally.

As in any nation, the "we" in the Indian nation involves exclusions and excisions. Climate change in an era of rising national chauvinism is already making these exclusions more acute and more dangerous. The rise of nationalist environmentalism—ecofascism—is a global phenomenon.[136] Ecofascism's response to climate change is a world of walls, of the self and its enemies, of dividing the planet into deserving citizens and those who want to corrupt or steal the birthrights of the deserving. The white supremacists who killed dozens in a mosque in Christchurch, New Zealand/Aotearoa, and in El Paso, Texas, offered arguments about climate change and overpopulation in their manifestos.[137] The El Paso killer murdered twenty-three people, claiming he was worried that Mexican shoppers, bargain hunting from across the border, were engaging in unsustainable consumption. That the wealthiest—and generally whitest—Americans have the most profligate lifestyles was not something that warranted consideration. It's much easier, as national zealots across the ages have done, to blame foreign women for producing too many children who consume too much, than to recognize one's own culpability in the formation of a crisis.[138]

Fascism turns everyone into police. Mobs stamping their notion of justice and order can be found from the US Capitol to state border patrols in India. There Narendra Modi's citizenship laws aim to disenfranchise and exclude Muslim Indians, drawing a Line of Control on the bodies of nearly 13 percent of the population, making more extreme the health disparities that already exist for minoritized groups, including Muslims.[139] Under climate change, diseases of pollution and climate will need to be far more widely treated.[140] Under ecofascism, the distribution of care will become a site of national policing, in which people denied citizenship will also be denied care, in the name of preserving the integrity of the nation, even as the world burns.[141]

Resource scarcity will be used as a pretext for violent nationalism, as mass migrations of millions of displaced and desperate people move within and between borders. But the only resource we truly need is care. It would be reassuring to point to a future in which deaths by fire, like Hina Pandey's, are entirely avoided. It would be a future in which her exposures to flames at her work on the municipal dump, at her work cooking for her family in the home, in the air on the street during her journey to the waste site, were eradicated. In that future, health care would be available to help her and her family recover from decades of air pollution, no matter her religion.

Unfortunately, we are rushing headlong into a crisis of colonial capitalism in which pollution deaths soar, driven by a climate crisis, like the Covid pandemic, in which a few profit greatly while billions suffer. Within the fortress of the nation-state, the *immunes*, those most disposable though identified now as "essential"—the Indigenous, the working class, women, people of color, the low caste, queer, religious minorities, and immigrants—will be those most exposed to the dangers of toxic air and a hostile climate. Absent a serious diagnosis of the climate crisis and its impact on the exposome and our bodies, medicine will continue to treat the symptoms but will miss the opportunity for a cure.

BREATHING TRUTH TO POWER

The physician Mark Mitchell uses a mnemonic to recall the multiple medical effects of climate change. HEATWAVE stands for "Heat effects; Exacerbation of preexisting heart and lung conditions; Asthma; Traumatic injury caused by climate-related severe weather; Water- and food-borne illnesses; Allergies; Vector-borne diseases, such as West Nile and Zika; and Emotional and mental health impacts from experiences like loss of property or life due to climate-related disaster."[142] The pharmacopeia has therapies to address each of these health threats, but nothing to address the diagnosis that reveals the connections between them.

In the face of climate catastrophe, we may feel able only to grieve. In English, there is an assonance between the words *grieve* and *breathe*. In a range of traditional medicines, the lungs are the seat of grief, of the breath of mourning and lament.[143] Health care and frontline workers have experienced a surfeit of grief during the Covid pandemic. The communities that have been hardest hit have been Indigenous, Black, people of color, poor, and elders[144]— the same people who are the most exposed to the effects of climate change.[145] It is wholly appropriate to grieve what we have done to the planet. One of the authors of the 2007 Intergovernmental Panel on Climate Change report[146] suggests that our grief must pass through Elisabeth Kübler-Ross's five stages: denial, anger, bargaining, depression, and acceptance.[147] But grieving—lamenting the damage—can be only the first step.

Public lamentations, especially by women, were restricted as part of the colonial civilizing mission. As one upper-caste Hindu reformer put it in his 1857 "The Madness of Crying and Beating of Breast":

> The Parsee says [on witnessing this] "how junglee these women are?" and the English people say "what stupid gypsies are they." Saying this, they hurriedly depart from the scene. This practice shows us to be worthless and after this they are not prepared to give any consideration to any of our virtues. . . . A household's prestige is dependent on the woman. The people of Europe take pride in their women.[148]

That women's loud grief was considered to be a marker of savagery, and something to be controlled, reflects the mores of British patriarchy. Restricting women's public laments, which were often laced with scathing social commentary explaining why someone had died and naming the appropriate consequences for those believed responsible, also fit nicely along the prejudices of upper-caste Hindu men. The challenge to this patriarchal worldview draws Indigenous youth to the political insurgency in India today.

In an important work, the anthropologist Alpa Shah noticed in India's forest-dwelling communities a commitment to equality where "not only did women work outside the household (with some women even going on hunts), it was common to find men cooking and doing other domestic work such as washing clothes, collecting water, sweeping and looking after children. And when there was drinking and dancing, Adivasi women participated alongside men with equal fervor. It often struck me that the communities that I lived with had a form of gender equality that surpassed the conditions in the West that decades of feminist movements had fought hard for."[149]

Even as governments attempt to displace them, Indigenous people's practices offer profound lessons in how humans might more equitably face the climate crisis.[150] A growing body of data shows that Indigenous systems of resource management are superior to those of both central governments and privatization schemes.[151] Indigenous land tenure often operates as a commons, for the good of the whole community, held outside the laws of private property. These systems are almost always democratic, run on the principle that every voice matters. The forest is treated not as a resource that can be divided and exploited for profit. It belongs to everyone and no one. It is the matrix of life in all its physical and spiritual dimensions.

We're not romanticizing indigeneity; nor are we pretending that tribes cannot be turned into agents of private property and capitalism.[152] We are well aware that, particularly in times of scarcity, individual greed and a mindset of scarcity can easily overwhelm even the most robust system of governance. Nor are we suggesting that more voices, even when some of them speak for the nonhuman world, will necessarily lead to better outcomes. We've been on Twitter and know better. But we are suggesting that certain principles of reciprocity and voice, the slow breathing in and out of views and ideas, can reframe how we humans understand ourselves, how we shape our breath into voice, and how we listen in turn. We've seen these processes of reciprocation work, in the slow deliberation of Zapatista meetings in the Lacandon jungle, in the shack settlements in Durban, and around the sacred fire at the Standing Rock prayer camp.

Over a lifetime, the writer Amitav Ghosh has told stories of the Sundarbans, the mangrove transitional zone that sits on the Bay of Bengal at the border land between India and Bangladesh, where the interface between ecosystems gives rise to new permutations of life and living.[153] From that fertile space of emergence, he observes that "great, irreplaceable potentiality of fiction is that it makes possible the imagining of possibilities."[154] Narratives both reveal and shape our cosmologies and our personalities.[155] Stories are an important part of our exposome, offering a means of persecution (as the narratives of ecofascism can do) and also a form of protection. The kinds of stories that we tell about our people and our place in the world, and about the planet, circumscribe our collective imaginings.

The voice, the oral tradition, has always been the central medium for the transmission of human culture and knowledge. Colonial administrators from antiquity through European colonization to modern nation-states, including India, have understood this, which is why enforced written literacy has been an essential element of the colonial cosmology, a weapon against the threat of Indigenous rebellion and sedition.[156] Whereas the written word is static, referenceable, and policeable, the spoken word is fluid and dynamic, changing between tellers becoming reflective of the time, place, context, and person uttering the narrative. These words become seeds, in the minds of the listeners, nestling into the folds of our being, germinating into a unique form in each person who then goes on to tell it again, bringing a story new life, new dimensions, and new dissemination. The United States prohibited Indigenous languages and traditions of orality in residential schools. When stories are silenced, the knowledge they transmit and relationships they encode remain hidden.[157] Fortunately, however, precolonial stories continued to be told, *sotto voce*, untracked by the colonial state.[158] These stories reveal how humans and the web of life are bound together, reflecting cosmologies in which breath is shared and borders are illusory.

The Tongan scholar and storyteller Fuifuilupe Niumeitolu identifies the subversive power of Indigenous knowledge and storytelling: the connection that is forged between the teller and the listener. That connection in Tongan culture is called *va*, which is roughly translated as "sacred relationality." The act of telling and listening to stories reinforces our humanity, Niumeitolu explains.

> When we tell stories, when you tell me your story, there's *va* there. There's a connection. Even though we might not know each other personally, and our histories might be different. I think, first and foremost, the difficult work is to find our own humanity within our own self. The humanity that colonization taught me to forget. To recognize my own humanity first starts with me. It's difficult and dangerous work.
>
> And that's how I can recognize yours. I hope that when I tell stories, it can connect me to you. That I can remind you that perhaps we don't know each other. We might even be enemies according to here in the West. I might even be seen as "other" to you or you might be seen as "other." But I hope by telling a story just for that one moment that we recognize the humanity within our own selves and within each other. I really believe that's the power of stories.

To tell different stories is to imagine a different world. As the Indigenous botanist Robin Wall Kimmerer explains in her masterpiece

Braiding Sweetgrass, stories from Indigenous communities should be understood not so much as "artifact[s] from the past but as instructions for the future."[159] They are not relics of lost or destroyed civilizations. On the contrary, they record in social memory the successful technologies of the planet's most resilient human survivors.

Colonial capitalism is animated by its own stories. In these tales, bold conquistadors discover and subdue the world and bring home riches for God's anointed, whether it's the god of the Bible or of GDP. The celebration of Columbus as a hero may be falling out of fashion, but his spirit lives on in Jeff Bezos's lunar colonization dreams and Elon Musk's Martian visions—and in the plans of leaders who clear land of Indigenous peoples and biodiversity in order to extract the Earth's resources. We know what happens to our lands when the Indigenous people who have been tending those environments for thousands of years are removed: essential knowledge about the world, and the stories that transmit it, are disrupted. But these aren't the only available stories.

Almost every culture has a story about the tree of life and its significance for humanity. The Bible relates the story of the tree of knowledge and the unfortunate consequences of eating its fruit. Rich agroecological science is embedded in tales about trees of life in other traditions. Indian sacred trees vary according to the ecosystem, but one of the myths shared across a range of faiths is *kalpavriksha*, the sacred tree that provides everything, which emerged from the divine churning of the ocean of milk that covered the planet at the beginning of time.

In southern India, a coconut tree provides water from the coconut, coir for rope, leaves for fans, and copra for oil. In other parts of the country, it's a fig tree, known as *pipal* or *ashwattha* or *Ficus religiosa*: it's also called the Bodhi tree because Buddha achieved enlightenment while sitting underneath one. With lifespans averaging a thousand years, fig tree are hubs for symbiosis. Wasps pollinate them. Bats eat the fruit and deposit the seeds in other parts of the forest. It's a tree from which old-growth forests can be renewed.[160]

It's a source of food, building materials, life, and medicine. Its leaves contain phytochemicals that prevent inflammation.[161] An extraction of the leaves inhibits the expression of pro-inflammatory cytokines.[162]

Indigenous forest knowledge is highly local and holistic, deeply empirical but also cultural, moral, and spiritual.[163] As such, it eclipses ecology in its holism, because it is a system of knowledge that integrates science, politics, economics (as the distribution of resources), sociology, medicine, and history. The result of this cumulative way of knowing is that the ecosystems tended by Indigenous groups for millennia are the most biodiverse on Earth. While Indigenous people make up less than 5 percent of the world's population, they manage 25 percent of the world's land surface and steward more than 80 percent of the world's biodiversity.[164] That figure doesn't even account for the human microbiome diversity they harbor or the soil biodiversity they tend. Yet colonialism requires that the landscape be denuded both of its stories and of their tellers.

The concept of untouched wilderness separate from human engagement is an invention of Eurocentric environmental movements. As Mark David Spence notes in *Dispossessing the Wilderness: Indian Removal and the Making of the National Parks*, "uninhabited wilderness had to be created before it could be preserved."[165] The romance of the wilderness was created through the erasure of the people who knew how to live sustainably in a specific place, often for thousands of years. In Yosemite Valley, genocidal tactics led by a man appropriately named John Savage were used to remove the Ahwahneechee from their traditional territories.[166] This murder and forced removal were inspired by the twisted notions of environmental luminaries such as John Muir, whose beliefs were foundational to the US National Parks system. Muir described Indigenous people as "most ugly, and some of them altogether hideous."[167] Removing this taint on the landscape would have severe consequences not only for the people but for the entire ecosystem: the invention of the pristine wilderness inaugurated an era of catastrophic forest fires.[168]

The newcomers, in their zeal to protect the forest as a wilderness untouched by human hands, suppressed the local fire ecology, which the Ahwahneechee had previously tended. California's tribes understood that fire is a medicine. And when this medicine was lost, the undergrowth took over, leading to gigantic, cataclysmic forest fires that burned faster and hotter than any before.[169] The colonizers did not know that fire was needed to keep the entire system in balance, and that it is essential to the life cycle of certain trees, such as the giant sequoia.[170] Now the practice of controlled burning is being reintroduced by tribal people, not simply as a tool for forest management but as a way to reconnect to ancient forms of knowledge.

When colonial rule silenced Indigenous voices and forced their stories underground, it silenced traditions of hearing other kinds of voices, too. In most Indigenous systems of knowledge, the world is not divided along hard borders, as it is in colonial capitalism, between minds and things, between the living and the dead, between those who can speak and those who cannot. The trees, the water, the rocks, and all the life they sustain have voices. To revive the stories that allow them to speak and to be heard is to restore worldviews that center reciprocity, worldviews that have been sidelined by the extraction of the Earth's gifts since the dawn of capitalism. To bring back the work of storytelling as a form of essential knowledge is in itself a deep medicine.

A story exists between two poles, a teller and a listener. A story is listened to with three ears: "two on the sides of our head and the one that is in our heart."[171] As important as it is to recognize the voices of those who still have contact with ways of being upon which our survival depends, their insights will be of no use if they speak and no one heeds their words. The art of listening is as important as the art of storytelling. Deep listening can have a transformative impact on both the storyteller and the listener, whether that storyteller is a person, the soil, a river, or an entire ecosystem.

As Covid spread around the world, it was people's stories that helped scientists understand how the virus was attacking different parts of the body impacting various systems—the dry cough, the lack of smell, the brain fog, the recurrent flushes of inflammation. Before there were tests and vaccines and treatments, there were stories. And it took a while for the medical world to catch on, because listening is unfortunately not a core competency of many physicians. The clinical encounter is, in microcosm, the centuries-long experience of having one's knowledge denigrated, and having one's story listened to only insofar as it comports with what the listener already knows. This ritual of diagnosis sits in a matrix of power in which a patient's own oral tradition is selectively turned into an official written record, which is hard to change once it has been put in the chart. In some health care systems, the United States prime among them, the patient will arrive in a specialist's office already humbled and broken by a bureaucracy characterized by this form of narrative violence.

In theory, doctors ought to develop a strong relationship with a patient by asking about their medical history, to understand how they became sick, and to understand the patient's agenda for seeking help. When a group of physicians was polled, only 36 percent asked for an agenda from a patient. And for those who bothered to ask what the patient wanted, the median time before interrupting the patient was only eleven seconds.[172] Listening is a skill that is neither honored nor modeled in a medical system in which the primary focus of the doctors' gaze is the screen on which they transcribe and code the record of symptoms. The rise of big data in medicine doubles down on the idea that the patient's words are mere noise hiding a signal, rather than a speech act in a dance of mutual knowledge and vulnerability. Listening requires humility, to acknowledge a state of not knowing. To listen is to inhale and create the delicate space for stories.

Learning to listen must be the work of settlers on colonized land, of modern societies that treat the Earth as a thing to be exploited, and of health care workers, as we increasingly encounter existential threats from forest fires, pandemics, catastrophic floods, and global warming—all signs that we are critically out of balance. As Joan Archibald writes in *Indigenous Storywork*, "The communal principle of storytelling implies that a listener is or becomes a member of the community."[173] Perhaps this is why doctors have such a hard time listening to their patients. The divisions between physician and patient—and even between physician and every other health care worker—rooted in the history of medicine and assumptions about the kinds of knowledge that matter, produce a chasm too wide for real hearing. To do this work of listening, physicians—and all settlers— must again establish community with one another and with those elements that support our very lives. We must reestablish these critical relationships so that listening and the transmission of stories can occur.

5

REPRODUCTIVE SYSTEM

REMATRIATING STRAWBERRY FIELDS

STORY #1 The Desecration

The desecration of the Sacred, violence against her Native
woman body
persistent upon his arrival.
he brought out all the instruments of progress
baptized and renamed her Berkeley
her body submerged under him,
he is heavy and unrelenting as Empire
her plaited black hair,
he wrangled into platitudes, singed the iridescent strands
  to silence
he is the weight of asphalt, a lonely parking lot,
his ownership of her, he terms as "freedom."

STORY #2 The Tongan Mormon Baptism Ceremony

I am an eight year old girl at my Mormon baptism Ceremony,
in a small chapel in Ma'ufanga, Tonga,
my hair plaited and split in two, a division so inconsolable,
my mother tenderly tied the wounds with bright white
  ribbons to mark this moment, the missionaries termed as
  the "coming of the light."
under a leaning breadfruit tree outside the Mormon chapel
hungry dogs mate, irrespectively, of the piety inside
his priesthood authority intrusive like the bleached baptismal
  water
surrounds me, my black hair contorted in their nets,
severing the cycles of memories,
until I am no longer able to discern my breath from drowning.
he renames me, declaring the Moana on behalf of his Gods,
bounded my feet with ropes made from woven human hair,
  lined with spears of whale bone tied with knotted fau,
  baptized and converted me
into a carcass of an obedient daughter and wife.
This moment, he proudly records in his missionary diary
  as "light."

STORY #3 We Are Still Here

The West Berkeley Shellmound,
her Native woman body rests under asphalt, luminous mana
  silenced by a parking lot, man-made and mundane,
she is their private property owned by a white settler family
  who refuse to negotiate with Indians.
On the battle grounds in Huichin and in 'Uiha,
Under the hands of missionaries and mercenaries,
our children's bones hung from trees like decomposed fekika
  fruit
the flagrant sour taste on our tongues

when we thought all was lost,

the Sacred was there, she picked up our memories, ancestors
left for dead

she fed our mouths with the flesh of sweet acorn and salt water
from her breasts until we grew strong,

fearless,

she weaves the circuitous dance of death and birth into her long
black hair, dreamtimes exchanged through collective breaths,
from our Moananui to Huichin,

she coughs origin stories, birthed before his arrival,
innumerable constellations, they grow in our altars like the
flowing yellow pua garlands in our hair

she is survivor, creation, Creator

always here

yes, we remember, the stories of us after the missionary and
mercenary are gone.

—FUIFUILUPE NIUMEITOLU,
"FROM THE WEST BERKELEY SHELLMOUND TO MOANA NUI"

Corrina Gould wakes up in the same place that her ancestors
inhabited for thousands of years. East Oakland, California, was
once marshland, populated by grizzly bear and tule elk and Indigenous people living in the villages of Lisjan. Today the nearby AB&I
Foundry spews toxic emissions and noxious fumes into the air. People who live close to the foundry die ten years earlier than people
who live in the hills above the flatland.[1] In 2020 the median price for
homes near the foundry was $452,000. Up the hill, the median home
price that same year was four times greater, $1.6 million. It's the cost
of breathing easy. Gould says:

The buying and selling of land is a new concept here. Real
estate was not a thing. If you can imagine two hundred
years ago, there was no concept of homelessness in the Bay

Area. Today we have thousands of people that are living on the streets, living in substandard housing. If the land were opened up, if the asphalt were to give away to land, and we were to open up all the creeks, and there was fresh water that was available and there was food that was abundant— two hundred years ago there was an abundance here where we live. There was enough for everyone here. The creeks were full of fresh water. They were not dirty or polluted, and nothing was thrown into them that would destroy them. There was fresh fish. Salmon and rainbow trout that would come up the creeks. There was enough tule to create boats and homes and mats to sleep on. There was enough deer and all kinds of other animals that lived in reciprocity.

Before colonialism, the San Francisco Bay Area was one of the most densely populated regions in the continent, home to some of the greatest cultural and biological diversity in North America. Europeans were surprised by how accustomed the animals were to human interaction. "Animals seem to have lost their fear and become familiar with man," noted a European captain. "Quail . . . were often so tame that they often did not start from a stone directed at them." Rabbits "could sometimes be caught with the hand." Another European attested that "geese, ducks and snipes were so tame that we might have killed a great number with our sticks."[2]

Gould wakes up early to go to the West Berkeley Shellmound, where she will hold a ceremony with hundreds of people who are joining her to defend the sacred site. It is the oldest continually inhabited place in the Bay Area, about five thousand years old. Shellmounds are where the Indigenous Ohlone people lived, conducting ceremonies and burying their dead. A survey from 1909 showed 425 shellmounds dotting the Bay Area, some of them up to three stories high.[3] They contained artifacts of daily living: shells, mortars, arrowheads, and remains. When this land became California, the shellmounds were raided and razed. Towns, roads, and shopping malls were built over them, and their contents were mined and mixed to make tennis courts, fertilizer, and pavement. "You're quite literally walking on my ancestors' remains as you're walking through those streets," Gould says.[4]

When she arrives at the West Berkeley Shellmound, she walks onto an expanse of asphalt. To the modern eye, it is just a parking lot, bordered on one side by a railroad that transports crude oil to the refineries that line the bay, and on the other, by the main road through a shopping district with an Apple Store. To Gould, however, this site connects her to her past and her future. She sees the shellmound beneath the parking lot, but not with what she calls "Western vision." She sees it with another kind of sight, something she likens to imagination:

> If you are able to soften your eyes and to maybe imagine. That's the word people would use. *Imagination*. For me, it's really being able to see past the layers of existence, across these different planes. You're able to see the village that was there, the water of the creek, now called Strawberry Creek, coming down. The freeway and the railroad tracks disappear. And you see the marshland and you can hear children's laughter, and you can hear people speaking in language. You can see tule homes and a landscape of abundance.
>
> This is the place where the roundhouse may have sat. A place where we can envision our ancestors leaving through the Western Gate, where the Golden Gate Bridge is, to be met by their ancestors. What would it be like to reimagine the sacredness of land, to reimagine the songs coming back, the sacred ways of being in a place that was a touchstone for my ancestors and through millennia continues to be a touchstone.
>
> It's amazing that at this place we now call a parking lot, people from all over the world have come and prayed. People from the Amazon and people from the Pacific. People have come and prayed. Indigenous and non-Indigenous people too. Because there is something that's magical.

And when we begin to reimagine this connection to the land underneath the asphalt, we understand that this energy that comes from the dancing and songs of my ancestors for thousands of years still remains there.

A real estate development group wants to build a six-story residential building on top of the shellmound, and to dig several stories down for an underground parking lot. A small group of locals gathering for prayers soon grows into large ceremonies with hundreds of people, crossing divides of race, class, and culture, to defend this sacred place. Born and raised in her ancestral homelands, Gould developed early on a capacity for seeing the spiritual spaces hidden beneath the urban landscape. As her relationship to her ancestors deepened, she would make a daily practice of defending Indigenous sites in the Bay Area. She began by rallying people to defend the shellmound, but she would ultimately come to a more expansive view:

> Sacred is about more than just sacred places and sacred sites. It is about who we are as human beings. It's the waters. It's the plant life. It's about being in relationship again with everything that's alive.
>
> What does it mean to be in a sacred relationship with all beings that are alive? I have grandchildren. And so if I don't do my responsibilities today, then they will cease to exist on their own lands. If we don't take care of the responsibilities of our relationships now, the sacred relationships between all living beings, we cease to exist as Indigenous people on our own homelands. And so that has to be solidly put back in place in order for the next seven generations and beyond to just survive.
>
> Sacred is about relationships between human beings. And the land, the water, the air, the fire. So it is about relationships and how we are all here and exist together. I think about what's happening in the world now with the climate crisis, with Covid sitting us down, with the Earth rejuvenating her-

self. I think about our sacred relationality with all living beings and our place as human beings in the circle of life.

Our creation story tells us that we were the last ones to be created. Everything else was created before us as human beings. And so what are our responsibilities as the youngest brother and sister? And if we look at human beings on this planet right now, Mother Earth, we see that we have come so far from that understanding. We have taken ourselves outside of the circle. And that has caused all kinds of confusion and chaos and destruction to everything that gives us life.

Colonization is definitely about taking the sacred first. They take the sacred away from the belief systems. Your ceremonies, your gods are taken away. Then they rape the women and take the sacredness of women as women. Indigenous women are held in high esteem because they are the life bearers. It's also our job to usher out those that are passing over.

The land is still stolen. It's not something in the past that people did a long time ago. People are continuing to steal land, continuing to extract things, continuing to pollute the waters. Colonization is a continuous process.

REPRODUCING COLONIZATION: WITCHES AND HEALERS ON THE FRONTLINE

If colonization were a singular event—an invasion, say—then its effects might be eradicated in the years and decades that followed, like an impact crater worn low over the centuries. But colonialism is a long, continuous process of consolidating and exercising power through violence and coercion and the manufacturing of consent. Colonialism is the invasion but also the subtle centuries-long dynamics of normalizing restructured relationships of power. In order to create a new normal, you need to control how society is reproduced. This is why colonialists have always held a deep concern for the institutions that shape the consciousness and behavior of colonial subjects: the school, the jail, the hospital, the workplace, and the household.

Reproduction involves both biology and hegemony. The processes that produce and reproduce order under colonial capitalism have historically been harnessed to the bodies of women. The subjugation and control of women's bodies are hallmarks of modern medicine, a system of knowledge and power that wouldn't exist without the knowledge, stories, and persecution of women. Women's medical knowledge has been stolen, and women have been used as laboratories for domination.

If this seems a little abstract, here's something that might help. In a 1974 issue of the *Journal of Geography*, two academics—one from the University of Chicago and the other from the University of South Carolina—offered a tool for fellow educators looking to teach high school and undergraduate students about Africa. It's a board game played like Monopoly, except the players represent European powers, in a classroom exercise entitled *A Game of European Colonization in Africa*.

Instead of Chance and Community Chest, there are cards for Fate and Fortune. Land on Fate, and you could "receive tribute from local chiefs; collect $10,000," or face a Native uprising and have to "pay $150,000 for deployment of additional troops." Alternatively, land on Fortune, and you might have to "pay each player $50,000 for wartime indemnities." Or your luck could turn: "American philanthropists provide a new hospital; collect $150,000."

The game is, if nothing else, refreshingly honest. It explores how colonial power reproduces itself and identifies the obstacles to this process, whether rival powers or Indigenous people resisting their subjection. In Monopoly, you build houses and hotels. In this game, called A Game of European Colonization in Africa, you win by collecting schools and hospitals: institutions for the production and reproduction of knowledge and power. But for certain institutions to prevail, institutions of education—and their educators—need to be silenced or even eliminated.

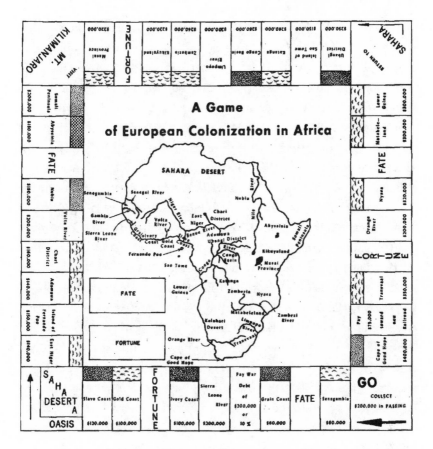

A Game of European Colonization in Africa[5]

One of the most important sources for understanding how co-lonialism lives today is Silvia Federici's masterful work *Caliban and the Witch*.[6] The transition to capitalism in Europe, Federici shows, in-volved the invention of twin monsters: the recalcitrant savage at the frontier of empire—Caliban, from Shakespeare's *The Tempest*—and the witch. Both are healers connected to systems of knowledge based in relationships with the web of life, independent of colonial authority and thus sources of danger to the forces that sought to dominate.

The process of dominating Indigenous people and women was an educational spectacle. If colonialism were to succeed, it had to be made normal in a publicly visible fashion. Colonial powers invented social technologies to make *known once again* that Indigenous people were savages, closer to nature than to society. Descartes had codified this cosmology in the seventeenth century, but words change the world only through constant performance. At the 1889 World's Fair in Paris, four hundred Indigenous people from across the French colonial empire were put on display for sightseers on the Champs-Élysées, in a kind of diorama called the Village nègre (Black Village). Across the Atlantic at the Bronx Zoo, Ota Benga, a central African man bought "for a pound of salt and a bolt of cloth," was displayed in the primate area.[7] He died by suicide in 1916, at age only thirty-two or thirty-three.

The subjugation of women was a public spectacle too. The Salem witch trials of the 1690s, familiar to most US high school students, were descendants of lesser-known European persecutions that began a century earlier. Just before Columbus's first voyage to the Americas, two Dominican Inquisitors published, in 1486, the *Malleus maleficarum* (Hammer of Witches), which laid the basis for this strange cultural ritual. At a time when Europe was bitterly split between Catholics and Protestants, its courts were unified in prosecuting witchcraft as a capital crime, even in the absence of harm to persons.[8]

Consider the witches of Warboys, a case that was reported at the time as something of a trial of the century.[9] In Warboys, a village on the English fens twenty miles north of Cambridge, the nine-year-old daughter of Robert Throckmorton had what appeared to be a series of seizures.[10] An elderly village neighbor, Alice Samuel, came to check in on her.[11] The girl joined her family in the parlor, pointed to Samuel, and according to the widely circulated official record, said, "Grandmother, look where the old witch sitteth." "Did you ever see," asked the child, "one more like a witch than she is?"[12] Her sisters reported similar symptoms and also identified Samuel as the source of their ailments. The following year a visiting noblewoman, Lady Cromwell,[13] administering a folk remedy for witchcraft, cut off a lock of Alice Samuel's hair and later that night experienced nightmares. She died two years later. At trial, Alice Samuel was found guilty of murder.

The Warboys case signaled a transformation in English society. The Throckmortons were part of a growing bourgeoisie, gentrifiers heralding the arrival of a new legal and economic regime in capitalist England. The Throckmorton daughters, and especially Lady Cromwell, were women of a higher class than Alice Samuel and her family. What was new in this trial wasn't that the testimony of the rich was heard differently than that of the poor but rather that it was the first major English case to link possession symptoms with witchcraft, connecting law, medicine, and religion using as rigorous a process of scientific reason as was compatible with a successful prosecution.[14] Alice Samuel offered her confession when her daughter, Agnes, was threatened with jail. The Throckmorton girls didn't relent: they extended their accusations to Agnes.

To prove their case, the Throckmortons conducted a series of public "experiments," including one in which fifteen-year-old Mary Throckmorton removed a coin-sized piece of flesh from Agnes's face. Throckmorton said that she didn't want to do it, but a spirit "told me that I should do it, and forced me thereunto."[15] Agnes's father, John Samuel, was arrested and accused by implication—he hadn't exercised sufficient dominion over his womenfolk and was therefore complicit in their witchcraft. This trial wouldn't just condemn Alice Samuel, her daughter, and her husband to death: it also augured deep changes in how working-class women's knowledge, symptoms, protest, and roles as healers would be viewed.[16]

After the Samuels were executed, the record of the trial notes that the jailer:

> stripped off their clothes and, being naked, he found upon the body of the old woman Alice Samuel a little lump of flesh, in manner sticking out as if it had been a teat to the length of half an inch; which both he and his wife perceiving, at the first sight thereof meant not to disclose because it was adjoining to so secret a place which was not decent to be seen. Yet in the end, not willing to conceal so strange a matter, and decently

covering that privy place a little above which it grew, they made open show thereof unto divers that stood by.

After this the jailer's wife took the same teat in her hand and, seeming to strain it, there issued out at the first as if it had been "beesenings" (to use the jailer's word), which is a mixture of yellow milk and water; at the second turn there came out in similitude as clear milk, and in the end very blood itself.[17]

This "witch's teat" became an excuse for the judiciary to look up women's skirts in search of the multiple nipples they might be hiding all over their bodies. Moreover, this monstrous body part entered medicine. The term *witch's milk* appeared in descriptions of infant breast secretions as late as 1950.[18] A medico-legal spectacle was performed with the "good intentions" to "fix" women's bodies and to make them proper subjects for state policing. The trial—conducted by men, in an independent judiciary performing a public act of peer review—was, after all, the only way to disentangle the magic and sorcery that victimized the accuser from the scientific facts of the case.[19] That Agnes Samuel's body was a laboratory through which the truth could be ascertained through the public dissection of her skin was a sign of the impartial, scientific integrity of the process. Agnes never confessed, but she didn't need to. Her words didn't matter in any case.

The Warboys case influenced England's new witchcraft law of 1604, which offered far harsher punishments for damage to persons and property than had the Elizabethan code.[20] In ramping up the persecution of women, the Crown made clear its allegiance to the forces that would turn common land into private property. Witchcraft trials were about renegotiations of local and state power, and conflicts between different kinds of knowledge and rights to property—contests that were written on the bodies of women, raising questions about who could do what to them, and what peasant women might do when the bourgeoisie came to town.[21] All because one peasant woman, a healer, visited a rich man's daughter to offer her care.

The Samuels were renters in a time when land rents were rising and tenancy contracts were shortening. Peasants across Europe were losing their rights to share the commons.[22] Commoners lost not only access to the land, food, medicine, and fuel they needed for their family's survival. In the enclosure laws and privatization of public lands, women also lost the possibility of practicing the work of care and medicine that had been an essential site of knowledge and power in feudal society.

The only immunity that offered itself to these injustices was class. Even as ostensibly influential an astronomer as Johannes Kepler found himself embroiled in an extensive court case in defense of his own mother against crimes of witchcraft.[23] Katharina Kepler, a former member of the aristocracy, had fallen on hard times and supported herself through her work as a healer and an herbalist. In 1615 she was accused of witchcraft. Her trial was a protracted affair, and by 1620 it had escalated to the point that she was imprisoned and shown the instruments of torture. She refused to confess. Johannes Kepler wrote an extensive brief in his mother's defense, which succeeded in winning her acquittal, though she died soon afterward. And even Kepler succumbed to the language that made it possible for his mother, and women like her, to find themselves persecuted by the state. In one letter, he described her as "small, thin, swarthy, gossiping and quarrelsome, of a bad disposition."[24]

Patriarchy used the term *gossip* to undermine not just women's words but women's knowledge and women's solidarity. Federici traces the history of *gossip*. In English, it used to refer to "god parent," a venerated carer and overseer.[25] That women might be keepers of knowledge and power was a threat to the patriarchy of the colonial social order. So it eroded the power of women's voices by attempting to trivialize them. Katharina Kepler's scientific knowledge of plants and medicine couldn't be permitted the same stature under the new regimes into which her son was published. Just as common land was being enclosed and privatized, and just as Indigenous land was being violently settled, so was medical knowledge. Women were banished from the domain of legitimate knowledge, their words rendered frivolous.

Tracking women's voices and stories is vital to hearing what poet and cultural theorist Fred Moten calls "the poetics of the undercommons."[26] One must strain to hear this language because of the sedimented history of disbelief that women face. The philosopher Miranda Fricker's insight on "epistemic injustice" points to two kinds of ways women are disbelieved. One is testimonial injustice, in which women's pain or trauma, for instance, is less likely to be taken seriously by those in power. Deeper is the idea of "hermeneutical injustice" in which "a collective hermeneutical gap prevents them in particular from making sense of an experience which it is strongly in their interests to render intelligible."[27] In other words, certain ideas and systems of knowledge have been extinguished, preventing women from naming their suffering and oppression. An example of hermeneutical injustice is the absence of a widespread understanding of postpartum depression. The cultural and medical failure to recognize postpartum depression as a biological reality is a form of injustice in which women are often blamed by their partners, or by themselves, for feelings that are common and treatable but cannot be known without a shared understanding.[28] The authority of women's experience is systematically diminished.

Witch trials were a performance of both testimonial and hermeneutical injustice. Persecution extirpated the *possibility* of women's understanding of, and advocacy for, a different mode of engaging with the web of life. This knowledge was driven underground, into a shared, fugitive commons. If certain stories transmit knowledge that sustains life, their systematic silencing under colonialism increases the exposure of women to damage.

The persecution of women and the poor at the frontiers of capitalist expansion continues today: around the globe we see mass incarceration of the working class, ongoing dispossession of farmers from their lands, and witch hunts in India, South Africa, and Brazil that often target female activists.[29] In a startling echo of early modern European history, in the Jharkhand forest in India, Indigenous women who protest the incursions of the state and private business interests (see Chapter 4) are labeled witches so that they can be stripped of their ancestral lands.[30] Commoners, women—and sometimes men—in Asia and Africa who resist the enclosure and privatization of land, are subject to violence, authorized by claims of witchcraft.[31] Despite this global hunt and its deep roots in the history of colonial capitalism, the radical commons of witchcraft persists. Silvia Federici records that "in a meeting on the meaning of witchcraft, the magic is: 'We know that we know.'"[32]

WHAT SKYWOMAN KNEW

It is no coincidence that the wealthy were expropriating common land in Europe at the same time that the first European colonies were established off the coast of West Africa. Witch trials attended the birth of the era called (in mercifully fewer circles) the Age of Discovery. If the new legal codes validated claims by the wealthy to common land in Europe, what—or who—would guarantee tenure on land at the frontiers of state power? In the mid-1400s, the answer was the pope. When Portuguese ships brought the first Black captives from the coast of western Africa to the Iberian Peninsula, Pope Nicolas V issued a series of bulls that granted Portugal the right to enslave sub-Saharan Africans. These writings not only formed the justification for the slave trade but laid the foundation for the Doctrine of Discovery, the dubious moral framework that legitimized Christian nations' seizure of other people's lands, from Africa to Asia to Oceania to the Americas. In 1455 Nicolas V instructed the Portuguese king Alfonso V

> to invade, search out, capture, vanquish, and subdue all Saracens [Muslims] and pagans whatsoever . . . [and] to reduce their persons to perpetual slavery, and to apply and appropriate to himself and his successors the kingdoms, dukedoms,

counties, principalities, dominions, possessions, and goods, and to convert them to his and their use and profit.[33]

The doctrine, summarized by a nineteenth-century Tennessee Supreme Court judge, was

the principle declared in the fifteenth century as the law of Christendom, that discovery gave title to assume sovereignty over, and to govern the unconverted natives of Africa, Asia, and North and South America, has been recognized as a part of the national law [Law of Nations], for nearly four centuries, and that it is now so recognized by every Christian power, in its political department and its judicial.[34]

The knowledge of Indigenous and non-Christian people fell before the civilizing and commodifying force of the invading discoverers.[35] Across the settler world, the Doctrine of Discovery, recognized by the United States Supreme Court in 1823, was cited as the basis for similar theft in Canada, New Zealand, and Australia.[36] In the twenty-first century, this doctrine remains in force, whether in Australia's Northern Territories or on the shores of Ngati Apa.[37] At a 2010 forum on the doctrine, Margaret Lokawua, an Indigenous activist from Uganda, summarized the principle thus: "You go stand over there, close your eyes and pray while we take your land."[38]

Every land grab, in dispossessing people of their ancestral home, is simultaneously an assault against the systems of knowledge and the social reproduction that bind people to the web of life in a particular place, and the stories that make those people who they are. The Doctrine of Discovery was a license not only to take land but to impose new systems of law, education, culture, and medicine in an attempt to indoctrinate locals out of their knowledge of their home. The historian Susan Hill (Wolf Clan, Mohawk Nation of the Haudenosaunee) points out that the links are directly inscribed in language: "Yethi'nih-stenha Onhwentsya is the Kanyen'keha (Mohawk) name for the earth. 'She-to-us-mother provides-[for our]-needs' describes the relationship between Onkewehonwe (humans) and the earth."[39] To suppress the language, and the stories told in that language, is to sever an umbilical connection to place.

One such story comes from Dish with One Spoon Territory, land that stretches across the Great Lakes in North America and has been recognized as a commons governed by Indigenous internation agreements since 1142.[40] The meaning of the name, Dish with One Spoon, is literal, signifying that the Haudenosaunee—or Iroquois— nations, in the northeast of what is now North America, are responsible for the land and life upon it. They should be mindful in their harvesting of its animals and plants and generous in eating with a shared spoon.

As retold in Robin Wall Kimmerer's *Braiding Sweetgrass*, the Ojibwe version of the story goes like this. In the beginning Skywoman, who birthed the people, was falling through darkness. Geese used their wings to soften her descent, and a turtle in the water below offered up his back as a safe place for her to land. All the animals gathered and saw Skywoman's need for solid ground in order to have a home. They offered to dive deep into the ocean to bring up mud for her. Each one tried to touch the bottom of the sea and failed. Finally, the tiny muskrat managed to get a pawful of mud but gave his life in the effort to bring it up from the seafloor. Skywoman spread it out on the turtle's back. She sang her thanks for the acts of generosity from the animals and danced her gratitude. With each step, the earth grew beneath her feet. She had brought a bundle of seeds with her, and now she sowed them, to grow all the plants that would support her and the animals with the food and medicine they would need.[41]

As Christian missionaries landed on the eastern shores of what is now the United States, they encountered the Haudenosaunee, whose women had equal rights to land, territory, and family and were powerful in stewarding the commons. This social order was perceived as a threat in the so-called Western Hemisphere as much as it was in Europe. As the Senecan scholar Barbara Alice Mann notes:

Since the Christian legend of Eve's responsibility for humanity's "Fall" prevented women from acting as instruments of creation or salvation, a good Grandmother . . . was out of the evangelical question. The missionaries therefore reposited Grandmother as Evil, a twist on the original story of Skywoman as a "Bad Medicine" woman. Since missionaries uniformly denounced medicine people as devil worshippers, they casually linked Skywoman, the original Medicine Woman, to their Devil, even as they linked "witches" to Satan in their own culture.[42]

Maintaining loving and treaty-bound relationships with plants and animals, as many Indigenous civilizations and nations still do,[43] prevents the transformation of those beings into resources. Jesuits in Europe and Peru hunted women who had sophisticated repositories of medical information, developed over the course of centuries, if not millennia—knowledge not only of how to administer plants but also of how to manage and be a nonextractive part of the ecosystems that produced them.[44] Tens of thousands of women who resisted the privatization of the commons were executed.[45]

It wasn't enough to displace ways of understanding the possibilities of worlds that existed without private property—bearers of this knowledge had to be put in their place: the household.[46] Although the nuclear family has been the norm for centuries, in the United Kingdom at least,[47] the legal creation of the household, with a man at its head, in charge of its private property and people, was a central project of early liberalism.[48] For Hobbes, the household was modeled on the state, in which a local Leviathan—the man of the house—would protect family members in exchange for obedience, just as the sovereign of state would do for society writ large.[49] Liberalism required a firm distinction between the public and private realms, the making of which was part of a global "great domestication" under capitalism in the seventeenth and eighteenth centuries.[50]

Men could be kings in the castle of their homes, just as kings

ruled over them in public. Crucially, though, the making of this order also demanded that men *be* men. When you make private spaces
in which men are judges, juries, and executioners of order, you also
make men in a particular image. A patriarchal household requires a
patriarch.[51] Installing one meant destroying other orders. In Yoruba
cultures, at the time of colonialism, hierarchies of age, not gender,
defined the social order. Gender, as a fixed category in a binary
structure, didn't exist. That was why, the Nigerian scholar Oyèrónké
Oyěwùmí argues, the British had to invent it.[52]

Many civilizations have rich and fluid understandings of the relationship between one's self and one's body: the Lyg'oravetl'a, Arctic
people in far northeastern Russia, for instance, have nine gender categories.[53] But colonialism forbade two-spirited and queer Indigenous
identities, so that households could be properly heterosexual and pa-
triachal.[54] Bodies that didn't already fit the binary mold were forced
to fit, sometimes through surgery and medicine.[55] In the process, the
medicalized disciplines of reading a body at birth, and writing its destiny as patriarch or housewife on a birth certificate, became ordinary
matters of law and medicine.[56]

The violence of making patriarchs and treating women as household resources for the extraction of labor, both biological and physical and emotional, is continually reproduced. Globally, 35 percent of
women have experienced either physical and/or sexual intimate partner violence, or sexual violence by a nonpartner, and of the 87,000
women intentionally killed in 2017, over 50,000 were killed by a family
member or partner.[57] One study found that "the proportion of women
reporting either sexual or physical partner violence [in the past year],
or both, ranged from 15 percent (Yokohama, Japan) to 71 percent
(Butajira, Ethiopia), with most sites falling between 29 percent and
62 percent."[58]

In every society, when survivors of sexual assault ask for justice
against their abusers, they are put on trial and their testimony is subjected to doubt. Moreover, in trying to escape from partner violence,
women continue to be hampered and harmed by regimes built around

the impossibility of women having freedom from the rule of men.[59] They become reinjured by a society that ensures that trauma is an inescapable part of too many women's daily exposome. Trauma leaves its impression in the body through inflammation.[60]

While the judiciary's complicity in retraumatizing women after domestic violence is familiar, the practice of modern medicine damages vulnerable women too. Medics who send women home to situations in which assault is taking place perpetuate the distinction between public and private space. In such instances medicine operates as an

"extended patriarchy" which functions . . . to reconstitute the diminishing sphere of private life and patriarchal privilege and to supplement the market's uneven regulation of female labor. . . . The private sphere is reproduced by [social] services not as a space where self-hood can be apprehended and developed but where it can be denounced, managed, and even eliminated. To this extent, far from extending the family's ideals into a liberating public space, the services achieve the opposite, the social construction of privacy as a living hell.[61]

Some US states and countries now have mandatory reporting requirements for physicians, who must tell the police if they suspect certain kinds of abuse. But this solution is far from perfect, particularly if a police intervention can inflame the situation and leave some survivors feeling that no real help is available.[62]

Pearla Louis, a fifty-two-year-old Black woman, was found dead in a suitcase floating in San Francisco Bay, the horrifying ending to a life shattered by abusers. She had encountered the medical system several times and had likely detailed the abuse she experienced at the hands of her partner to social workers and her medical team, who would have been mandated to report the violence, but could not give her options that could ensure her safety. Louis felt trapped between a known dangerous partner on one hand and the racial trauma inflicted by the San Francisco Police Department on the other.[63] The year her partner killed her, 2010, also marked a peak of officer-involved shootings in San Francisco.[64] These killings were and still are disproportionately of people of color.

Patriarchy and gender violence are ancient. Colonialism has turned them into policy, and standard operating procedure, and men are expected to enforce it. The subjugation of women isn't expressed only through rape and murder or the threat of it. Colonization uses sexual violence as a tool of conquest. Indeed, the language of colonialism creates women so that they might be dominated: land is often gendered as female, a virgin landscape ready for conquest. Tacitly invoking the Doctrine of Discovery, European explorers delighted in using the language of "penetrating the dark continent,"[65] and more recently Brazil's president Jair Bolsonaro referred to the Amazon as "like a virgin that every pervert from the outside lusts for."[66] In the United States, when petroleum pipeline or mining projects enter regions near territories still held by Native Americans, they bring an influx of well-paid, predominantly white male workers, who settle in temporary housing called "man camps." The men working in these encampments have been implicated in the sexual assault and disappearance of Indigenous women along pipeline paths.[67] In some rural counties where man camps are prevalent, the murder rate of Indigenous women is ten times higher than the national average for women of all races.[68] The proliferation of these camps at the forefront of extractive industries is so pervasive and so global that the World Bank even has guidelines on how to make camps a little more acceptable to its critics, if not to the women who bear extraction's most horrific consequences.[69]

Indigenous women continue to bear a disproportionate share of violence. In 2016 a National Institute of Justice study showed that more than four in five Native American women have experienced violence in their lifetime, and over half have survived sexual violence. Over a third have experienced sexual violence, a rate double that of white US women.[70] Unlike US women of other racial groups, Native American women are most often raped by someone not of their race,[71] a parallel with the racial violence perpetrated on Black women during chattel slavery: many were raped by their white oppressors, sometimes in front of their own families.[72] Not only were enslaved women more likely to suffer this fate than white women, but their bodies, considered property, were treated as medical laboratories, sites of violence and exploration and theft, without which modern medicine would have been impossible. In the name of modern scientific knowledge, capital accumulation, and the Christian God, the exploitation of Indigenous peoples, slaves, nature, and women has been continuous.[73] This violence remains central to the reproduction of colonial capitalism.

THE AGONIES OF OB/GYN

Colonial medicine has generally proved very ready to extend patriarchy, and we live with the consequences today. Although we'll deal with this more fully in Chapter 6, it's important to note here that medical outcomes for Black and Indigenous women are systematically worse than for other women.[74] This is the case not just in the United States but everywhere. In Australia, Indigenous women are more likely to die from breast cancer than are their non-Indigenous sisters.[75] In Mexico, Indigenous maternal mortality rates are six times higher, and in Yunan, China, where there is a large Indigenous population, the maternal mortality rate is two to five times the national average.[76] Black and Indigenous women's experiences of pain and suffering were—and still are—the most systematically muted by the intersections of racism and patriarchy. Nowhere is this clearer than in the field of obstetrics and gynecology. One of its early nineteenth-century pioneers, William Potts Dewees, claimed that wealthy white women suffer more from childbirth than poorer white women or

Black women do, because civilization makes the brains of the former more sensitive. An 1819 reviewer of Dewee's *Essay on the Means of Lessening Pain* writing in the *London Medical and Physical Journal* agreed, noting that "the call made by the uterus in that act on the cerebral system . . . in the savage, is either not experienced, or so slightly perceived as only to cause an effort with no more sensation of pain than what ordinarily takes place in the expulsion of the faeces."[77]

The inability to empathize with Black women's pain remains a critical problem in medicine today. Since the nineteenth century, the direct testimony of Black women has been treated with suspicion, because believing it would open the door to having to listen, take seriously, and reconfigure the racial order.[78] Class offers little reprieve. Dr. Susan Moore, a Black physician who was hospitalized with Covid, complained to the hospital that her pain was not being treated adequately because of racism. She died a few days after being discharged home, her testimony ignored—a victim of the colonial mentality that continues to dominate medicine.

The link between enslaved women and the cosmology of private property is foundational to this mentality. Forcibly removed from their own homelands, they were introduced into stolen lands as private property, bodies from which labor was extracted to expand production and profitability. Their physical labor kept the plantations and households running. And their reproductive labor was integrated into a global system for the circulation of people, goods, natural resources, and capital. Enslaved women were sources of new workers, treated very literally as livestock—referred to as "increasers" by the men who traded them.[79] To the slave owner, Black women of reproductive age served one main purpose: to birth new slaves. They were forced to reproduce the traumatic exposome of slavery through their own wombs. Slave owners raped enslaved women in order to harness their body's reproductive cycle to match that of white women's pregnancies, so that the Black women could serve as wet nurses.[80] For as long as their reproductive power has been subjugated across the intersecting lines of race, class, and patriarchy, Black women have been practicing deep medicine, birthing the resistance to colonial oppression, planning and executing the most dangerous parts of escape. They were integral to making the Underground Railroad function, turning spaces like churches and schools into places of care: to shelter, feed, and help fugitives escape.[81] They contributed important medical knowledge, even while their own voices were being silenced and written out of history.

In the early days of United States, white practitioners of what was known as "slave medicine"[82] made their careers through a mixture of theft from and experimentation on their patients. Enslaved women were on the front lines of care work on plantations, and slaveholders deployed their knowledge of traditional herbs and remedies—passed from mother to daughter—in the maintenance of enslaved people's health.

The historian Martia Graham Goodson recounts the example of Francis Peyre Porcher, a celebrated nineteenth-century Confederate doctor.[83] Porcher's doctoral thesis on the medical botany of South Carolina is filled with knowledge stolen from enslaved people. *Eupatorium perfoliatum*, a plant commonly known as boneset in the southern United States, was "very extensively used among the negroes of the plantations," Porcher recorded.[84] It has since proved to be a potent anti-inflammatory.[85] The theft of this knowledge made Porcher's name in the medical world, and his *Resources of the Southern Fields and Forests* was said to have "saved the Confederacy for two years" with the information it put into the hands of resource-strapped white physicians working to help the side that fought to maintain slavery.[86] Techniques stolen from traditions of African medicine made it into the US medical canon.

Enslaved women had not only their milk and their knowledge stolen from them but also their DNA. The much more recent theft of the cells that became the HeLa line—taken from the cervical tumor of Henrietta Lacks without her knowledge in the 1950s, reproduced in laboratories around the world today, and made famous by

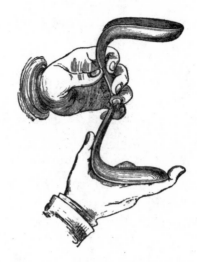

Sim's speculum.
Note the cuff and
shirtsleeves in this drawing
from an 1876 catalog of
medical devices.[87]

Rebecca Skloot's brilliant *The Immortal Life of Henrietta Lacks*—is
another case in the history of this larceny.

Black women's bodies have been used as laboratories of scientific knowledge and racial capitalism: not only have their cell lines
been stolen, but their flesh has been extracted in the name of progress, even at the birth of modern gynecology. J. Marion Sims, long
hailed as "the father of gynecology," is one of the most celebrated
surgeons in US history and was the president of the American Medical Association in 1876.[88] In his autobiography, he reported having
a eureka moment while attending Betsey, the enslaved woman of
another local doctor, who suffered vesicovaginal fistulas.

> I said, "Betsey, I told you that I would send you home this
> afternoon, but before you go I want to make one more ex-
> amination of your case." She willingly consented. I got a
> table about three feet long, and put a coverlet upon it, and
> mounted her on the table, on her knees, with her head rest-
> ing on the palms of her hands. I placed the two students
> one on each side of the pelvis, and they laid hold of the
> nates [buttocks], and pulled them open. Before I could get
> the bent spoon-handle into the vagina, the air rushed in
> with a puffing noise, dilating the vagina to its fullest extent.

> Introducing the bent handle of the spoon I saw everything,
> as no man had ever seen before.[89]

It's another echo of the Doctrine of Discovery: with the use of a spoon, Sims conquered a previously unseen world. He would later develop the spoon into the modern speculum.

Fistulas are openings that develop at the interface of two body parts. Vesicovaginal fistulas connect the bladder and the vagina, allowing urine to leak through the vagina, which can be a deeply distressing experience. They have a range of causes, from injury in childbirth or surgery to inflammation due to gynecological malignancies or recurrent urinary tract infections.[90] Sims's experiments made it possible to treat the discomfort, embarrassment, and possible infection that accompany these fistulas.

By his own account, his patient agreed to the operation. But for things that did not appear in his autobiography, Sims's statue was removed from New York's Central Park in 2018.[91] While Betsey might have "willingly consented," the measure of consent is whether she was actually free to say no. Like Sims's other patients, she was an enslaved woman whose owner had brought her to him. He installed these women in the ramshackle eight-bed hospital, or "laboratory," that he erected in his Montgomery backyard,[92] promising the owners that

> he would repair their laborer, making her fit for her duties. In a slave economy, this surgery held particular value. Not only did it repair the slave capital, so she could work, but by ridding her of the fistula's "loathsome" and "disgusting" attributes the surgery also affected her likelihood to reproduce, a vital aspect of her role as slave.[93]

To compound the horror, Sims didn't use anesthetic on the enslaved women on whom he developed his techniques and tools. His defenders point out that this decision was free of racial animus, since he didn't use anesthetic on white women either, thinking that their agony under surgery wasn't as severe as they let on.[94] Giving consent requires having a voice that can be heard. To be denied having one's pain heard is to be deeply silenced. Medicine is guilty, then and now, of being deaf to Black women's voices.

In the United States today, reproductive health is marred with the signs of a racist society, and markers of racism are visible even before birth.[95] One study tracked Black mothers born in Africa and the Caribbean whose children and grandchildren were born in Illinois, and compared their birth weights to the children and grandchildren of white women born in the United States.[96] While foreign-born Black women were more likely to have children with birth weights similar to white Americans, their children were more likely to have babies with lower birth weights, more akin to those of US-born Black women. Preterm birth is associated with an intrauterine inflammatory state. Stress in a pregnant mother creates epigenetic changes in her baby and her grandchildren, and those changes result in shorter pregnancies, or higher rates of preterm birth.[97] Ancestral trauma and the allostatic load of being Black in the United States is transmitted in the womb, accumulating over generations. The biological warfare of racism shapes health even before a baby takes their first breath.

In the United States, although infant mortality rates have fallen, the gap between Black babies and white babies is actually greater today than it was under antebellum slavery.[98] Historical demographers estimate that in 1850, enslaved infants died before one year of age at a rate 1.6 times higher than white infants (340 versus 217 deaths per thousand live births). In comparison, Centers for Disease Control and Prevention figures from 2016 show that today non-Hispanic Black infant mortality is 2.3 times higher than mortality among non-Hispanic White babies (11.4 deaths and 4.9 deaths, respectively).

As of 2016, the US infant mortality rate was 71 percent higher than that of comparable high-income countries.[99] While socioeconomic inequalities play an important role in this disparity, the difference between life and death may also be embedded in the attitudes of doctors.[100] In the United States, when Black physicians care for Black newborns, the mortality difference from white babies is halved. Phrasing this data another way, Black babies are three times more likely to die in the United States when they are cared for by white physicians.[101]

Changing these dire outcomes will require dismantling white supremacist patriarchal power structures in society. In a recent study, Black women identified the racist structures impacting their reproductive health. Better birth outcomes, they clarified, would require changes in housing, in negative social attitudes toward Black women, in medical care, policing, employment, education, access to community resources, and community infrastructure.[102] As that work is done, little changes also have a big impact. In a study where health care researchers asked women of color what can improve disparities in reproductive health, one simple recommendation floated to the top: listen to Black women.[103]

ON STRAWBERRY FIELDS
AND SEEDS AND SCHOOLS

Medical dehumanization isn't easy to bear. It's difficult for medical workers to shut off their feelings for and duties toward their fellow human beings. A study of burnout found that rates among women and men were similar across professions, but the reasons were different: women were generally exhausted from caring and fighting unfairness, while men were exhausted from psychological distancing in order to maintain a lack of compassion.[104] The contours of caring and not-caring follow the shape of the terrain of power and injustice. It takes institutions to normalize the work of dehumanization, and these institutions must be created and recreated. From the household to the corporation to the clinic to the school, such work continues today.

The work of dehumanization relies on the repetition of epistemic injustice, sedimented through denying women's experience about, knowledge of, and authority over their own bodies. The journalist

Maya Dusenbery, in *Doing Harm*, notes that women have been systematically left out of research studies, in one case "because there
wasn't a women's bathroom at the research site."[105] The exclusion
of women from drug trials has been justified for two contradictory
reasons: either women's bodies are functionally identical to men's,
so it shouldn't matter, or they're so vastly different from men's that
they'll confound the results.[106] In both cases, what's at work is the
construction of what is normal and natural, and the contortions necessary to sustain it. In one study, which concluded that aspirin might
help lower the risk of heart attacks in everyone over forty, every
single one of the 22,071 participants was a male physician.[107] There
is nothing new here. This is how colonial cosmology is reproduced
as common sense.

   Clinical trials in which bourgeois men's bodies are a metonym
for everyone's bodies is the reductio ad absurdum of modern medicine's history. For such an outcome to have passed unnoticed required a great deal of work. Women's medical knowledge had to be
stolen and suppressed; Indigenous science had to be deemed super-
stition; women's bodies had to be turned into laboratories of power
(but not laboratories for health-giving pharmaceutical trials). Although women now outnumber men entering medical schools in the
Global North, the institutions that reproduce doctors remain firmly
rooted in the practices that denigrated medicine women and burned
witches.[108] The consequence for all our bodies, not women's alone,
is continuing inflammation.

   Consider a therapy for the heart: the strawberry. When Skywoman
fell to Earth, she brought seeds with her, including tobacco, corn, and
strawberry. The strawberry, the first Haudenosaunee medicine, is an
anti-inflammatory.[109] Wounds heal faster with berry ointment,[110] and
the sharing of strawberry drink—mashed strawberries, sometimes
with maple syrup—is a hallmark of Haudenosaunee ceremony. Harvesting berries was a source of economic and agricultural power and
knowledge, and a means of creating and reproducing Haudenosaunee
sovereignty and independence. For this reason, the Indian Boarding

School system targeted it, transforming it from an activity for the entire community into gendered work for women.

In 1838 the Ogden Land Company used chicanery, bribery, and forgery to con the Seneca and other Haudenosaunee peoples out of their traditional upstate New York territory.[111] The federal government offered the Seneca plots in Kansas and sent them there while tribal elders stayed in New York to appeal the mishandled treaty. In 1842 a compromise was hammered out, in which Ogden took only some of their allotted parcels. The journeys from New York to Kansas and from Kansas to New York exposed the displaced families to immense suffering and disease. By the time the Seneca returned to western New York along Lake Erie, many of the parents had died.

Enter the Thomas Asylum for Orphan and Destitute Indian Children, which was established in 1855 and named for Philip Evan Thomas, the first chairman of the Baltimore and Ohio Railroad.[112] His philanthropy contributed to the founding of the school, which was one of 350 such private and federally funded institutions in the United States. By way of comparison, Canada had 130 residential schools for First Nations children; in Australia at least one of every ten Aboriginal children in the Stolen Generation was taken from their family and placed in a state-run facility or white household; in Ireland, some children were cast into a system of state reformatories and church facilities throughout the nineteenth and twentieth centuries. Nonsettler colonies in Asia and Africa experienced kindred kinds of institutional violence against children in the name of civilization.[113]

Residential schools were designed to interrupt Indigenous kinship, knowledge, and sovereignty.[114] The Federal Indian Boarding School program's founder, Captain Richard Pratt, famously articulated the schools' goal: "Kill the Indian, and save the man." But this goal could not be achieved if young Native children could stay with their families on their lands. "Isolate the child, steal the land," might have been more apt a slogan. The schools taught boys and girls the labors and expectations of domestic life, preparing them for a permanently junior position in white society. Ni:mi:pu: scholar Beth Piatote writes in her excellent *Domestic Subjects* that the kind of education administered at the asylum was the corollary of "the legal invention of Indians as wards of the nation and perpetual minors under law."[115]

The Tuscarora Haudenosaunee scholar Meredith Palmer's research on the Thomas Indian school shows how the reproduction of colonial society required the transformation of relationships between humans and other living beings. Part of Haudenosaunee girls' kinship with other women lay in the practice of harvest. When aunts and mothers wrote to the school, asking that girls to be sent home to join such activities, the administration denied the requests. Girls were taught that their work picking strawberries should be done not as healers but as biddable labor that local farmers might hire seasonally.

These berries are "a symbol of cyclical time," Palmer told us. "Capitalist temporalities are overthrown by Indigenous understandings. The strawberry ceremony every year is a reminder of the woman who brought that medicine to us." Strawberry-leaf tea is a powerful cardiac pharmaceutical: its nitric oxide dilates blood vessels, which increases blood flow to critical muscles like the heart and lowers overall blood pressure.[116] In some tellings, *strawberry* means *heartberry*.[117] Contrast that with the understanding of strawberries as products that are harvested every year to be snacked on mindlessly. By turning the berry harvest into a commercial activity, the Indian school was an attempt to destroy the reproduction of an entire cosmology around the strawberry, Skywoman, and cyclic time.

The privatization of the strawberry went hand in hand with the enclosure of the land on which it was grown. Berries from Dish with One Spoon Territory were cross-bred with varieties from California, where they were featured in Karok foodways, and with varieties from Chile, where they were part of Mapuche and Picunche traditions.[118] The resulting genome was privatized: the knowledge of Indigenous people was stolen and their prior art denied.[119] Driscoll's—a brand popular in North America, responsible for 29 percent of 2017 global strawberry sales—licenses its berries under its own name.[120]

Like many plants, strawberries can reproduce both sexually and asexually. In the wild, their asexual reproduction involves growing long stolons, or runners, from which daughter plants emerge. But this happens too slowly and inefficiently for the market. The rhythms of industrial agriculture require dense annual plantings. In order to maintain maximum productivity, plants and their ecosystems are wiped clean every year. To create a sterile earth, to clear the soil of pathogens that might harm their harvest, farmers fumigate it with methyl bromide, a potent ozone-depleting chemical. In the barren exposome of strawberry monoculture, pests can spread untroubled by most predators, and the chemical arsenal of the landowners has expanded to keep up.

Studies have yet to compare the nutritional characteristics of wild and proprietary crops. We do, however, know something about the differences between conventional and organic strawberry cultivation. The more diverse the soil, and the less exposure to pesticides, the higher concentrations of phenols and ascorbic acid—two vital nutrients that give strawberries their anti-inflammatory properties.[121] Conventionally grown strawberries have lost their heart medicine.

Organophosphate pesticides used in the strawberry industry were originally a dividend of biological warfare research—they're acute neurotoxins that enter the circulatory systems of people on and near the farms.[122] The children of women who were exposed to the pesticides while pregnant suffer a seven-point drop in IQ compared to those whose mothers weren't exposed.[123] We are still learning how the poisoning of the soil and the damaging of its microbiome by these industrial processes affects long-term health outcomes via the human gut microbiome.[124]

Those hoping to counter all this at the supermarket checkout by purchasing organic berries are likely to be disappointed. Debts imposed on the Global South are technologies to create landlessness and communities of workers ready to migrate to sell the only thing they have left: their labor. In the United States, around three-quarters of farm labor is done by people from Latin America.[125] Because growers pay the workers by volume, they earn much less picking naturally grown than conventionally produced strawberries. As every worker knows, *"la fresa orgánica no crece grande"*—organic strawberries don't grow big.[126]

California strawberry fields are a part of a global assembly line of high technology, land theft, and human disposability. Toiling on unceded and occupied Ohlone territory, workers are exposed to pesticides that will scar their children's bodies. Pregnant workers are exposed to organophosphates that risk their unborn children. In their turn, male farmers exposed to pesticides have chemicals in their semen, some of which have been linked to childhood cancers.[127] Exposure to pesticides also damages sperm DNA, thus reducing male fertility.[128] Pesticides have been found in the amniotic fluid surrounding a fetus, in umbilical cord blood, and in mothers' breast milk. Children are conceived and born bathed in chemical exposure.[129] Crops grown in this chemical stew are less nutritious.[130] The soil, like the people, becomes less fertile.[131]

The obvious protagonist in this transformation of land, cultural practices, and bodies are the corporations at the hearts of the international chemical distribution and supply chains. But other institutions that reproduce colonial power are also responsible. National universities are hubs for the discovery and promotion of knowledge about seeds. In the United States, one such university in Haudenosaunee territory has long offered advice to local growers and now seeks to disseminate their expertise more widely: Cornell University.[132] There the Gates Foundation has funded an Alliance for Science, with a vision to promote industrial agriculture in the Global South.[133]

Philanthropists traditionally use their money to project their visions onto foreign places, replacing Indigenous forms of knowledge with new Western categories and practices. Philanthrocapitalism is the latest in a long series of technologies for the social reproduction of colonial power. In the first half of the twentieth century, the

Rockefeller Foundation funded the idea of "international health," which was characterized by "agenda-setting from above; use of budget incentives; a technobiological paradigm; narrow interventions to max-imise efficiency and success; consensus through transnational profes-sionals."[134] The Gates Foundation follows the same pattern, offering its own equally imperial visions of science, knowledge, and appropri-ate technology.[135] A cornerstone of this vision is capital investment and larger land holdings: an early draft of the Gates agriculture plan called for "land mobility"—in which the land stayed where it was but its owners sold it to more efficient farming operations.[136] There's plenty of evidence—and organizing—against this idea. Somewhere be-tween 170 million and 255 million people are members of organiza-tions committed to different visions of sustainability, with different relations to land and life.[137] Chief among them is the international peasant movement, La Via Campesina, whose women have drawn on their lived experience of both patriarchy and agricultural capitalism to demand transformations not just in agricultural production and reproduction but also in humans' relations with the web of life.[138]

Gates's celebrity and cachet remain alluring, and his widely shared prediction about the coronavirus—that there would be a pan-demic and that money would be required to prevent it—has legiti-mized a philanthrocapitalism that helps to line a pocket or two of the right players. Through his investments, Gates owns 97,933 hect-ares (242,000 acres) of arable land, making him the largest farmland owner and occupant of stolen territory in the United States.[139] Or as the Game of European Colonization in Africa puts it: "American philanthropists provide a new hospital; collect $150,000."

CONDOLENCE AND REMATRIATION

Exposure to trauma and the development of PTSD are strongly associ-ated with inflammation, and the effect adds up over a lifetime.[140] This is not about individual choices or lifestyles; it is an inherently systemic social and political process.[141] These experiences are stamped onto our genes, passed through our microbes, and transmitted from one generation to the next.[142]

Here the literature is growing, and we must tread carefully. White supremacy has been furthered, as we'll see in more detail in Chapter 6, by pseudoscience. Pointing to the actual biological scars of trauma in the bodies of BIPOC people, and naming the medical consequences of structural violence, runs the risk of rationalizing and naturalizing racism, mistaking social cause for biological effect. Yet trauma's fingerprints last for generations. Studies of survivors of the Nazi Holocaust and the Tutsi Massacre have found epigenetic markers at specific sites on genes. Terror in the exposome leaves its marks inside the body, on predictable parts of survivors' DNA.[143]

Domestic violence and child abuse leave similar traces and run similar risks of misinterpretation. In repeating the story of broken families, state agencies can potentially point to methyl groups added by trauma onto DNA as an index of poor parenting, deflecting analysis from the social structures and histories that break those families and make it close to impossible for some families to ever remain whole. Medicine can be used as a tool to disconnect the body from the exposome, to dislocate and then relocate the origins of intergenerational trauma in the dysfunctions of one body passed along to another. Medicine, in service to colonial state institutions, often mistakes social reproduction for biological reproduction. Epigenetic markers are signs of the deeper disease—the social, economic, political, and ecological conditions that manufacture trauma, which is passed on, generation after generation.

Deep medicine here involves breaking the cycle of reproduction. It requires, at its core, the abolition of patriarchy, including the gender categories and gendered violence it has created.[144] While modern social institutions make it hard to imagine such a world, it isn't impossible. Oyèrónkẹ́ Oyěwùmí reminds us that age-based, nongendered social organization in Yorubaland has not been entirely extinguished. A recent study of women in the matriarchal

Mosuo community in China shows that women who are in charge of their lives have less than half the level of elevated CRP compared to women who live under patriarchy, and those women with less inflammation had better health outcomes.[145] Long before the suffragist movement fought for white women's right to vote, Haudenosanee women enjoyed centuries of political power and equality in their communities.[146] The Haudenosaunee Confederacy is the longest-functioning participatory democracy in the Americas. Through Benjamin Franklin—who represented Pennsylvania at Iroquois meetings, published Iroquois treaties, and attended at least one Iroquois condolence ceremony—the spirit and practices of the Confederacy's form of self-government influenced what would become the US Constitution. That this fact is unknown and even held in disbelief outside Haudenosaunee territory is a mark of the success of the colonial narrative about the founding of the United States.[147] The historian Barbara A. Mann describes Haudenosaunee women's social power:

> Women were in charge of both the literal birth-naming of children and the figurative naming of men to federal political office. Women might impeach any man (or woman!) found unworthy of public office. Women likewise had a gatekeeping authority over warfare. . . . The Jigonsaseh [head clan mothers] . . . allowed or disallowed passage of war parties, thus giving them tacit veto power over warfare. Because federal officials could be put forward *only* by their respective Clan Mothers, and could be impeached by them, Clan Mothers effectively controlled the national agenda.[148]

Franklin did not hear these women's voices; nor did he recognize their power to name new generations and wage war and constitute a political community. He recorded being especially moved by the condolence ceremony, a practice that continues to this day.[149] In this ritual, the grief-stricken and those who have come to console

them gather around a table. Together they make community deci-
sions about reparation and restitution, acknowledging that grief can
cloud judgment but should not lead to silence. On the contrary, the
ceremony places the acts of mourning and restoring justice in public,
where they must be done for healing to begin.

Some Indigenous women healers in North America, particularly
in social work, are finding the rituals of condolence to be effective
in managing the "unresolved historical grief, stemming from centuries of genocide and assimilation, . . . still being passed down from
generation to generation."[150] These rituals are not a protocol so much
as a process that recognizes, names, and collectively explores the
history and continuing sources of that trauma. Haudenosaunee condolence rituals, even as recorded by Franklin, demand a transformation through shared grieving.[151]

As the scholar Saidiya Hartman puts it, "The issues of loss and
our identification with the dead are central to both the work of
mourning and the political imagination of the African diaspora. And,
for this reason, *grief* is a central term in the political vocabulary of
the diaspora."[152] To grieve is to weave the narrative of the past and
present mourning together, in order to begin to imagine a future
with healing in it. The purpose of grieving rituals is to mark loss and
to build the social bonds needed to see a future together. It is the first
step toward a deeper reproductive medicine, a way of producing and
reproducing society without domination.

Collective grief over loss has sometimes spurred action at an international level. The massacre of nineteen peasants in Eldorado dos
Carajas, Brazil, inspired a mobilization that led to the international
Declaration on the Rights of Peasants.[153] A number of United Nations
documents, with origins in loss and violence, recognize the protection of lifeways: the Convention on the Elimination of All Forms of
Discrimination Against Women (CEDAW), and the Declaration on the
Rights of Indigenous Peoples, sit alongside codes on pesticides, on
racism, and on workers' rights.[154] There are also ways to address the
testimonial silencing not just of women but of the planet. The planet

has been speaking in the language of wildfires, hurricanes, and sea-level rise. Hearing that grief, Indigenous movements in Ecuador have led the world in recognizing the rights of Pachamama, the Earth goddess that is the same being as the Earth to the people of the Andes.[155] These are floors, though, not ceilings, and we're very far from reaching even them, because declarations don't make change—actions do.

For Corrina Gould, the way to heal the wounds created by colonialism is to reawaken those connections to the sacred, which she views as those things that are necessary for life to proceed in health and wellness. And only rematriation can do this. The back of the shirt she wears as she stands in a circle that has assembled around her reads "Rematriate the land." To overcome the legacy of violence toward women and the Earth, we must correct our relationships. As Gould explains:

> The rematriation of land is about giving the land back to the Indigenous people from whom it was stolen. It's about the sacred responsibilities that we have to the land. The sacred responsibilities that women have to the land are different than those of men. Our sacred responsibilities are our songs for the water, our songs for the children, our ability to take care of the plants in a different kind of way. The medicinal plants that we are able to gather and tend to, the songs that we have for those plants, the umbilical cords of our babies being buried for thousands of years in our own land.
>
> Rematriation is the bringing back of all those plants, to allow for Indigenous cultures to thrive and to grow and to be where they're supposed to be, to allow for our responsibilities on the land that we were intended to take care of and live in reciprocity with. Rematriation is really a spiritual journey as well as bringing that culture back, bringing those songs back, bringing those ceremonies that need to be on this land back. In order for us to heal, Indigenous ceremonies on the land have to come back, because it doesn't just help the Indigenous people—it helps everyone who now lives here. It's the

responsibility of the guests on our land to help us to figure out
how to do that as well. Rematriation is also about working on
reciprocity with the guests that are on our territories.

It's about acknowledging whose land that we're on, no
matter where we go in the world. Acknowledging whose
ancestors are there. And then how are we as guests? Because
I will be a guest if I go past a certain county close by. Then
what is my responsibility to those First Nations people that
live there and all of their ancestors that have been there for
thousands of years? How do we make sure that we're able
to take care of it?

For me, rematriation is really about women taking their
rightful place in the world right now, taking care of the land
and the ceremonies and the songs and the language. It's
about looking at what men have done to the world in terms
of land. When we talk about real estate speculation, when
we talk about wars that are created over land and resources,
when we equate land and the destruction of what has happened to the land, we can equate it to women's bodies and
what has happened to us through the ages.

We're talking about the buying and selling and extraction
of land, and they're buying and selling and extracting
women's bodies. And so I think that what we are hearing
through our ceremonies is that it is time for women to take
their rightful place to bring balance back into the lands,
back into the world again. There's been an imbalance for
so long that our mother, the Earth, is sick. And so our songs
and our ceremonies and coming back into that way, it's a
different way of being.

There's a privilege of being a man in this world, whether
they know it or not. And women don't have that same privilege. So we need allies that are men and that are going to
allow for this balance to come back. I'm not talking about
hating men or not including men, but rather having our
voices uplifted so that we can bring the balance back. When
I think about what's happened with Covid right now, I think

about all of the leadership of women in other countries and how they have taken care of the people first. That's what rematriation is. It's about taking care of the people and the needs of our brothers and sisters first, instead of corporations and greed.

Rowen White is a farmer, mother, artist, Earth tender, and seed keeper from the Mohawk community of Akwesasne. The Mohawk are one of the six nations that make up the Haudenosaunee Confederation. In her culture, the women protect the seeds and ration the food to ensure that everyone has enough to eat. Today, through her work at her farm, Sierra Seeds, White sees the path toward a better way of living together on the Earth, starting with reawakening the ancient bonds between people and these nourishing germs of life. That process of reconnecting involves rematriation, which to White means making space for the mother again, in all areas of life:

We are rematriating seeds, back to the land, back to the people. We are rehydrating that understanding that seeds are mothers, that the land is a mother. There's a fundamental core understanding and a core relationship that has atrophied. So that's why we call it rematriating, because it's putting the mother back into things, making sure that people understand that fundamental relationship.

We're making place for mother again, the big mother to be in our lives, to relate to her in our lives, to create that possibility that people don't just say, "Oh, Mother Earth," as, like, just mere words upon their lips, but that they understand in all the ways they act, that the Earth is their mother. That those seeds are their mother. That we have been adopted by plants. We've been adopted by corn, and we've been adopted by beans, and we've been adopted by squash. Because we humans, we're dependent on all these beings to feed us. We would be nothing without them.

And so they've adopted us into their family and have said that they will continue to nourish us. And that comes through in our stories. The corn grew from the grave of Original Woman's daughter. The corn grew from her breast. The beans came from her hands, and the squash came from her belly button. It came from her body. In the sense of "My body is going to nourish you from now until the end of time." The Earth is going to nourish you in these ways.

So that's the real concept of rematriation. It is making space for mother again in our lives, because we've denigrated the mother for so long in Western society. In native communities, we've kept that center of mother alive. But we've also been in a fight-or-flight trauma response for five hundred-plus years, trying to keep this cultural sanity alive amid the madness. Trying to protect the mother in all her forms, trying to protect our connection to the land, trying to keep our seeds alive, trying to keep the waters clean, and all the ways in which we're protecting how mother shows up. So this is the rematriation movement. It's a big movement. It's bringing that place of mother again, because it's been so off balance for so long we have to name it. We have to name where the corruption has happened.

It's this banishment of the mother that has produced a society deeply out of balance, but to White, the pathology responsible for this process emerged in Europe long before Europeans set foot on Turtle Island, the land that grew under Skywoman's dancing feet. Turtle Island is the Haudenosaunee name for what is now called North America. She continues:

Colonialism, from my understanding, is a spiritual virus. It's a horrific pathology that is an outgrowth of trauma and disconnection. It grows over the generations as that trauma and that violence gets internalized and then projected outward.

And I feel there is no culture that worships and is in reverence of the divine feminine, that acknowledges the power of the feminine, that would be capable of doing what those countries and those powers have done through the hands and tools of colonialism. And I think it's deep. Whatever trauma happened in the Middle Ages or in the Dark Ages in Europe, that really violently dismantled the matriarchy that existed there, and the understanding of the balance of feminine and masculine, infected a whole lineage of people with this spiritual virus, to do unspeakable things, to allow the patriarchy to grow in such a pathological way.

For White, the path to healing runs through reconnecting people to their ancestral seeds. Reawakening these vital relationships deepens the understanding of what power truly is. Reconnecting to seeds centers power in a life-giving context:

The inherent value of seeds is in the relationship we have to them. They are these keepers of memory. They link the past and the future and the present all together. They weave this intergenerational web. They are life-giving beings. And they represent lineage for us. As Indigenous people, we are intimately interconnected with the seeds that have been passed down through the generations. Through cosmogeneology, we see ourselves as direct lineal descendants of the foods that have offered themselves up for us to eat, for us to nourish ourselves. These seeds, both wild and cultivated and some of the ones that lie in between, we learn about them in our creation stories. We learn about them playing significant roles in our cosmology. And we learn through the upkeeping of our cultural memory and our cultural traditions that we are blood relatives to them. It's not a metaphor. It's a relationship that's real. And it's enlivened by the way in which we continue to uphold our ceremonies and our culture. It's how we relate to them.

And so for me as a seed keeper, as somebody who came to

seeds as a young woman, and reestablishing and rehydrating my relationship to them at a very critical point in my life, they're showing me a blueprint and helping me to understand the map of what it means to be an Indigenous woman, of what it means to uphold my responsibility to feed and nourish, what it means to always show up in alignment with many of our cultural values that are represented by seeds: reciprocity, interdependence, generosity. All the ways the seeds help us to understand what it means to truly be in a reciprocal and co-evolutionary relationship with the world around us.

And so for me, seeds are a reflection of the people that carry them. And they sit at the very center of real cultural sanity. The wellspring of culture comes from the way in which we feed and nurture ourselves. If you look at all of the ways in which culture has kind of grown and expressed itself, in all the diverse ways across the globe, at the very center of that wellspring is the way we feed and nurture ourselves and have our basic needs met. It's through this beautiful, storied, sacred, spiritual, cultural relationship that we have to these seeds, because we see them as no different from ourselves. There's no separation, in that their good life means our good life.

When our seeds are healthy and strong and we're taking good care of them, then the people are healthy and strong and are well taken care of. And because of colonization, acculturation and displacement and all of the things that came in the last two centuries, our people were violently disconnected from these time-honored relationships to seeds, and you see that reflected. You see the people suffering. You see the people are not in good health. You see the people in all kinds of ways that this disconnection ripples out into our collective well-being.

For me as a seed keeper, there are many pathways to what we call dignified resurgence. But for me as a seed keeper, I see that one would be the reseeding of the people. When people begin to have a complex understanding of their place in the world as it relates to their relationships to those beings that feed and nourish them, there's the revitalization of cultural sanity. A revitalization of real humans, not the kind of humans that are walking the Earth right now, because a lot of the humans that are walking the Earth right now have been so splintered from any cultural intactness or any sense of cultural sanity for so long that they're not really human. They're trying to be human, but they don't have an understanding of what it means to really be human, in the sense of upholding our relationships to all of our relations around us.

Through my apprenticeship to seeds and through my apprenticeship to the land and these relationships, I'm gaining the tiny glimpses of what the new world coming might look like. They offer their creativity and their incredible imagination to even be able to get a glimpse of what cultural sanity on Turtle Island might look like. And because these seeds and these foods—they go inside our bodies when we eat them, they inform the very cellular level of our bodies in a way that gives us an understanding of who we are and what we stand for and how we should be as real people of the Earth. They go inside us and inform us in ways that we can't necessarily always think into those places or use our brains to sort of think into those places. That to me is the value of seed. They give us a pathway to such a dignified resurgence of Indigenous peoples in this time.

Since time immemorial, we've seen these seeds as talismans of hope and also just real, true power. Our word in Mohawk for seed is *ganna*. And at the beginning of the word is the sound *ga*. It's feminine in nature. So it's a feminine word. It encapsulates this idea that there's this divine feminine essence that moves through things and animates the world around us. And seeds are an embodiment of that essence, that life-giving feminine force with the endless capacity to just give and give and replenish and multiply exponentially.

That's where true power is: not like the corrupted

power that we think of when we say the word *power* now, but the true power of the essence of life. It's that same essence that grew you in your mother's womb or that allows a flower to turn into a pod and then turn into a seed—that essence runs through all of us. When we reconnect to seed and understand that it's our true source of power, then dignified resurgence is possible.

And the colonial powers knew that food and connection to land was where our spiritual power was rooted. That's why they specifically manufactured a very violent dismantling of those systems, in order to cripple the Indigenous peoples of Turtle Island, in order to continue their merciless death march of colonization, which ended up morphing into the current face of capitalism that we see today.

For me, I feel like the power and value of seed is that we, as Indigenous people, see the true source of our power through this ever-changing, ever-adaptive entity that is seed. Because they are always forever changing and forever adapting. Our life is dependent on that adaptability and that generosity that comes with seeds. I think that, for me, one of the only pathways to a dignified resurgence is to reseed ourselves, to reclaim seeds as part of our bundle and part of our way forward.

6

CONNECTIVE TISSUE

BEYOND BORDER MEDICINE

James Baldwin: I'd seen what white people had done to the world and I'd seen what white people had done to their children. Because in gaining the world they had lost something.

Nikki Giovanni: Their life.

Baldwin: No. They lost the ability to love their own children.

Giovanni: Or the ability to love themselves.

Baldwin: Which is the same thing. And I didn't want that to happen, if I may say so, to you. . . . As I said once, you know that a cop is a cop . . . and he may be a very nice man. But I haven't got the time to figure that out. All I know is that he's got a uniform and a gun and I have to relate to him that way. That's the only way to relate to him because one of us may have to die.

—NIKKI GIOVANNI AND JAMES BALDWIN[1]

The plague of racism is insidious, entering into our minds as smoothly and quietly and invisibly as floating airborne microbes enter into our bodies to find lifelong purchase in our bloodstreams.

—MAYA ANGELOU[2]

I can't breathe.

—ERIC GARNER, JAMES W. BROWN, WILLIE RAY BANKS, BYRON WILLIAMS, BALANTINE MBEGBU, CALVON REID, FERMIN VINCENT VALENZUELA, HECTOR ARREOLA, CRISTOBAL SOLANO, VICENTE VILLELA, CARLOS INGRAM LOPEZ, ROBERT RICHARDSON, RODNEY BROWN, DAVID MINASSIAN, MARSHALL MILES, JAMES PERRY, CRAIG MCKINNIS, DANIEL LINSINBIGLER, MANUEL ELLIS, JUSTIN THOMPSON, MATHEW AJIBADE, BEN ANTHONY C DE BACA, LASHANO GILBERT, JACK MARDEN, FRANK SMART, LUIS RODRIGUEZ, HERNAN JARAMILLO, ELIJAH MCCLAIN, BYRON WILLIAMS, RAKEEM RUCKS, BRANCH WROTH, INDIA CUMMINGS, ELEANOR NORTHINGTON, JAVIER AMBLER, DERRICK SCOTT, MADELYN LINSENMEIR, PAUL SILVA, DIAMOND ROSS, CHRISTOPHER LOWE, QUAM AHMODU, ZACHARY BEAR HEELS, ALEJANDRO GUTIERREZ, MOHAMMED MUHAYMIN, ANDREW KEARSE, STEPHEN SCHENCK, THOMAS PURDY, TROY GOODE, TERRAL ELLIS JR., MIGUEL RAMIREZ, HERIBERTO GODINEZ, BARBARA DAWSON, JONATHAN SANDERS, ROY NELSON JR., ROBERT MINJAREZ JR., FREDDIE GRAY, MICHAEL SABBIE, JOHN GLEESON, FRANCISCO CESENA, KENNETH LUCAS, ANTHONY FIRKINS, LUIS SOLANO, JORGE AZUCENA, ALESIA THOMAS, CASEY BABOVEC, NATHAN PRASAD, RAUL ROSAS, KELLY THOMAS, DEREK WILLIAMS JR., STANLEY STREETER, EARL BROWN JR., RODNEY BROWN, GEORGE FLOYD, JOHN NEVILLE[3]

Skin is the human body's largest organ. On average, it weighs about 4 kilograms (9 pounds) and covers 1.85 square meters (11.23 square feet).[4] Skin delineates the outer bounds of our physical selves—our borders. It defines us. It sets our boundaries and is the organ that most allows us to experience embodied intimacy. But in the modern exposome, the organ that connects us to one another by touch divides us by sight. What we are getting at, of course, is racism.

All modern humans have been taught how to read one another's skin to assess race. The various conclusions that are drawn from that assessment shape our every move. At the level of simple biology, however, there's no such thing as race.[5] There is no genetic basis on which to sort humans into different kinds. Yet as we've seen, the social fiction of race making was a key justification for the colonial profit motive. A long history of exploitation and colonial conquest codified a global racial order—and created an exposome hemmed in by racist social structures. The trauma experienced by people of color living under these structures is written into our cells and DNA. The colonial fictions of race has been a centuries-long campaign of biological warfare. As Friedrich Engels wrote in 1884, it is a form of "social murder" because it places people of color "under conditions in which they can neither retain health nor live long."[6]

Recall that stress is the main mechanism that the body has to mobilize resources to address a perturbation in homeostasis. When something has been damaged or is under threat of being damaged, the stress response activates the nervous, endocrine, and immune systems, mobilizing pro-inflammatory cytokines and hormones to allow us to adapt in the short term. When those systems are chronically activated, the body experiences increasing wear and tear.[7] Chronic stress's cumulative toll is called *allostatic load*, and the biological expression is *chronic inflammation*.[8] Racial discrimination brings a high allostatic load and turns on genes to keep the body constantly prepared for threat.[9]

What this means is that the health disparities we see globally along the color line are driven not by biological difference between fictional races but by the realities of rac*ism*—ancestral trauma, daily acts of discrimination, extrajudicial killings by police, PTSD, forced family separations, land theft, environmental poisonings, lower socioeconomic status, hotter neighborhoods, less access to clean water, crippling debt, forced exposure to a deadly pandemic, food deserts, and a medical system that fails to heal the body as these impacts take their cumulative toll.[10] Reality actually alters our biology.

In the United States, Covid unmasked the realities of a society built on stolen land and stolen labor, as the dead reflected those bodies who bore the highest cost of maintaining the current social order during their lifetimes. The Navajo Nation, where at least 30 percent of the population lives without access to running water, had the highest per capita infection rate in the country, surpassing the epicenters of New York and New Jersey in May 2020.[11] Essential workers, who keep our societies functioning in health care, agriculture, meatpacking factories, grocery stores, manufacturing, and transportation, are more likely to be Black and Latinx.[12] In California, the frontline workers most impacted by Covid are Latinx. About 70 percent of New York City's health care workers are also Black, Latinx, and Asian.[13] Latinx people comprise 60 percent of the frontline cleaning staff.[14] It's no surprise that Covid killed Black and Latinx people at twice the rate to white folks in New York City in the spring of 2020.[15] Nightly applause from New Yorkers on their balconies at the height of the pandemic afforded no safety to such exquisitely vulnerable people on the ground.

In the United States, Covid was always going to hurt people of color worse. Remember that social oppression alters which genes are switched on, increasing the expression of pro-inflammatory cytokines, such as IL-1β and decreasing the expression of protective cytokines, such as type I interferons.[16] Low circulating levels of type I interferons are linked with a life-threatening course of Covid infection.[17] It wasn't simply poor access to health care that drove the racialized disparities of Covid infection and death. It was the preconditioning of bodies over centuries to be ill prepared to handle the challenge when it came.

Many studies confirm how disproportionately Covid killed people of color in the United States and Europe and how it was racially inflected worldwide.[18] While leaders from Frantz Fanon to Monica McLemore to Camara Jones have long fought racism within medicine and while today's BIPOC medical students are actively rewriting the Hippocratic Oath to include the fight for racial justice before they even don the white coat, scientific racism is morphing in the twenty-first century. New forms of digital medicine, for instance, rewrite racism into algorithms for assessing risk of disease. One study examined a health-risk algorithm that had been trained on data that drew on Black and white people's health care costs as a way of predicting in future how sick they might become.[19] But because Black people in the United States have historically been discriminated against, the algorithm itself repeated that racism. An independent audit of the proportion of Black people needing medical help wasn't at the 17.7 percent level stated by the algorithm—it was 46.5 percent. With deadly irony, the racial fiction of colonialism demands that our bodies be read by the color of our skin. Then, through the medicalization of suffering caused by racism and the science fiction of artificial intelligence in medicine, it erases the testimony of people of color altogether.

THE SKIN'S BORDER PATROL

The skin is a liminal space. It is a dual site of protection and intimacy; it is both finite and totally porous. But like the history of immunity, colonial cosmology has taken the living complexity of skin and turned it into another violent metaphor—a highly regulated national border, with patrols, passports, and persecutions. Every nation-state has borders that are accompanied by technologies that read bodies—are you self or other?—and thereby determine their fate. What happens at the national border is always articulated with the rest of the body politic. The activist theorist Harsha Walia observes that "borders are an ordering regime, both assembling and assembled through racial-capitalist accumulation and colonial relations."[20] Colonialism has ascribed our most sensual organ a police function, using it to apply a social order of inclusions and exclusions.

The engine of this national racial order is the economy. Across a number of countries, class and race intersect profoundly through the living legacy of the colonial profit motive. The political theorist Cedric J. Robinson, who coined the term *racial capitalism*, points to the centrality of race in making class, right from the beginning: "As an enduring principle of European social order, the effects of racialism were bound to appear in the social expression of every strata of every European society no matter the structures upon which they were formed. None was immune."[21] Colonialism by design assigned people of color to lower income levels for generations to come, because racism justifies exploitation. This is what the Black British academic Stuart Hall means when he observes that "race is the modality in which class is lived."[22]

Although every country experiences race differently, the bodily consequences are always inflammatory. From Finland to New Zealand/Aotearoa, the poorer someone is, the more C-reactive protein there is in the blood.[23] To live as a BIPOC person in a white supremacist society, as Dalit in a society structured through Hindu caste, as a West African in South Africa, as a Muslim in Burma, or as a migrant or refugee anywhere is to live under constant stress. Black Americans in the United States carry a chronic allostatic load,[24] showing consistently higher levels of C-reactive protein compared to white Americans.[25] British Asians' blood also runs with higher CRP than their white counterparts.[26]

Racial capitalism orders the entire world, given the global reach of colonialism's legacy. But as we continue our discussion of skin color as a sorting function, we will concentrate on the United States, which has been built on a foundation of racial capitalism. No matter how long ago 1619—the date of the first landing of enslaved people to the English colony of Virginia—seems, slavery and its patrols still live on.

Today residents of Black neighborhoods experience a greater prevalence of chronic illnesses, such as cardiovascular diseases and diabetes, greater disability with earlier age of onset from these illnesses, and lower life expectancy than other groups in the United States.[27] The chronic illnesses that disproportionately impact Black families all have inflammation involved in their pathogenesis.[28]

Discrimination, PTSD, and adverse childhood events all set adults up for chronic inflammation, mediated through pathways of stress.[29] Notably, sources of that trauma stem from the civilizing institutions of the state, patrolling the borders of race. Consider, for example, disciplinary violence in school systems, in which "zero tolerance" policies disproportionately target Black students. Teachers and school administrators are deputized as border patrol agents, knocking Black children out of school and into the juvenile detention system. Patterns of racial segregation, in the United States, are connected to a process that brings together many of the institutions of social reproduction we discussed in Chapter 5: the school-to-prison pipeline.[30] These daily exposures make it far harder for Black people's bodies to regain homeostasis, because it's hard to heal when under constant assault. And harder still when chronic racism becomes acute.

In the United States, police kill 2.8 people a day on average.[31] They are 2.5 times more likely to stop Black people, leading to more overall encounters between law enforcement.[32] Black people are also more likely than white people to be killed by police, but how much more depends on location, reflecting the cultural attitudes of the police departments. Regionally, in the Northeast it's 2.98 times, while in Chicago it's 6.51.[33] This variability has nothing to do with the level of violent crime in an area.[34] At the neighborhood level, a Black person is more likely to be killed by police in a white neighborhood.[35] Police kill four times more unarmed Black people than unarmed white people. For Black men in the United States, being killed by police is the sixth leading cause of death,[36] about the same lifetime risk as dying of measles.[37] Black women in the United States have to worry about being shot by police while sleeping in their own bed.

When a person survives a police shooting, officers accompany them to the hospital. The victim is often shackled to their bed, the police guarding them and at times restricting who can visit. After San Francisco police shot Jamaica Hampton in the leg, necessitating its amputation, they stopped his mother from seeing him while he was in the hospital.[38] In 2016 Sophia Wilansky's arm was blown up by the explosive launched at her by police when she was assisting Water Protectors protesting the Dakota Access Pipeline. Seven federal law enforcement agents refused to let her leave her hospital room for surgery until her father surrendered her clothing to them. Her jacket had residue of explosive chemicals in it, evidence that could identify her attackers. The federal agents were hoping to bring domestic terrorism charges against *protesters* for creating IEDs.[39] No such charges were ever brought. Instead, Sophia is suing the police for their violence and is trying to get her jacket back from the FBI; the proceedings are ongoing, with grand juries being called even in 2021, to try to break the solidarity of the Water Protectors and to deflect the attention from holding law enforcement accountable for their violence.

Unlike in physician-patient relationships, the preponderance of evidence suggests that racial concordance between police and the people they interact with appears to make little difference for outcomes. White and nonwhite police are equally likely to use lethal force against Black people, pointing to the deep encoding of anti-Blackness and the maintenance of white supremacy in the culture and institution of policing.[40] The infiltration of departments across the United States by officers involved in white supremacist, far-right militant organizations doesn't help.[41] It explains why on January 6, 2021, when a white supremacist mob stormed the US Capitol in an armed insurrection, the police were seen taking selfies with the insurrectionists, opening the doors, and letting them in. Infiltration of law enforcement has also occurred across Europe, where policing originated.[42] But the problem runs deeper, to the institution's very core: in the United States, the police played a central role in capturing runaway slaves.[43] Escape into underground networks of care and exchange has always been a response to colonial capitalism. Enslaved people achieved freedom not merely by refusing to be property but by embracing practices that uplifted the commons instead.

In the moment of its formation, the western part of the border between the United States and Canada offered some hope to Indigenous communities looking to escape the regime of private property and its enforcers. For Indigenous people and Métis on the lands that were coalescing into the United States and Canada, the forty-ninth parallel offered a kind of magic. The border came to be known as "the Medicine line" because its magic seemed to prevent the troops of one nation from pursuing fugitive Indigenous people into another country. But this medicine has side effects—borders are instruments to demarcate ownership, power, and sovereignty. The historian Michel Hogue points out, "The forty-ninth parallel began as a political fiction, but it was soon made real by the actions and investments of state agents and borderland peoples."[44]

With national borders comes state sovereignty, and with the modern capitalist state came its most sophisticated racial weapon: individual private property. The theft of Indigenous land was central to the making, and financing, of the United States.[45] As the Settler (originally from the traditional territories of Albannach) Canadian scholar Sam Grey put it, "How do you steal a continent? You redefine stealing."[46] The Dawes Act of 1887 carved up Indian reservations, formerly held in common by all the tribe members, into private allotments, forcing Indigenous people to assume an identity that had never existed before in their societies: the individual landowner.[47] Rather than grant communal property rights, settler governments insisted on individual land titling as the path to civilization and wealth. Property that can be managed only by a single head of household is an institution that has torn communities apart across the world.[48]

Policing has always been about protecting not just private property but the racial order that supports it. The Black congressional representative Cori Bush correctly identified the welcome that US Capitol Police gave the white supremacist mob in January 2021 as "the America Black people know."[49] As the law professor Cheryl Harris has argued, whiteness developed at the same time as private property and can itself be viewed as a form of it, based on "a [shared] conceptual nucleus . . . of a right to exclude."[50] Following the genocide of Indigenous people and enslavement of Black people at the foundation of the United States, whiteness was the basis of racialized privilege. the rationalization of how some were allowed to own things while others could be owned.[51] To participate in care along the Underground Railroad or to dance in a potlatch was to subvert this order by offering a different regime of love and exchange.

Potlatches—ceremonies of nonmonetary generosity and celebration, deriving from the Chinook jargon term "to give"—were so dangerous to the ideology of the market that the Canadian government banned them in 1885. That the commons was the enemy of colonialism was observed clearly by a commissioner of Indian affairs: in 1838, T. H. Crawford wrote of the virtues of foisting individual property rights on Native Americans. Common property and civilization cannot coexist because in a commons, a surplus of wealth is soon redistributed. Under regimes of private property, it's accumulated. By turning Indigenous economies into capitalist ones, Crawford suggested, it'd be possible to create an Indigenous bourgeoisie who'd shore up the colonial order.[52] A century later Frantz Fanon saw the idea made flesh in anticolonial struggles, as erstwhile antagonists of colonial rule swiftly became proponents of colonial-era property relations, and of the police to defend them, as soon as those relations proved personally lucrative.[53]

There's a straight line running from the police to Wall Street. But owning private property doesn't itself confer a change in social status. Texas's Harris County, which includes Houston, is the most racially diverse in the United States. There a home worth $289,000 in a white neighborhood would be valued at $127,000 in a Black neighborhood or $120,000 in a Hispanic one, even after controlling for "individual home characteristics, neighborhood housing stock, community socioeconomic characteristics, neighborhood amenities, and consumer housing demand."[54] Painfully, people of color know to erase themselves from their houses when the white appraisers visit. With each family photograph portraying a lineage rich with melanin, home values plummet.[55] BIPOC communities have long been familiar with the economic geography of housing segregation.[56]

If that makes you hot under the collar, try living in a redlined neighborhood. In the language of policing, high-crime areas are known as "hot spots," terminology that naturalizes crime as a disease—think: fever, inflammation—and disclaims any racial bias.[57] But here, too, the fiction has become a reality: these spots are *actually* getting hotter. A survey of 108 urban areas throughout the United States found that 94 percent had an average disparity of 2.6°C (with a maximum of 7°C) across the borders between majority-white and formerly redlined neighborhoods.[58] Denser housing, housing with more concrete and less grass, and lower rates of investment in trees and green space have transformed the social fiction of race into the physical fact of climate change.

Sweating is the body's way of maintaining its temperature at around 36.6°C.[59] Moisture on the skin's surface cools as it evaporates. Therefore climate change wrought through racism will be felt through the skin—though some people will feel the heat more than others.[60] A heat wave in Chicago in July 1995 caused the deaths of six hundred people. Temperatures ranged from "33.9 to 40.0°C, and on 13 July, the heat index peaked at 48.3°C."[61] Of the fifty-eight people admitted to Chicago hospitals with heatstroke, the majority were Black people who lived in homes without air conditioning, lacked private health insurance, and had preexisting medical conditions. Soaring rates of heatstroke are an inevitable hallmark of emergency rooms under climate change.[62] But as the sky scalds, it will be disproportionately BIPOC communities in the United States and those in the undercommons around the world who get burned.

The institutions that reproduce this climate of inequality have also spawned a sprawling carceral system. The prison-industrial complex, the heart of American racial capitalism, reached its full expression as neoliberalism was restructuring the economy. The recessions of the 1980s called for new fiscal solutions. Neoliberal "shock doctrine" ideology prohibited the kinds of Keynesian government intervention and investment that had previously spurred economic recovery.[63] Unemployment rates soared. The expansion of the prison complex was the quick fix, disproportionately incarcerating low-income people and people of color as a swift response to broken windows. Draconian policing was coupled with draconian sentencing. "Three strikes" laws kept people in prison for life for minor infractions and provided sources of employment, in the prison-industrial complex, to parts of the country experiencing deindustrialization.[64] Throughout California, for instance, even as the number of crimes was falling in the mid-1980s, the number of prisons increased: from 1984 to 2000, the state built twenty-three new prisons despite having built only twelve from 1852 to 1964.[65]

Think of neoliberalism as a kind of biological extraction, finding new and profitable uses for bodies that have always been regarded as disposable under colonial capitalism's cosmology. The prison industrial system provided an economic stimulus that trickled down to poorer white communities hollowed by industrialization.[66] In other cases, Black people were used directly as sites of profit.

In 1951 Albert Kligman was a young professor of medicine at the University of Pennsylvania, specializing in dermatology. When he was called to Holmesburg Prison in Philadelphia to treat an outbreak of athlete's foot, he was overjoyed: "All I saw before me were acres of skin. It was like a farmer seeing a field for the first time."[67] He turned those acres into profit, plowing deep and reaping vast rewards. In addition to performing product trials for cosmetics and pharmaceutical companies, he developed Retin-A, an acne treatment—literally on the backs of prisoners who were disproportionately poor and Black. In exchange for fees ranging from $10 to $300, inmates subjected themselves to chemical scars, biopsies, and blisters. In later experiments, they were also dosed with hallucinogens, radioactivity, and dioxins, all for a modest fee. Kligman died a multimillionaire in 2010, made rich through his Retin-A patent. He had destroyed the records of prisoners in his experiments in 1974 after the program was exposed.[68]

The United States has of late seen something of an awakening to the injustices of the prison-industrial complex. Incarceration rates, which have generally been exponentially higher than in other countries, have been falling. This trend is to be celebrated, even if the industry is not. But a bipartisan consensus remains that incarceration and policing are a central tool in solving economic problems. The budget for US Customs and Border Patrol rose from $5.9 billion in 2003 to $17.7 billion in 2021, and Immigration and Customs Enforcement (ICE), responsible for the detention of immigrants at the border, saw its budget increase from $3.3 billion to $8.3 billion over the same period.

The growth and global deployment of military forces to police crises of migration are part of the economic and cultural strategies that produce nations.[69] In the United States, ICE is the nation's largest police force. Its law trumps workers' rights. "La Migra" monitors employees who speak out against their employers. In one case, a Cessna Aircraft Company worker slipped off a ladder, injuring himself, for which the corporation fired him. He went on record, despite being undocumented, saying, "I don't care if they deport me, I want people to know how big companies use people up."[70] He and his wife were arrested and indicted soon afterward, and Cessna was commended for reporting them to the authorities.

If you believe this to be harsh but deserved justice for the "crime" of living in the United States without papers, then consider how Customs and Border Protection treated a US citizen. Tianna Spears, a diplomat who had passed extensive background checks, was a consular official in Ciudad Juárez. During her trips into El Paso, she invariably suffered the indignity of being stopped and searched by the border patrol. No convincing explanation was ever given for why she was routinely pulled aside while her colleagues were waved through the fast-track lanes. She developed PTSD from being repeatedly harassed and humiliated at the border and ultimately left her job because of it. In a searing essay, she made a convincing case for the reason: it was because she's Black.[71] Angela Davis anticipated Spears's experience, which was echoed in the January 6 insurrection at the US Capitol: "We knew that the role of the police was to protect white supremacy."[72]

The expansion of border police in the age of counterterrorism is an international one, and it sits alongside another trend: in the global crackdown on immigration, police and military budgets are expanding, and their roles at the border are increasingly blurred.[73]

THE COLOR OF MEDICINE

Like all humans, physicians are readers of skin. According to a study conducted in 2016, 58 percent of the general white US population believed that Black skin was thicker than theirs. This view was shared by 40 percent of first-year white medical students. By their fourth year, 20 percent of white students *still* believed this to be true.[74] White physicians in the United States are less likely to take Black pain seriously.[75] According to colonialism, Black skin is legible, but Black pain is invisible. This is a crisis of empathy.

The most exquisitely sensitive skin in the human body is the small membrane that covers our aural canal, the eardrum. Through it, we feel the music, as well as howls of pain. When sounds become too loud, the body involuntarily responds: the acoustic reflex tightens the muscles in our ears. To experience the reflex, and then to ignore the pain that lies behind it, takes a long history of institutional conditioning and desensitization.

Medical racism isn't merely an unfortunate accident. We've noted how enslaved, colonized, and Indigenous women and their knowledge were used in the making of modern biology. From Newton to Linnaeus, Enlightenment science wouldn't have been possible without the transatlantic slave trade in *Home sapiens afer*. Newton's tidal calculations depended on data from the slave port of Martinique. Linnaeus's students found passage on slave ships and formed part of a global network of wildlife trafficking by slave mariners.[76] An apothecary and naturalist in London, James Petiver, was able to amass one of England's most important collections of plants and animals through the cultivation of friendships with ship's captains and surgeons. As historian Kathleen Murphy notes, these naval officers were expected by their employers to be able "to discern relative value and potential profits rather than humanity in the captives before them."[77] The history of medicine and racism are as intertwined as the snakes on Hermes's staff.[78]

The grim natural history of Enlightenment medicine is reproduced in the practices of modern doctors, nurses, orderlies and janitors, administrators, and patients alike. Power is defined and concentrated along lines of gender, race, and class—between hospital leadership and workforce, between doctors and patients, between physicians and nonphysician staff. Medical students chronicle discrimination as part of the unwritten curriculum of their training, with 33 percent experiencing gender-based abuse and 17 percent experiencing racism.[79] As physicians of color enter the workforce, they quickly learn that advocating too strongly for Black patients can put them at risk for being harassed by their colleagues and superiors for being unprofessional, as if centering Black health were antithetical to medical professionalism.[80] In the United States, people of color make up 44 percent of the physician workforce,[81] yet only 14 percent of the board members and 11 percent of the executive leadership of health care systems. And this despite minorities' constituting a third of the patient population served. Additionally, while the percentage of minorities in midlevel management increased from 2011 to 2015, the percentage of minority board members remained the same, and the percentage of minority executive leaders actually decreased.[82]

For patients, racism in medicine influences who has access to care, how much care they receive, and the financial burden they will carry as a consequence of that care.[83] It is present in how the health care team perceives their pain and evaluates their medical conditions.[84] Glomerular filtration rate is a parameter that indicates how well the kidneys are functioning. It is followed to assess timing for kidney transplantation for those with end-stage kidney failure. Up until recently, a weighting value was ascribed to Black patients, as if their kidneys filtered blood differently because of the color of their skin—a practice rooted in eugenics.[85] The race-based calculation of this value falsely overestimated their kidney function, leading many people to die waiting for a transplant.[86] Black nephrologists like Dr. Vanessa Grubbs worked inexorably to overturn this practice in the hospital where she worked. Race may be a fiction, but racism in medicine has real consequences for real bodies.

Racism is even embedded in the technology that physicians use to diagnose their patients. Pulse oximeters monitor red blood cell saturation by detecting slight changes in color below the surface of the skin. Because they have been tested predominantly on white people, many overestimate the amount of oxygen in the blood of Black people when its level is low.[87] At 88 percent O_2, most hospitals recommend supplemental oxygen to stop organ failure, but if the oximeter reads 92 percent, then the protocol says "wait and see." Black people can have readings that falsely register above 92 percent, when their blood oxygenation taken by a blood sample—the gold standard—is actually much lower. Going by the oximeter alone, they wouldn't get oxygen or be admitted to the hospital for further care. For Covid patients, this can spell the difference between life and death and may be contributing to why US Black patients are more likely to die from infection.[88]

"Silent hypoxia" is a harbinger of clinical deterioration from Covid, in which people do not appear to be in distress, are able to speak normally, and lack the classical symptoms of low oxygen levels, but when checked with a pulse oximeter, they are found to be in dangerously low territory.[89] Early oxygenation improves survival outcomes. A pulse oximeter that does not make accurate readings in Black people's bodies because it is calibrated to whiteness will not document their hypoxia, and lifesaving treatment will be postponed until it is too late.[90]

Not surprisingly, the field of dermatology is whitewashed. In the United States, 3 percent of the profession's physicians-in-training are Black and 4.2 percent are Latinx, while these groups constitute 13 percent and 16 percent, respectively, of the general population.[91] Nearly half of US board-licensed dermatologists don't feel comfortable diagnosing skin issues in people of color, attributing the lack of preparation to medical training.[92] When Dr. Jenna Lester—who is currently the University of California, San Francisco (UCSF)'s only Black dermatologist—was a second-year medical student, she noticed something that she believes explains why her colleagues have a hard time diagnosing common skin conditions in people of color. On her dermatology rotation, she saw a range of photos of different diseases, from psoriasis to cancer, but always in white skin.

She reviewed thousands of educational dermatology photos in textbooks and teaching sets and found that fewer than a third of them had skin of color.[93] This is a problem because skin conditions appear differently in darker skin, and if physicians are not trained to see the differences, they will miss the diagnosis. Lester remembers a Black patient "who had these plaques all over his body, and everyone was hemming and hawing about what it could be. And they took a biopsy. It was psoriasis. This is something we consider a clinical diagnosis that couldn't be made without a biopsy in a man with dark skin." This clinical ineptitude has far-reaching consequences and continues today. With Covid predominantly impacting communities with more melanin across the United States, Lester saw the same trend in the medical literature: over 92 percent of the images demonstrating skin findings caused by the virus—hives, red blotches on the toes with blisters and other rashes—were in white patients. Not a single image was of a Black patient.[94]

There is an exception to the teaching of skin conditions exclusively from white case studies. Lester recalls from her student days:

> When you get to the sexually transmitted infections, all of a sudden it's only black genitalia that you see. These diseases have manifestations outside of the genital area, but they always show these unceremonious pictures of black genitalia. It is reminiscent of slave auctions, looking at their muscles and reproductive potential, humiliating them.

Dr. Lester's review of dermatology education images confirmed this: while only 20 percent of photos of common skin conditions showed skin of color, as many as 58 percent of photos of STD manifestations showed skin of color.[95] Her solution was to create the Skin of Color Clinic at UCSF, where she is able to offer care specific to patients who have skin with more melanin.

Currently, the amount of melanin in your skin is inversely proportional to the likelihood that you will leave a US hospital alive after suffering cardiac arrest.[96] Just as women survive heart attacks more often when they are treated by female physicians, race concordance between physician and patient may lead to better health outcomes.[97] Black men with Black doctors were more likely to select every cardiovascular prevention measure, even those that were invasive, suggesting that simply having Black doctors care for Black patients could reduce the Black-white cardiovascular health disparity by 19 percent.[98]

To understand why it's so hard to find Black doctors to care for Black patients, we must look back to the beginning of the twentieth century, when the US medical profession wasn't yet recognizably professional. Debates raged around who could and couldn't accredit, who might treat and prescribe, who was a doctor and how one might know. Abraham Flexner was an unusual arbiter of these questions. In the late 1880s he instituted a school in Louisville, Kentucky, that had no grades, exams, records, or curriculum. But he had his eye on a position at the Carnegie Foundation, and his 1908 criticisms of US education, published as *The American College: A Criticism*, cited a senior official at the Carnegie Foundation repeatedly and approvingly.[99] The strategy landed Flexner a job at the foundation. He visited all 155 medical schools in operation at that time in the United States and Canada. In 1910 he wrote a report disseminated by one of the first modern philanthropic organizations, the Carnegie Corporation. Published as the last word in the debates over medical professionalization, philanthrocapitalism would decisively alter the course of US medical education and practice.

The Flexner Report argued for standardizing medical education across the United States by promoting the scientific rigor found in German university-based medical schools.[100] He criticized the mediocrity of for-profit, proprietary schools and the inadequate curricula and facilities of certain others. His report was particularly brutal toward Black medical colleges and Black physicians. The chapter entitled "The Medical Education of the Negro" "strongly accentuated" that "the more promising of the race . . . be sent to receive a substantial education in hygiene, rather than surgery."[101] Flexner's dim view of Black medical education in the United States had immediate consequences. In 1900 there were seven Black medical schools. In the aftermath of the Flexner Report, only two remained: Howard University and Meharry Medical College.[102]

The Flexner Report impacted not only Black medical colleges but also schools that taught herbalism, homeopathy, and chiropractic, which were popular modes of maintaining health at the turn of the century. Schools of eclectic medicine that taught European and Native American herbal traditions were told to drop these courses or risk losing their accreditation.[103] Those that refused were cited as being run by "unconscionable quacks" and soon closed.[104] While

Flexner did indeed sweep out quacks from the field, his criteria for differentiating between good and bad owed little to peer review and much more to the prejudices of his day and to the racially inflected agendas of his philanthropic sponsors. Among them were the Rockefellers, who were newly rich from the inauguration of the petroleum industry and eager to see its products insinuated into every aspect of modern life—including medicine. Philanthrocapitalists shaped modern medicine and brought their pursuit of profits and prejudices to bear on the process. The political theorist Tiffany Willoughby-Herard points out that the Carnegie Corporation was involved in the promotion of "global whiteness," particularly through its support of Afrikaner white nationalism in South Africa.[105]

Flexner's racist legacy has been long. Today Black patients report greater satisfaction with their care and more trusting relationships with Black providers.[106] But in the United States, finding a Black doctor can be challenging thanks in part to the Flexner Report. Whereas Black people make up 13 percent of the general population, they constitute only 5 percent of working physicians.[107] Over the past thirty years, moreover, the number of Black men in medicine has dropped, the only underrepresented minority of whom this is true.[108] This outcome is not simply a matter of chance. It was engineered.

MEDICINE'S MASTER RACE

Prior to colonialism, Europeans ascribed differences in the color of people's skin to the climates in which their communities lived. Under colonialism, those geographic and climatological explanations morphed into ones shaped by shifting relationships to religion, state, and property. Recall that Columbus set foot on the Western Hemisphere just as Jews were being expelled from Iberia. As Cedric Robinson, and Aimé Césaire before him, have observed, the process of colonization overseas was articulated with a project of persecution aimed at Europe's "others," be they Jews or Romani communities or other migrants.[109]

Debates about how biology might account for differences among peoples were particularly lively in the eighteenth century. The botanist Carl Linnaeus, in his 1758 edition of *Systema Naturae*,[110] had subcategories of *Homo sapiens* with annotations about physiology and character. According to that foundational text for modern biology, *Homo sapiens europaeus* was, among other things, orderly and governable. Americans, Asians, and Africans had their own character traits: *Homo sapiens americanus* was regulated by customs, *Homo sapiens asiaticus* by opinion, and *Homo sapiens afer* by caprice. In a residual category, the Calibans of different sorts were grouped together as *Homo sapiens monstrosus*.[111]

The Linnaean system classified life-forms into hierarchies of kingdoms, classes, and orders—a rather direct transposition from the language of colonial domination. Linnaeus's taxonomy of human beings provided a scientific reasoning for the destruction of Indigenous medicine, knowledge, and ecosystems. Indigenous people were inferior, and it was the manifest scientific destiny of the new US state to eradicate them and to replace them with principles of government, knowledge, and order that were in closer harmony with the racial European science.

In the war on the Indigenous people of the Great Plains, the United States explicitly targeted the buffalo, their spiritual cornerstone and staple of food, medicine, shelter, and clothing. Toward the end of the nineteenth century, the US military sponsored the killing of millions of buffalo, inflicting starvation and dependency on the tribes. While it was never officially announced as the army's policy, the Montana land baron Granville Stuart noted in his journal in 1879 that "slaughtering the buffaloes is a government measure to subjugate the Indians." Colonel Richard Irving Dodge summed up the spirit of the massacre: "Kill every buffalo you can! Every buffalo dead is an Indian gone." Before 1800, an estimated 30 to 60 million buffalo ranged the Great Plains. By 1900, only a few hundred remained, the survivors of the most violent genocide of any mammal ever documented.[112] With the buffalo gone, Plains Indians' bodies suffered trauma, cultural erasure, and starvation. Depression, diabetes, and drug dependency became endemic—all diseases characterized by chronic inflammation.[113]

Sundering people from their sources of food and medicine, from one another, and from their lands are preconditions for poor health for many Indigenous people in the United States. As the Indigenous scholar Nick Estes explains, "What was once a subsistence economy based on wild harvesting and small-scale agriculture was transformed almost overnight into dependency on USDA commodities. White flour, milk, white sugar, and canned foods replaced formerly protein- and nutrient-rich diets. Diabetes rates skyrocketed, and its spread can be contact-traced to a single public works project."[114] On Pine Ridge Reservation today, the rate of diabetes remains 800 percent higher than the national average.[115] Food insecurity is rampant—40 percent of families report having no access to healthy food.[116] The long-term impact of these colonial strategies, destroying the knowledge in which food *was* medicine, rendering access to medicine impossible through extinction and displacement, has been to ascribe a rigid limit to Indigenous land and life.

Replacing Indigenous medicine required investment. In the nineteenth century, schools of tropical medicine boomed, paid for by colonial merchants (Liverpool) or governmental colonial offices (London) so that white men might survive in the tropics.[117] This branch of medicine, geared toward the frontier of capitalism, was expressly intended to further colonial domination. As one journalist put it in 1911, "Australia is a big blank map, and the whole [white] people is constantly sitting over it like a committee, trying to work out the best way to fill it in." The historian Warwick Anderson notes that through the application of laboratory techniques, "medicine was not just a means of knowing a territory, it offered in this case an opportunity to reshape it."[118]

Medicine reshaped the colonial world both at home and abroad.

Remember Charles Darwin and his impact on modern medicine? The integration of medicine and racial biology crystallized in the work of Francis Galton, Darwin's cousin. His book *Hereditary Genius*, published in 1869 by Macmillan,[119] combined theories of inheritance, reproduction, and racial hierarchy. Galton marshaled his knowledge of statistics to claim, for instance, that if fathers were of "literary stock," then their sons were likely to be similarly talented.[120]

Galton codified a definition of race that would come to have wide legal significance. The logic of hypodescent—in which one drop of blood from an ancestor of a minority race would permanently affix that category to all their descendants—found a scientific and medical home in his work.[121] *Hereditary Genius* accentuated the positive consequences of *eugenics* (a term he derived from Greek to mean "of good stock"). If those of good stock, whether literary or political or artistic, were to reproduce abundantly, the world would be populated with the best kind of people—and science would be able to provide direction.

Darwin enthusiastically supported his cousin's thoughts on the improvement of the human race.[122] In his 1871 *Descent of Man*, he offered that "at some future period, not very distant as measured by centuries, the civilised races of man will almost certainly exterminate and replace throughout the world the savage races."[123] Galton himself explored the hierarchy of races, offering the usual assessment of the inferiority of Black to white but also a nuanced ranking of the relative merits of "lowland Scotch, North Country English and the Englishman of the Midland," people separated by a distance of less than 300 kilometers (200 miles).[124] By 1877 he was able to refine his prejudices sufficiently to present them to a meeting of the British Association for the Advancement of Science, in a discussion about the "hereditary moral weaknesses" of some races.[125] The popularity of such views spread not only through British colonies but globally, and so did ideas about what governments might do to manage "racial enfeeblement," from Japan to the United States to Brazil.[126]

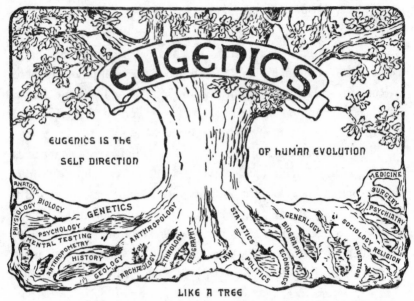

EUGENICS

EUGENICS IS THE
SELF DIRECTION

OF HUMAN EVOLUTION

LIKE A TREE
EUGENICS DRAWS ITS MATERIALS FROM MANY SOURCES AND ORGANIZES
THEM INTO AN HARMONIOUS ENTITY.

An illustration from the Second International Exhibition of Eugenics[127]

Eugenic science guaranteed the idea that some "bloodlines" were inferior to others. The policies that it spawned were patterned on public health ideas about infection control, with its vocabulary of protection, defense, and security. It styled itself as a harmonious and ecologically well-considered approach to the improvement of humanity: the print in the illustration—showing a 1921 New York exhibition on eugenics—presented the program as a mighty tree with roots of medicine, history, biology, and economics, among others: one science to unite them all. Visual metaphors like this were deployed to make the artifice of racial science common sense. The logic of white supremacy reproduced itself just as colonialism did, from these origins within the academy, state, and economy, normalized through consent and coercion, into the norms of the modern hospital.

Rooted in the soil of British colonialism, eugenics blossomed under the Nazis, reaching the nadir of the concentration camps and Joseph Mengele's medical experiments.[128] In the United States, from 1932 to 1972, the Tuskegee Syphilis Experiment, run by researchers from the Public Health Service, offered to treat Black men in Macon County, Alabama, for "bad blood," a term for syphilis.[129] No treatment was actually administered, despite penicillin's indication and wide availability starting in the 1950s. By 1972, when the story broke, between twenty-eight and one hundred of the men in the study had died from lack of treatment, wives had been infected, and children had been born with congenital syphilis. These are the politics of racial hygiene made flesh.

TOKENISM VS. TRANSFORMATION

Disregard for Black doctors and disregard for Black pain are outcomes of the same system. One of the ways that clinicians might learn to take Black pain seriously is through "epistemic humility," a willingness to listen.[130] The philosopher Miranda Fricker contends that good listening is done by "someone whose testimonial sensibility has been suitably reconditioned by sufficient corrective experiences."[131] The idea is that it's possible to learn humility. This, however, begs the question: what constitutes a suitably corrective experience?

An entire industry of diversity consultants are offering ideas about what sorts of mandatory training should be instituted to combat white supremacy.[132] The data suggest, though, that requiring employees to attend a course tends to have long-term negative impacts on diversity in a workplace.[133] Significantly more effective than subjecting employees to a two-hour diversity PowerPoint presentation, evidence suggests, is facilitating a transfer of power and authority to BIPOC people, through mentoring, active recruitment, and providing access to leadership. But such efforts are rarely sufficient when the structures of medicine itself are left unchallenged, and only performative gestures are offered as the solution.[134]

In the wake of the uprisings ignited by the murders of George Floyd and Breonna Taylor, medical schools across the nation issued statements committing to antiracism. Actions soon belied these words. At the University of California, San Francisco, faculty of color and their allies banded together to demand that the university publicly condemn the research of dermatology professor Howard Maibach, who, following in the footsteps of his mentor Albert Kligman, had tested chemicals on Black prisoners.[135] In 1974, conducting his own research at San Quentin prison, Maibach injected pesticides and herbicides into human subjects to assess their toxicological impact.[136] Rather than publicly denouncing Maibach's work and forcing him into retirement, the university did nothing.[137] Perhaps this was because its Institutional Review Board—the regulatory entity created to protect human research subjects after the horrors of Nazi experimentation on Jews were revealed—approved the research. Asking the university to hold Maibach accountable simultaneously forces it to reckon with its own legacies of racist practices. The professor, now in his nineties, continues to attend monthly department meetings, much to the chagrin of faculty and students who are eager for systemic change.

Antiracism is a process of changing the dynamics of power in a transformative manner. It is not a declaration or a seminar. It is not a training session you can attend or a book you can read. It is structural change that redefines practices. At an institution that offers its workers a mindfulness stress-reduction class, it's the workers coming together to tell the institution to reduce burnout and workplace stress by dismantling the systems of white supremacy within its own power structures. It necessarily requires removing some folks from positions of power and inviting others to assume those roles. It is reimagining those roles altogether, understanding that systems that were created to uphold architectures of domination cannot simply be tweaked to become vessels for equity. It is creating an environment where low-wage workers are not predominantly people of color and the C-suite is not predominantly white. Hospitals with more people of color in their leadership meet their diversity benchmarks more readily.[138] But having Black and brown people in positions of power in oppressive structures is not enough. Abolishing the C-suite altogether may be a first step. The very foundations of the structures in capitalism must be changed. It's far easier to just hire liberals and Black people to take care of the racism thing and carry on as usual.

Medical antiracism must be driven by the communities most impacted by racism's horror. It must include the allocation of money and other resources to address health impacts of racism with the same urgency as treating cancer. Antiracism is hiring and retaining faculty of color who stay because the work culture is not racist. Antiracism is rifling through an institution's past and making reparations for perpetuating racist lies, such as the biological differences in kidney function. Antiracism is cultivating pipelines that offer young underrepresented minorities opportunities to train and excel in the best medical institutions, and through their radically engaged presence, allowing the institutions to be forever changed. Antiracism in medicine is decolonizing work, extending the borders of healing to include honored traditions from those communities who have been oppressed under medicine's histories. Antiracism in medicine must start from the beginning, and for many places that means at the dawn of the colonial era. It is acknowledging the stolen land upon which one practices. It is giving the land back and asking Indigenous people for permission to bring one's medicine into another's territory, because a people and a territory already have their specific medicines and to add another one requires asking and granting permission. This is what the practice of humility can look like.

Antiracism centers the knowledge, inquiry, and methodologies of minority faculty and staff, who are the experts when it comes to the toxic exposome of their communities. It prioritizes ways to knowledge that may not necessarily fit into Eurocentric scientific conceptualizations. It includes listening to people as they identify why they feel they are sick, believing their testimony, and applying tools of research and scientific inquiry to examine their concerns. It is teaching the historical and structural underpinnings of poor health, the social forces that are produced and reproduced along racist lines of power, instead of allowing them to remain invisible and therefore inevitable. It is making health care a right, available to all. In this respect, medicine could do itself a favor by taking a page from the communist playwright Bertolt Brecht, who used the theater to expose the ways injustices can be turned on their head: "The purpose of our investigation was not merely to arouse moral misgivings about certain conditions. . . . The purpose of our investigation was to make visible the means by which those onerous conditions could be done away with."[139]

Empty gestures—as when police took a knee with protesters, feigning solidarity—entrench the idea that the structure is static, stable, and inescapable. Officers who reckon deeply with policing's racist roots should walk off the job and find other ways to serve communities impacted by racism.

In hospitals especially, diversity training will never be enough, because the problem isn't simply about an institution and its inadequacies. A hospital isn't just, as Ruth Wilson Gilmore writes of prisons, "a building 'over there' but a set of relationships that undermine rather than stabilize everyday lives everywhere."[140] Deep medicine will require the abolition of the colonial hospital itself.

HOW TO DECOLONIZE A HOSPITAL

The expulsion of Indigenous Americans from their ancestral land was viewed with approval by Hitler, who said that the Volga would be the Nazis' Mississippi.[141] But the US genocide had global repercussions long before Germany launched its ill-fated assault on the Soviet Union. In 1830 France invaded Algeria. The two volumes of Alexis de Tocqueville's *Democracy in America*, published in 1835 and 1840, spurred conversations among French colonists in Algeria, who soon began referring to Algerians as *indigènes*—a term previously reserved for Indigenous people on the other side of the ocean.[142] It was the colonial mentality of the American conquest that animated France's imposition of brutal colonial rule in Algeria. The Algerian liberation struggle was bloody, and by the time independence was won in 1962, after an eight-year war, hundreds of thousands had been killed.[143]

Frantz Fanon, a psychiatrist and philosopher, was born under French colonialism in Martinique in 1925. His middle-class family was able to afford the fees for him to attend the most prestigious school on the island, where he came to admire one of his teachers, Aimé Césaire. After Vichy rule arrived in Martinique in 1940, during World War II, Fanon escaped to fight fascists in Europe, where he was wounded and awarded the Croix de Guerre. During this period, he saw European racism up close: at emancipation celebration dances, white women preferred to dance with white Italian fascist prisoners rather than with the Black soldiers who had freed them.[144]

Fanon submitted *Black Skin, White Masks* as his medical thesis in 1952 at the University of Lyon. It was rejected as "inappropriately subjective."[145] In haste, he dictated a replacement dissertation on the most common genetic disease, Friedreich's ataxia. It affects one in fifty thousand people, and its symptoms range from slurred speech to scoliosis.[146] The range of those symptoms, Fanon argued, called for not just physiological explanations but cultural ones, too. He developed this idea after securing a post at the Blida-Joinville Psychiatric Hospital in Algeria in 1953. There he treated soldiers who tortured Algerians as part of France's counterinsurgency strategy against the local independence movement as well as victims of torture themselves.

Fanon came to see colonial violence as embedded not only within the bodies and minds of his patients but within the institution of the hospital itself. He doubted that the hospital could be an instrument of therapy when it was so often an accomplice to the arbitrary exercise of power: "Without warning, the police office of the doctor unexpectedly meets with the head of ward's decision to cut dessert or the orderly's threat to transfer a patient to the ward of agitated or senile patients."¹⁴⁷ Fanon was given supervisory power over two psychiatric wards. He deinstitutionalized the treatment offered there, creating film and music clubs and a hospital newspaper and appointing his clients to run them.

Once patients were given autonomy and power over their own mental health, it quickly became clear that many didn't require the straitjackets into which they'd been strapped for years. Turning the hospital into less of a prison worked well for the white women in Blida but not for the Algerian men there. Fanon and his team came to understand that it wasn't enough merely to loosen the straitjackets—once again, culture was important. Only after he embraced local customs and rituals and built a football field and a café, in what the Fanon scholar Jean Khalfa calls "a complete reversal of the prevalent ethnopsychiatric gaze,"¹⁴⁸ did his Algerian male patients see themselves in their rehabilitation and take charge of their treatment.

His therapeutic victories did little to undermine the coloniality of the hospital institution or to stop the pathologizing of the women and men under his charge in the first place. He observed that "behind 'the doctor who heals the wounds of humanity' appears the man, a member of a dominant society and enjoying in Algeria the benefit of an incomparably higher standard of living than that of his metropolitan colleague. Moreover, in centers of colonization the doctor is nearly always a landowner as well."¹⁴⁹ And no matter what kind of regime ran the hospital, if the nation outside the clinic remained colonized, the long-term prognosis for those living within it were dim.

In 1956 Fanon resigned his hospital position to dedicate himself full time to the liberation of Algeria. He was diagnosed with leukemia soon afterward and died in 1961. In his final years, he wrote *The Wretched of the Earth* and *A Dying Colonialism*, both of them meditations on violence, its toxicities, and its uses. He foresaw the betrayal of liberation struggles at the hands of new national bourgeoisies, whose interests in private property and police were on a par with those of the colonizers whose offices they'd occupied.[150] His philosophical legacy on power and race has guided generations of revolutionaries in Africa and beyond.

Among the groups that have been inspired by Fanon's insights on colonialism and liberation is today's Black Lives Matter. It proposes a range of treatments for the ills of the US-Mexico border. It calls for an end to the war on Black migrants (as part of a broader alliance to defund the CBP and ICE).[151] It notes that one quarter of Black people in the United States have some form of documented disability.[152] The remedy is an accountable form of socialized medicine. But it is in the movement's herstory, written by one of the three founders, Alicia Garza, that we may find the most potent approach to racial borders.

Black Lives Matter, Garza notes,

> goes beyond the narrow nationalism that can be prevalent within some Black communities, which merely call on Black people to love Black, live Black and buy Black, keeping straight cis Black men in the front of the movement while our sisters, queer and trans and disabled folk take up roles in the background or not at all. Black Lives Matter affirms the lives of Black queer and trans folks, disabled folks, Black-undocumented folks, folks with records, women and all Black lives along the gender spectrum. It centers those that have been marginalized within Black liberation movements. It is a tactic to (re)build the Black liberation movement.[153]

The deep medicine in Black Lives Matter is the knowledge of built-in struggle against multiple forms of social division: not just racism, but class, documentation status, and membership in the LGBTQIA2+ community.[154] An important part of that herstory, as Garza notes, is that two of the founders of Black Lives Matter identify as queer. To queer the border between these categories is to dissolve them, to mock their absurdity, to undo the hegemony that seeks to make racial categories common sense.[155] Political queering works for the borders of heteronormativity just as it does the invented categories of race. Whiteness, a construction made to marginalize and control nonwhiteness, will one day be as unthinkable as apartheid.

Black radical feminists and queer writers, from Audre Lorde and Angela Davis to Akwugo Emejulu, laid the foundation in our imaginations for the most direct route to justice in health care: abolishing the police.[156] The Anti Police-Terror Project's outline, the Black New Deal, offers clear policy on how this would work.[157] Funds currently used for policing—which in Oakland, California, for example, consume roughly 44 percent of the general budget, amounting to $300 million annually—should be used to create jobs, housing, improved schools, lush parks, and greater access to healthy food: to build the foundations for the community to thrive.[158] Together with devising new systems of safety based on mental health and social services, as well as community-based responses to violent crime, these proposals can transform historically harmful practices into ones that further the possibility of well-being.

Abolition means changing the very circumstances that prioritized incarceration instead of a culture of care. Material inequalities in private property reproduce the injustices that prevent white doctors from hearing Black pain as well as the police forces that create systemic social damage in protecting that property. Decolonizing hospitals means changing the material arrangements that profit from colonized people, their knowledge, bodies, and labor, and shifting toward radical equality. Doing so demands a better understanding of how humans can communicate across borders and ultimately escape borders altogether.

This project ought to be understood not as an onerous task but as a dance of liberation, for white people as well as for those over

whom white supremacy has dominated.[159] The project of emancipation and abolition from white supremacy is one that will, necessarily, involve a loss of security and power, as relationships are
renegotiated with repair and care. Like the undoing of patriarchy, it
is a project that will last a lifetime. Yet the gains of real equality, the
joys of mutual recognition and love, are far greater than the loss of a
precarious and illusory dominion.

There is joy in liberation. From the undercommons comes a music that cannot be owned, which carries that joy.[160] It points the way
forward if we are ready to listen.

THE EDGE EFFECT

Unlike rigidly enforced political borders, the world around us can
teach us about the deep medicine of fluidity, as when two ecosystems encounter each other, mingle, and form distinct new communities. Where they intersect is a third space—a transition zone. It
is neither here nor there but somewhere in between, with its own
particular resonance. This liminal space is called the ecotone. Derived from the Greek roots *ecos* meaning "home" and *tonos* meaning
"tension," it gives way to greater biodiversity. A classic example is a
wetland, the area between terrestrial and aquatic ecosystems, which
serves several crucial hydrological functions to keep water—and the
life sustained by water—filtered and healthy.[161]

Ecotones are characterized by a change in physical environment,
which brings with it a change in the flora and fauna of two distinct
systems. The transition between one landscape to the other can
be sharp or gradual; it can span continents or just a hundred meters.[162] Ecotones tend to have greater population density and species
richness—what is called "the edge effect." With that biological friction comes more diversity, as new encounters, genetic selections, and
habitat change the course of development for living creatures.[163]

Though its name has changed from *cline* to *hybrid zone* to *intergrade* to *ecotone*,[164] the idea remains that the shift from one kind of ecology to another opens rich possibilities for new kinds of life to evolve. The transition can be simple, from one kind of climate and topography to another, or sophisticated, involving interactions between and within species and microclimates, genetics, and physiology.[165] Ecotones exist across very different scales, from the borders of our digestive system to the shores of ocean and land. They provide environments for exchange and, for the right kinds of species, opportunities for evolutionary transformation.

The transition zone where the African rainforest meets the savanna is often more than one thousand kilometers wide. In this ecotone, differences in the amount of annual rainfall between the rainforest and the grasslands lead to a divergence in food availability for birds, in birds' habitat structure, and in the presence or absence of aerial predators. The ecotone provides unique selection pressures for evolution, as predators and prey negotiate their relationships. Bird species living in the ecotone, compared to the same species in the rainforest, developed morphological changes that increased their ability to survive, such as longer wingspans to make it easier to avoid aerial predators and longer beaks to access hard-to-reach foods. These birds can then move from the ecotone back to the rainforest, where these newly acquired traits are genetically shared.[166]

Note that the border between ecosystems is a living, moving boundary—not a wall. As any first-grade science book makes clear, the definition of life includes the phenomenon of movement. In motion, species find new relationships to the Earth, to water, and to each other, generating new possibilities of expression. These changes, these forces of life and movement, are rooted in biology—unlike race, a fixed and rigid fiction whose only purpose is to enforce a social order supporting the agendas of colonialism.

• • •

The ethnomusicologist Martin Stokes explains that music "provides [the] means by which people recognize identities and places, and the boundaries that separate them."[167] Music can be a tool for people in diaspora to negotiate their identities, occupying and moving between several cultures and spaces at once.[168] One of the best examples is jazz.

The origins of jazz are subject to debate, but in the conventional telling of the story, jazz was created in the 1880s in New Orleans.[169] Others believe it's not that old, while the composer Sun Ra says it was created billions of years ago. What historians do agree on is that jazz is a music of intermingling and improvisation, a mixture of African musical influences, played on African and European instruments. The European American pianist Dave Brubeck once described jazz is an "improvised musical expression of European harmony and African rhythms."[170]

New Orleans in the mid-1800s was a confluence of worlds, exemplified by the unique culture of Congo Square, just outside the French Quarter, where West African, North American, and European influences harmonized to create an ecotone of languages, including Wolof, French, English, Choctaw, German, and Spanish.[171] The Indigenous Choctaw name for the place now called New Orleans is Bulbancha, translating to "the place of many tongues." Even before European colonists arrived, the area attracted linguistic diversity. In the alluvial fan where the largest watershed in the continent empties into the gulf, over forty distinct Indigenous tribes would gather, trade, and intermingle.[172]

Congo Square has been a cultural transitional zone for several centuries. It remains a sacred site of the Indigenous Houmas people, who used to celebrate their annual corn harvest there. After the arrival of colonialism, the space became a market where Indigenous and Black people would trade goods they had grown, hunted, and foraged. As such, it became an important site of cultural and economic resistance for enslaved Black people.[173]

Jazz is a Black artform that grew out of the pressure-cooker reality of segregated slavery and then Jim Crow in the South. Long before the birth of jazz, enslaved Africans used musical instruments from Africa and Europe as weapons to push back against the oppression of racist colonial structures. In 1675 in Barbados, enslaved Africans intended trumpets to signal a revolt and would "beat drums, blow shells, or use any other loud instruments" as means to communicate with their fellow revolutionaries. The music of enslaved Africans, like women's speech and Indigenous forms of storytelling, was often a threat to the social order.

The one place in the entire antebellum South where enslaved people were allowed to have their drums and congregate, at least for several uninterrupted years, was Congo Square, where on Sunday afternoons dance parties emerged with the drumming. The physical space for gathering in this manner was a critical ingredient for the emergence of the revolutionary ecotone of jazz. As the New Orleans-born jazz composer and educator Wynton Marsalis proclaimed, "The genealogy of all important modern American music can be traced to Congo Square."[174] The scene was described by the music historian Ted Gioia:

An elderly black man sits astride a large cylindrical drum. Using his fingers and the edge of his hand, he jabs repeatedly at the drum head—which is around a foot in diameter and probably made from an animal skin—evoking a throbbing pulsation with rapid, sharp strokes. A second drummer, holding his instrument between his knees, joins in, playing with the same staccato attack. A third black man, seated on the ground, plucks at a string instrument, the body of which is roughly fashioned from a calabash. Another calabash has been made into a drum, and a woman beats at it with two short sticks. One voice, then other voices join in. A dance of seeming contradictions accompanies this musical give-and-take, a moving hieroglyph that appears, on the one hand, informal and spontaneous yet, on closer inspection, ritualized and precise. It is a dance of massive proportions. A dense crowd of dark bodies forms into circular groups—perhaps

five or six hundred individuals moving in time to the pulsa-
tions of the music, some swaying gently, others aggressively
stomping their feet. A number of women in the group begin
chanting.[175]

One important distinction between jazz and European classical
music is the former's participatory nature, which is epitomized by
New Orleans's "second line," a crowd of people accompanying the
band in a parade of dancing and what the jazz historian Bruce Raeburn
described simply as "fun."[176] Contrasted with the separation between
audience and performer that is characteristic of European music, jazz
invited a blurring of boundaries, an "emotional expression and release
for both musicians and audience."[177] These fluid sounds invited mixing
in a society that was otherwise strictly segregated according to the
color of people's skin:

> The subversive impact of this new form has been said to
> "subvert racial segregation, musically enacting . . . [an]
> assault on white purity," and the music was said to have
> "encouraged racial boundary crossings by creating racially
> mixed spaces and racially impure music, both of which al-
> tered the racial identities of musicians and listeners."[178]

Upending the political boundaries of identity is part of the evolutionary and liberatory force of jazz. Marsalis notes:

> The fact that the slaves could play the drums in New Orleans
> at Congo Square when they weren't permitted in other parts
> of the South allowed the drums to become the centerpiece
> of the style. Now the drums, while rooted in Africa, is Afro-
> American, which is American. To be Afro-American is also
> to be part Anglo-American. That is at the root of many of
> the problems related to race in America. It's hard for us to
> come to grips with that notion. We have been conditioned
> into making a false binary choice, an either/or, when life isn't

that cut and dried. Often times it's both/and. But it's hard for us to reconcile that both/and when we are so used to having to choose sides.[179]

Just as birds of the savanna ecotone fly back to the African rainforest, bringing newly adapted traits, jazz was brought back to Africa and served as an important aspect of the freedom fighters' language against white minority rule in apartheid in South Africa. The jazz legends Hugh Masakela and Miriam Makeba transmitted the sounds of resistance to racial oppression through their songs, and those subversive sounds of South African jazz became important drops in the mighty river that would end apartheid. For historian Gioia, not just jazz but the entire history of music can be told as a four-thousand-plus-year-old story of resistance, upheaval, and change, brought through the songs of those pushed to society's margins.[180]

To the composer and bassist Marcus Shelby, all Black American Music has this liberatory force, which is grounded in the spirituals, work songs, field shouts, and blues hollers of the slavery-era South. These sounds encoded information for the resistance and sowed hope of freedom. "Early blues, blues ballads, jazz, rock and roll, soul music, hip hop, rap, R&B, funk—these are all just really beautiful fruits hanging on the same tree. The DNA that runs through all American music is authentically, at the roots, Black American Music."

Even the word *jazz* is undergoing its own evolution, as contemporary Black artists look with a critical eye into how legacies of white supremacy have confined and defined their artforms within an industry dominated by Eurocentrism. The trumpeter Nicholas Payton outlines the contradictions carried in the name:

To speak of "jazz tradition" is like to speak of "racial justice." It's not possible to have justice within the confines of race because race was specifically designed to subjugate certain people to an underclass so that the "majority" thrives. Injustice is inherently built within the racial construct. There has never been any tradition within jazz other than to ensure Black cultural expression is depreciated and undervalued.[181]

Undervalued is an understatement when you look at the balance sheets of the modern music industry and compare the percent of top streaming songs created by Black artists to the percent of industry dollars Black people actually control.

White cultural whiplash emerged as soon as the artform did. Early critics of Black American music were those who were most invested in maintaining and reproducing forms of white dominance. To most white Southerners, the seductive sounds that caused some of their own to break ranks indicated that a supernatural force was at play. So they called it "devil's music."[182] Thomas Edison, who famously hated Black American music and also invented the phonograph, said it sounded better when he played the records backward.[183] Pope Pius XI, chafing at the notion of Black people emancipating themselves from the mental chains of the Doctrine of Discovery, "spoke of the 'discordant cacophony, arrhythmic howls and wild cries' of the new music."[184]

Black American Music has its roots in Black resistance, and its evolution was also nurtured by transgressive white participation. Back at the turn of the last century, the music created a place for encounter, in what the historian Richard Sudhalter sees as a "tale of cooperation, mutual admiration, cross-fertilization; comings-together and driftings-apart—all *despite,* rather than because of, the segregation of the larger society."[185] As adventurous white music lovers sought out the speakeasies and underground spaces where mixed groups of people could revel together in sweaty exchanges, Black American Music was creating—through its relentless joy and its insistence on breaking European musical and social conventions—an immeasurable force of liberation. Then and now, the music crossed borders of race and class, making it possible to imagine a new, more just social order, one that abolished constructed notions of race.

But the racial border patrol attempted to police the static hierarchies that the music upended. In the days of early Big Band music, terrorist groups like the Ku Klux Klan threatened to tar and feather a band of Black musicians "just because we were playing for white people."[186] Local cities and music venues tried to ban the music, ban "mixed dancing," and enforce antimiscegenation laws; they worked hard to reaffirm the binaries of Black and white, master and slave, "self" and "other." Hip-hop artists today experience the modern versions of this policing, quite literally. The New York Police Department had dedicated an entire unit, called the Rap Intelligence Unit, to gather information on performers and their entourages, coordinating their efforts with similar operations in Miami.[187] The social borders that made colonial rule possible continue to exert their presence today.[188] Luckily, music transcends borders. Our bodies are far richer than the fiction of race could ever contain.

7

ENDOCRINE SYSTEM

BUILDING A NEW NORMAL

Human beings are not built in silence, but in word, in work, in action-reflection. Saying that word is not the privilege of some few persons, but the right of everyone. Dialogue is the encounter in which the united reflection and action of the dialoguers are addressed to the world which is to be transformed and humanized, this dialogue cannot be reduced to the act of one person's "depositing" ideas in another, nor can it become a simple exchange of ideas to be "consumed" by the discussants. It is an act of creation; it must not serve as a crafty instrument for the domination of one person by another. Men and women who lack humility (or have lost it) cannot come to the people, cannot be their partners in naming the world. For the truly humanist educator and the authentic revolutionary, the object of action is the reality to be transformed by them together with other people.

—PAOLO FREIRE[1]

f you've been lucky enough to take a relaxing vacation away from your home, you've experienced a little of what it's like for your body to be in a different relationship to the world around you. For the duration of exposure to a holiday, markers of inflammation fall, telomeres are maintained, and healthy cell metabolism increases.[2] This "vacation effect" fades as we return to our routine exposures of stress and unhealthy routine, but the effect is real nonetheless.[3]

There are ways of making a vacation stick. Allow your body and mind to connect more deeply to your new environment by leaving your phone behind.[4] Meditate.[5] Most of all, get outdoors and engage with the web of life.[6] For people with multiple sclerosis—an inflammatory autoimmune disease of the central nervous system—a nature-and-meditation retreat left participants feeling better at statistically significant levels five years after attending.[7]

Our bodies have evolved a kind of innate intelligence, the capacity to synchronize with the world around us: the air we breathe, the microbial life in the soil, the rhythm of sunrise and nightfall, affection from a partner, and the pressure of work. Our histories, our stories, and our languages modulate the tempos of our bodies. When your exposome changes and your body adjusts to its new environment, it's the endocrine system, a liquid network of chemical messengers, that is playing a central role in this recalibration. Stimuli from the world are translated into molecular conversations between our cells and our organs, leading to coordinated responses that can leave us in good health or suffering in illness. The US military is a good student of human biology. During the War on Terror, they made it official policy to use the body's rhythms against itself.

Guantánamo derives from the name that Taíno people called the bay in what is now Cuba.[8] Columbus, on his second voyage, renamed it Puerto Grande. The British in 1741 renamed it Cumberland Harbour.[9] Spain continued to govern the island until the Spanish-American War in 1898—part of the US peace treaty involved the US payment of a lease from the newly independent Cuban government for land around Guantánamo. (Post-revolution Cuba has cashed the check for $4,085 just once, in error.) On the bay is located the US Guántanamo Bay Naval Base, including a detention facility where doctors and psychologists are experimenting with ways human bodies can self-destruct.[10]

Mohammed Jawad's family report that he was twelve when he was detained in 2002, in the wake of the 9/11 attacks.[11] At the camp, Jawad was subjected to "enhanced interrogation techniques," tortures defined by the US government as "safe, legal, ethical, and effective."[12] Among them was a practice dubbed "the frequent flyer program" in official documents,[13] although the government denied its existence. In May 2004, he was moved from cell to cell 112 times over fourteen days, once every two hours and fifteen minutes—more often at night, in order to maximize sleep deprivation. At a hearing about his treatment, a Harvard sleep expert testified over videolink. Jawad asked why the expert was needed—"they should give me time to talk about my sleeplessness" instead, he said.[14] In a reprise of the logic of the witch trials, his voice and his testimony about his own body and experiences didn't matter.[15]

Under normal circumstances, our body's sleep rhythms are determined by an axis that runs from the eyes to the pineal gland situated deep in the brain. When the sun is out and the light enters our eyes, the pineal gland suppresses the production of melatonin and continues to create serotonin, a hormone that helps to buffer our mental resilience.[16] When the sun sets and darkness surrounds us, an enzyme converts serotonin to melatonin, which is released into the bloodstream. There this anti-inflammatory hormone[17] coordinates the symphony of neurochemistry that results in restorative sleep.[18] The pineal gland releases melatonin throughout the night. It serves as a principal biological clock in mammals.[19]

Melatonin is also made in immune cells, in the gut, in the gonads, in the bone marrow, in the placenta, and in the skin. Our skin creates a whole suite of other hormones, including endorphins (our body's endogenous pain reliever) and vitamin D, another anti-inflammatory hormone whose best effects cannot be replicated by simply popping a pill.[20] New understandings of skin are framing it as an endocrine organ, demonstrating once again how antiquated concepts of anatomy fail to describe the intertwined relationships within our own bodies.[21] Deprivation of both sleep and sun disrupts melatonin production, knocking biological time out of synchronization with astronomical time. For actual frequent flyers—flight attendants, for example—low levels of melatonin have been linked to higher rates of breast cancer.[22]

The importance of melatonin to health reveals that the immune, endocrine, and nervous systems share a common chemical vocabulary.[23] This anti-inflammatory molecule has multiple functions across these systems, behaving like a neurotransmitter, a hormone, or a cytokine, depending on what secretes it (a nerve cell, a gland, or a cell in the periphery) and where it acts (between nerve cells, in a distant organ, locally, or systemically).[24] At the molecular level, melatonin inhibits the production of reactive oxygen species, protecting tissues from damage.[25] It also stops the production of pro-inflammatory cytokines, pushing back the onset and progression of inflammation.[26] In animal models, it has been shown to help restore homeostasis in the face of the overwhelming inflammation of septic shock.[27] During the Ebola outbreak, melatonin emerged as a useful treatment because it targets the inflammation that leads to the life-threatening hemorrhaging seen in this disease.[28] And during the Covid pandemic, melatonin supplements led to a 30 percent reduction in testing positive for the virus.[29] It is being explored as an adjuvant treatment to counteract the profound inflammation seen in critical Covid cases.[30] It is one of the human body's most effective antioxidants, reducing the damage wreaked by oxidative stress.[31] Intriguingly, melatonin is also present in fruits, seeds, vegetables, and grains, serving a similarly protective role. This versatile molecule appears to be present across the web of life.

Sleep deprivation torture deprives the body of melatonin.[32] It activates our cells' damage response pathways, leading to the development of the senescence-associated secretory phenotype, that pro-inflammatory cytokine profile that we discussed in Chapter 1.[33] This process is causally linked to accelerated biological aging. Rats totally deprived of sleep die within 11 to 32 days.[34] Reactive oxidative stress caused by sleep deprivation plays a damaging role.[35] Over time, sleep deprivation of the kind Jawad was subjected to leads to shorter telomeres and other forms of internal damage.[36] As a form of torture, it doesn't leave visible marks on the skin but ignites the body to consume itself through systemic inflammation, resulting in decreased longevity. This most toxic exposome of the torture chambers of Guantánamo Bay reveals what we might be facing, not under the eyes of torturers and doctors, but under the dysfunctional rhythms of the open prison of everyday life in a colonial capitalist society.

Descartes thought the connection between the material and the spiritual worlds lay in the pineal gland, the principal seat of the soul. While he was certainly wrong about this, he was right to sense that the system of glands and hormones have a kind of alchemical power. The pineal gland may not be the bridge between matter and mind, but the endocrine system of which it is a part can transmute cellphone light into inflammation and chronic stress into diabetes.

LIQUID ANATOMY

When the endocrine system is taught in medical school, it's often described as the complement to the nervous system. If a nerve cell firing is the lightning of immediate action, the endocrine system is the swell of the tides, taking longer and reshaping the landscape of the body. If the nervous system is fast, the endocrine system is slow. Although the biologist E. O. Wilson dismissed endocrinology as "concerned with the cruder tuning devices of nervous activity,"[37] our endocrine system is, in fact, a complex orchestration of regulation that keeps our body synchronized with itself, setting the different rhythms of sleep, growth, digestion, lactation, reproduction, metabolism, respiration, and mood. The endocrine system also attunes our bodies to our surroundings—responding to light, food, and social interaction—by matching internal conditions with external cues. It is exquisitely sensitive and thus deeply susceptible to disruption.

Imagine the endocrine system less as a tuning device than as a rhythm machine, producing a series of overlapping and intersecting beats that regulate our bodies through the complex communication of hormones. A hormone is a molecule that acts as a regulator for processes in other parts of the body. When you think of hormones, you're likely to think of the teenage years, when puberty leads to many body changes and a new preoccupation with sex. That's as good a place as any to start understanding them.

We communicate with others through chemistry. For many animals, from rodents to wild pigs, the scent of an ovulating female signals the time for mating. Likewise, some men swear they can tell when their partner is ovulating based on her scent. To test this idea, men were given T-shirts that were worn by women who were ovulating, worn by women who were not ovulating, or not worn at all (the control group). Men who smelled T-shirts worn by ovulating women produced a testosterone surge.[38] Gay men given shirts worn by anonymous men preferred the scents of other gay men over those of heterosexual men, heterosexual women, and lesbians.[39] Newborns are able to distinguish the scent of their own mother's breast.[40] Even our tears have chemical messengers. Men who sniffed odorless tears from women who had cried in response to a sad movie experienced a drop in testosterone and sexual arousal. Crying signals both visually and chemically that this is no time for fooling around.[41]

This system of chemical communication doesn't connect humans only to each other. The microbes in our gut interact with our cells by way of hormones in acts of interkingdom communication. Stress hormones such as epinephrine and norepinephrine produced by host cells can activate receptors on the surface of microbes living in our gut, impacting the virulence of the organism. Hormone-like molecules produced by bacteria can act on our cells and modulate the body's immune reaction.[42]

The plant kingdom speaks a kindred language. Sagebrush that is being eaten by an insect sends chemical warning signals to nearby plants, which cause those neighbors to increase the production of compounds that can attract predators against that insect.[43] Cashew trees signal that they're being eaten by pests and guide hungry African weaver ants to the sites where they're being attacked, showing us how ecological pest management works.[44] Plants communicate with each other and respond to other cues with their own hormone changes. They grow their roots under the influence of root hormone toward the sound of water, even in the absence of moisture. The presence of noise in the environment hampers their ability to tune in to their surroundings.[45]

Many organs produce their own hormones that act locally, such as the brain, kidney, heart, lungs, skin, and intestine. But the classically taught endocrine organs—the pancreas, placenta, pituitary, adrenals, thyroid, testes, ovaries, and pineal—secrete hormones systemically and serve as metronomes that regulate our life's rhythms. Within our bodies, the molecules that act as hormones can do double duty. What we think of as hormones, such as the reproductive hormone oxytocin, also function in the brain as neurotransmitters, sending signals between nerve cells. Nerve cells send their projections from the brainstem traveling along the vagus nerve onto the very cells of the pancreas that release insulin into the bloodstream.[46] Hormones and cytokines act in the same way, but the former are secreted by glands, while the latter are secreted by cells such as white blood cells, not organized into glands. Like melatonin, these chemicals are redundant in different regions of the body, serving multiple roles.

The history of understanding the endocrine system stretches back centuries, and like teenagers, the early investigators were compelled by the vicissitudes of sex. In the tenth century, Chinese physicians, who early on associated the testes with secondary sexual characteristics such as beards, isolated sex hormones from human urine and used them medicinally. They also employed estrogen-rich placenta medicinally, as documented in the pharmacopeia *Pên Tshao Shih I*, compiled by Chhen Tshang-Chii in 725 CE.[47]

Further back, the medicinal use of testes from various animals was documented in the first century CE by the Greek botanist Dioscorides and in ancient Ayurvedic healing texts.[48] In modern Europe, early attempts to harness the power of the endocrine system were prompted by the demands of music and the demand to keep women's voices out of church. An edict of Paul the Apostle in 67 CE was written into the New Testament: "Let your women keep silence in the churches: for it is not permitted to them to speak; but they are commanded to be under obedience as also said the law. And if they will learn anything, let them ask their husbands at home: for it is a shame for women to speak in the church" (1 Cor. 14:34–35).

The early Christian church developed chants that were always performed by all-male choirs. Not until the 1400s was polyphonic choral music created with the addition of the treble voice. With women effectively gagged, someone needed to cover the soprano range. Young Italian boys from poor families were mutilated by castration to keep their vocal range from dropping as they entered puberty.[49] These *castrati* were deemed essential for religious music and European operas through the eighteenth century.[50]

In the 1880s, the physician Charles-Édouard Brown-Séquard reported, at age seventy-two, that he had had a "rejuvenated sexual prowess after subcutaneous injection of extracts of dog and guinea pig testes."[51] Quite how this worked, though, was a mystery. At the time, people believed that any invisible signals in the body must be communicated through the nervous system, which was understood in rudimentary terms. If it wasn't exactly clear which nerves were being used, it was only because they were too small or had yet to be found. The Russian physiologist Ivan Pavlov had proposed that just such a network of nerves existed in the stomach, and that this network helped to regulate digestion.[52]

In 1649 Descartes wrote in a letter to the mathematician Marin Mersenne, "I don't explain the feeling of pain without reference to the soul."[53] Since animals didn't have souls, it made no sense to imagine them actually in pain. About 250 years later, two British physiologists, William Bayliss and Ernest Starling, put Pavlov's idea to the test in a controversial experiment, which would, in Britain, set feminist antivivisectionists against the scientific establishment. They anesthetized a dog, scraped the nerves away from around its stomach, and fed it. Digestive juices flowed from the pancreas. Since there were no nerve signals to cue digestion, they wondered whether there was a signal in the blood. They injected some of the animal's ground intestine into a vein far from the stomach and watched as the pancreas responded as though the dog had eaten. Since they hadn't fed the animal this time and had made their injection far from the stomach, they couldn't have excited any of its nerves, visible or invisible. Yet the dog's stomach behaved as if it had just been fed.

The body clearly had mechanisms of communication and regulation that medicine hadn't yet imagined. Bayliss and Starling called this mysterious substance "secretin." We now know that secretin is a hormone that is created by the specialized cells in the small intestine and circulates by way of the blood to the pancreas, where it stimulates the release of digestive enzymes.[54] Starling described hormones as "the chemical messengers which, speeding from cell to cell along the bloodstream, may coordinate the activities and growth of different parts of the body."[55]

Like any medical field, endocrinology has followed the contours of power over time. One of its particularly dark chapters was "chemical castration": the use of sex hormones to "cure homosexuality."[56] This treatment was controversial from the beginning. But the potential to medically intervene and change another's sexuality remains a live debate in public policy and continues worldwide.[57]

YOU GIVE ME FEVER

On the other side of the Atlantic, William H. Welch, one of the founders of Johns Hopkins Hospital, also experimented on animals in the name of advancing scientific understanding. Investigating the physiology of fever in the mid-nineteenth century, he created a box in which he could heat up a rabbit by degrees, documenting what happened to its various systems along the way. He admitted that slow-cooking living animals for several days doesn't really approximate a real fever in the human body, but this didn't stop him from his gruesome work, to attempt to understand how fever happens and how it's linked to the body's healing process.[58]

Fever and its causes have long been a source of mystery and wonder. One of the oldest extant records of a medical symptom, carved in Akkadian cuneiform in the sixth century BCE, is a flaming brazier, representing both fever and inflammation.[59] In Hippocratic medicine, fever was a sign of excess in one of the principal humors, yellow bile. The heating up of the body was viewed as beneficial, a way of cooking out an illness.[60] Hippocrates's writing is so precise that it is possible to recognize different diseases by the timing of their fevers: pneumonia's fevers are persistent, typhoid's escalating, and malaria's intermittent.[61]

Welch hypothesized that fever originates in a thermoregulatory center in the lower region of the brain. To prove it, he injected dogs and rabbits with infected pus after transecting their spinal cords. When their brains were cut off from the rest of the body, there was no fever.[62] From this he theorized that fever occurs when a host's white blood cells acting to fight off infection produce a chemical that acts on the central thermostat in the brain. He was right, at least in part. White blood cells in the blood and in the tissues, sent out to target inflammatory lesions, trigger the creation of a hormone called endogenous pyrogen, which acts on the hypothalamus in the brain to initiate the physiological process of fever.[63]

We now know that endogenous pyrogen is actually a cytokine,

one that is central in the innate inflammatory response and that we saw in our discussion of immunity in Chapter 1: interleukin-1. This molecule plays an important role in the body's attempt to restore homeostasis. In tissues it can act as the cell-membrane-bound version IL-1α, where it causes localized tissue inflammation. When it enters the bloodstream as IL-1β, it behaves like a hormone, setting off changes that impact multiple body systems. In the first few hours after infection, the biological effects of IL-1 can be seen in every tissue of every organ in the body.[64]

In Western medicine, although many questions remain about the underlying mechanisms of fever, its benefits are becoming clearer. It is part of the body's intelligent design to mobilize greater immune resources to address the cause of disrupted homeostasis. Suppressing high fever is critical to preventing acute brain injury, but more data is emerging in the "let it ride" camp to support letting a fever do its thing. With critical illness and infection, suppressing fever does not beneficially alter the course of an illness,[65] but aggressive suppression of fever in critical illness can be harmful.[66]

Bridging the immune, endocrine, and nervous systems, IL-1 not only acts on the thermoregulatory center of the brain to initiate fever but also induces the release of a whole range of hormones from the hypothalamus and its neighboring pituitary gland, such as endorphins, plus others that drive the production of stress steroids such as cortisol.[67] It is the signal that trips the HPA axis into mobilizing in response to psychological stress.[68] With acute stress, the HPA axis coordinates a neuroendocrine response to mobilize adaptive resources to manage the threat or damage. With chronic stress, however, these systems continue working, creating fever and inflammation—responses meant to heal the body but that now turn against the body. The potential consequences include neurological changes such as memory loss and depression and the death of insulin-producing cells in the pancreas, leading to conditions such as diabetes. The exposome we have built—defined for many by chronic stress—is a world in which the body synchronizes with a damaging environment, and the result is illness.

This is how a damaging exposome creates the wear and tear we see in the bodies of those who are forced to endure it. IL-1 induces insulin-producing cells in the pancreas to make more insulin, but overstimulation can result in the death of those special cells.[69] This suggests one mechanism by which chronic low-grade inflammation could lead to conditions such as diabetes. Not unsurprisingly, Indigenous people who share similar patterns of colonization are transmitting diabetes through the generations.[70] The ways in which our exposomes impact our cells are being programmed into our biology. No amount of insulin can reverse this pattern. The exposome must be restructured for health to be a possibility.

THE NEW NORMAL

When the world is in balance, we are too. But the modern world in all its structures is out of balance, leading to bodies that are badly damaged by chronic inflammation. The biological cost, in the face of ongoing damage, is the allostatic load the body carries.[71]

The abnormality of the modern world makes it incredibly hard for us to get back to a healthy equilibrium. The fast food marketed to us most frequently is unhealthy and contributes to damage that makes it harder to return to health.[72] The air we breathe carries noise and particulate pollution that presents a cognitive and biochemical load for our brains.[73] Living in a low-income neighborhood means carrying biomarkers of a higher allostatic load.[74]

To be Black in the United States is to be confronted with daily acts of discrimination—sources of stress that manifest as higher blood pressure even while we are asleep.[75] Instead of the restoration that sleep and melatonin afford, the allostatic load that racism brings effectively leaves Black people sleeping with one eye open. Differences in allostatic load are contributing to the disparities between health outcomes for cardiovascular death between Black people and white people.[76] Increased allostatic load may explain why most people in modern industrial societies develop hypertension as they get older—beginning even in childhood.[77] People in hunter-gatherer and agrarian societies don't experience this same age-related hypertension and have lower rates of hypertension altogether.[78]

We also live in a world steeped in industrial chemical noise. Signals from some of the thousands of products of the pesticide, plastics, and manufacturing industries are already interfering with our bodies' own biochemical conversations. Endocrine disruptors mimic or interfere with our own hormones, leading to a wide range of problems from developmental disorders to cancer. The disruptors, found in everyday products such as children's plastic toys and foods, range from the bisphenol A (BPA) in canned food lining to industrial solvents (dioxins) to pesticides and fungicides.[79]

One study calculated the economic impacts of industrially manufactured endocrine disruptors in Europe and the United States in 2010.[80] By looking at the range of pathways through which endocrine disruptors are known to cause disease, from testicular cancer to diabetes to loss of IQ, researchers computed the health care costs that might be connected to endocrine disruptors. In the United States, that cost was $340 billion (2.33 percent of GDP); in the EU, it was $217 billion (1.28 percent of GDP).

Despite the cataclysmic burden of disease they cause,[81] regulating endocrine disruptors has proven difficult, not least because of the power of the chemicals industry.[82] Lobbyists from the European Centre for Ecotoxicology and Toxicology of Chemicals (ECETOC), a think tank funded among others by Bayer, BASF, Dow, DuPont, and Syngenta successfully obstructed a range of public health initiatives that might have reined in their profits.[83] One of ECETOC's former experts testified that "synthetic EDCs at the present exposure are no risk for human health," especially when compared with the endocrine disruptor that features most often in our diets, sugar.[84]

In spite of the evidence that the structures around us are causing these health problems, medicine often treats endocrine conditions as something patients have done to themselves. One of the most troubling and widespread examples is type 2 diabetes. When your body is deficient in insulin or when your cells grow insensitive to it, blood sugar levels can fluctuate harmfully. The possible dire consequences include blindness, tissue necrosis, cardiovascular disease, and kidney failure. One in eleven adults on Earth now has the disease, with the highest concentrations in Asia: China and India lead the world, with 110 and 70 million cases, respectively.[85] The main drivers are generational poverty, chronic stress, and ultraprocessed foods.[86] Predictably, Black, Indigenous, and other people of color suffer the most from the colonial diet's scourge, with higher diabetes rates than settler populations across the world.[87] This happens not by magic but by design. In the United States, advertising for sugary drinks increased by $1 billion from 2013 to 2018, with Black and Latinx youth as the primary targets.[88]

When societies *do* take collective action against the food industry, it fights back. Mexico in 2011 had the world's highest per-person soda consumption: 163 liters per year.[89] Three years later a range of public health activists scored a victory with the passage of a 10 percent tax on sweetened beverages. The victory was made possible in part because the tax funds were to be used to install water fountains in schools, a remedy that would help low-income and Indigenous groups in particular.[90] The projections were that the resulting decreased consumption would lead to 189,300 fewer cases of diabetes and 18,900 fewer deaths over ten years.[91] But it would also lead to reduced profits for the soda industry.

In 2016 three of the leading public health advocates started to receive odd text messages, just as they were preparing for a legislative battle to increase the tax. Dr. Simón Barquera at the National Institute for Public Health, Alejandro Calvillo of Poder del Consumidor, and Luis Encarnación at Coalición ContraPESO were being targeted by military-grade spyware, sold by the Israel-based technology firm NSO Group exclusively to governments, according to a detailed investigative report published in *The New York Times*.[92] Their communications pathways were hacked so that industrial sugar vendors might do the same to our endocrine systems. (To date, no one has been prosecuted.)

Were this an isolated incident, we might dismiss it as an example of the food industry's being unusually powerful in Mexico. (Vicente Fox, the Mexican president from 2000 to 2006, was also the president of Coca-Cola Mexico.) But endocrine disruptors have been pushed across the planet by industries reluctant to see their sources of profit come second to concerns of human health. The sugar industry, like the tobacco industry, has long been in the business of obfuscating science for profit. It has a history of funding medical conferences and professional association meetings and publications as part of a sophisticated suite of ways to buy off incriminating science.[93] In the EU, the chemical and biotechnology industries fund experts to cast doubt on a well-established body of science showing the dangers of endocrine disruptors.[94] Globally, vendors and users of endocrine disruptors continue their war on science.[95]

The power of these chemical companies is changing young people's bodies. Hormones control menses. The age at which girls have their first period has been falling across the planet.[96] The reasons range from exposure to endocrine disruptors in hand sanitizer and plastic bottles, to the ubiquitous presence of artificial light and increased sugar consumption.[97] These disruptors are social problems, catalysts in the circulation of global capital, but the illnesses that they cause are increasingly blamed on the individual.

THE TRAGEDY OF
THE BUILT ENVIRONMENT

The allostatic load is greatest where humans have done the most to transform the world around them. Since 2009, for the first time in history, more humans are living in cities than outside them, exposed to artificial light and constant noise.[98] Although the global shift from majority rural to majority urban happened only recently, England

and Wales hit that milestone in the 1850s.[99] London's West End night sky was forever changed by a gaslighting system that began to be installed in 1806.[100]

Millions of years of evolution had shaped the web of life's circadian rhythms, but it didn't take long for them to be jolted sideways. The impact of artificial light at night was first tracked by an ornithologist who noticed that the same technology that had been used for over a century indoors to make chickens lay more eggs was also affecting undomesticated birds: comparing finches and other migratory birds inside and outside London's glow, William Rowan observed that those in a city aviary reproduced earlier than their rural counterparts.[101]

The skies haven't just become brighter. The color of night has also changed. From the warm flicker of candles, to gas lamps, to the orange low-pressure sodium lamps that lit our walks home from school as children, to the white of modern LED streetlights and the glow of our smart phones, our nights are now bluer. This is, as we're learning, the color of light that creatures have evolved to use as a signal for the beginning of the day. When lights are off or warm yellow, the pineal gland will marshal the processes of sleep through melatonin. When blue wavelengths that signal the beginning of the day hit the retina in the eyes, the direct window to our brain, hormone production is dramatically changed.[102] Turn the blue lights on, and melatonin levels drop.[103] When rats, hamsters, and salmon are constantly exposed to bright blue lights, they exhibit signs of stress and decreased immune function.[104] Exposure to light, in other words, has an impact not only on individuals but on entire ecosystems.

Just as light causes changes in the endocrine system, so too does noise. Tree frogs, which have evolved so that the loudest are the most attractive, have had their romances upended by traffic noise.[105] This background noise has profound effects on humans—disrupting sleep and producing knock-on endocrine disruption that can activate the stress response, causing a rise in circulating cortisol and adrenaline.[106] Activated stress leads to inflammation, which can in turn upset the endocrine system: a dangerous feedback loop. A 10-decibel increase in road traffic noise five years before diagnosis can lead to a 1 percent increase in diabetes for those within earshot.[107] A noise level consonant with good sleep is 40 dBA—any louder is disruptive.[108] One study found that in the United States, noise levels in areas with 75 percent Black residents average 46.3 dBA, whereas those in areas with zero Black residents average 42.3 dBA.[109] The problem is worldwide: in one Indian city's silence zone, ambient bedroom noise levels range between 65 and 75 dBA—and that's typical across all India's cities.[110]

All this noise and 24/7 illumination would seem to suggest that cities are hubs of social activity. But the promise of more social connection in the bright lights and big city is not borne out. In fact, a sense of loneliness in cities is common. Even though rural spaces afford more opportunity for social distance, residents of cities experience higher rates of social isolation, an experience that was dramatically heightened during the Covid quarantines when millions of people isolated themselves from friends, family, colleagues, and neighbors.[111] Quarantine, self-isolation, is an extreme situation, but it reveals something essential about the nature of our urban environments.

For the first time in human history, an unprecedented level of people are living alone for an extended period of time—a trend seen most starkly in cities. The paradox of loneliness in the midst of a crowd defines life in urban environments where people do not have adequate paths and time to build authentic relationships with one another, in third spaces that are neither their homes nor their workplaces. Forging community is more challenging in urban spaces that are not designed for people to gather and encounter one another. Although we can exist as individuals completely on our own, it appears we cannot thrive. Humans evolved to live as social animals constantly exposed to one another and very rarely alone. It has been suggested that the subjective feeling of loneliness is an adaptive trait, a kind of warning signal that our web of social interactions has become unhealthily frayed.[112]

The impact of urban loneliness on our health is seen in how cities are associated with 40 percent more depression and 20 percent more anxiety than rural spaces, as well as double the rates of schizophrenia.[113] Social isolation is associated with elevated rates of cardiovascular disease, dementia, and mortality.[114] When early humans were separated from their tribes—whether by a rite of passage, the need to hide from enemies, or an accident—it was a temporary condition.[115] Nowadays we're steeping permanently in the long-term chemistry of social isolation: the activation of the HPA axis and the downstream inflammation that the stress response creates. Our built environment is designed, intentionally or not, to cause depression, cognitive decline, dementia, and other illnesses—all mediated by inflammatory cytokines.[116]

Feelings of isolation create a vicious circle between the body and the environment. In cities, people have more access to the kinds of foods that will provide both a short-term uplift and a longer-term predisposition to diabetes.[117] A full spectrum of products exploit the disruptions of modern life to help us cope with this stress, to make us temporarily less unhappy—and to hook us with a promised return to some imagined state of bliss. The physical environment drives us, through anxiety and opportunity, to the kinds of behaviors that generate more inflammation: overeating, drug use, and self-isolation.[118]

Chronic stress makes the body vulnerable to addiction,[119] increasing levels of emotional stress cause decreased impulse control,[120] and the more chronic the stress becomes, the more maladaptive the behavior becomes.[121] Chronic stress dampens activity in the prefrontal cortex—the part of the brain responsible for rational decision making and self-control—and heightens activity in the limbic system, which includes the amygdala, an ancient center of the brain that guides impulsive behavior.[122] Global industries intuitively understand this connection between the endocrine and nervous systems, encouraging addiction and overconsumption as a path to happiness, a dynamic that David Courtwright calls "limbic capitalism."[123] As Facebook co-founder Sean Parker explained, social media are engineered to hijack our need for social connection, offering "a little dopamine hit" to the reward centers of the brain through likes and retweets and views.[124] This is not exactly an accurate description of the complex neurobiology at play, but it is a fair assessment of how Facebook keeps us coming back for more.[125]

A string of epidemiological studies has connected early-life exposure to stress or trauma with addictive behavior, through the activation of the HPA axis, the endocrine superhighway that is intimately connected to the nervous system. Unsurprisingly, inflammation plays a role.[126] Drugs such as opiates and alcohol induce the expression of a transcription factor that turns on the genes that make inflammatory cytokines in the brain *and* noninflammatory targets such as opioid receptors. This transcription factor plays a central role in the inflammatory response and also mediates complex behaviors involved in drug reward, learning, stress responses, and depression.[127] These systems are interconnected on the molecular level and provide a possible framework to understand how opiate addiction modulates the stress response, leading to more inflammation.[128]

As these drugs and the story of fever itself reveal, systems that were once considered separate are in fact tightly bound together. As we saw above, IL-1 was understood as a hormone known as endogenous pyrogen before it was relabeled a cytokine, a feature of the immune system. All these chemical signals keep the nervous system, the immune system, and the endocrine system tightly interwoven and in constant communication as they respond to our environment, interact with organisms inside and around us, and optimize our readiness for the challenges ahead.

THE OPPOSITE OF STRESS

Something as seemingly trivial as having a plant in a hospital room reduces pain, anxiety, fatigue, and blood pressure in patients compared to those in rooms without them. It's not surprising. One study found that remission from depression was significantly higher among those who walked in nature (61 percent) than among those who were treated in a hospital (21 percent) or left untreated (5 percent).[129] The sprawling literature on forest bathing points to an urban route for deep medicine: the web of life is already in cities, even if its attenuated compared to rural areas.[130]

Central to the story of how human well-being is regulated in nature is the chemical language of hormones. Even though we're at the early stages of understanding the human-web-of-life boundary, we are a little further along in understanding how human bodies create hormones that react to being in harmony with their surroundings and in relationships. One such hormone is oxytocin, made by the hypothalamus, which plays a role in reproduction of all vertebrates. It is also made by the uterus, the testes, and the heart. This important hormone is responsible for the smooth-muscle contractions of the uterus that push a baby out into the world and for the contractions of lactiferous ducts that bring milk to an infant's mouth. It also plays a central role in spontaneous erections and ejaculation.[131]

Oxytocin is essential to social cooperation and empathy and to modulating the impact of stress.[132] Called "the love hormone" because of the feeling of connection it engenders, oxytocin enhances an organism's responsiveness to socially relevant stimuli.[133] It boosts the action of endogenous feel-good molecules, like anandamide, that help cannabis promote a sense of well-being and social reward.[134] It is also involved in the complex behavior of bonding, which makes you want to cuddle your partner or kiss your children even after they've drawn on the walls with permanent markers.[135] Oxytocin levels rise when one feels strong social support and when one gives or receives a massage.[136] Its presence drives down the amount of circulating cortisol, even in the face of psychosocial stress, creating a calming effect.[137] It also has an anti-inflammatory effect through direct modulation of the immune system.[138]

Although one study showed that oxytocin may be involved in developing in-group bias, Jewish Israelis who were given a dose expressed more empathy toward the pain of Palestinians.[139] When taken intranasally, oxytocin makes people more generous, more trusting, and even better at anticipating and understanding others' emotional states.[140] It enhances social cooperation, but only when participants are not overwhelmed by greed or self-interest.[141] It also acts differently depending on an individual's cognitive approach, whether intuitive or more reflective.[142]

Listening to music increases our oxytocin levels, and when the music gives us chills, dopamine is released in the deep reward centers of the brain.[143] Singing together in groups also stimulates oxytocin release, and improvised singing promotes higher levels.[144] In birds, singing plays a crucial role in bonding and mating, often for life in pairs—and these behaviors are also mediated through this hormone. Research is ongoing into how language acquisition in humans might be tied to the action of this incredible molecule.[145]

Oxytocin acts on different centers in our brain to release dopamine. It also prevents serotonin from being taken up, which leads to an overall sense of well-being.[146] But lest we fall into the trap of advocating cuddle chemistry, it's important to note a few things.[147] The studies that tout the positive effects of oxytocin are far from definitive, and good science avoids sweeping generalities.[148]

Deficits of oxytocin are, we suggest, symptoms not of an underdeveloped pharmaceutical approach or of a personal failure to find happiness—an endorphin deficiency for which something might be prescribed—but of a world that has severed human connections to the web of life. The exposome is, by definition, not something for which there can be a pill. No chemical can erase the cumulative burden of exposures from before birth or remove social, ecological, or economic injustice. The solution to stress isn't an oxytocin pill, just as the solution to a denuded microbiome isn't a poop transplant. If oxytocin is like happiness, then the answer isn't a Brave New World with happiness dispensed to all for the profit of a multinational corporation. It's reimagining and reconfiguring how we live, so as to fill our lives with the opportunities to naturally enjoy oxytocin by connecting with other humans and the rest of the web of life.

A POLITICAL ANATOMY

Cartesianism makes for bad physiology and bad politics. Descartes knew that if he posited two separate realms of mind and body, he'd need a bridge between the two. As we'll argue more fully in Chapter 8, this philosophical problem disappears. We appreciate that mind and body aren't hermetically sealed, as Cartesian logic and so much of colonial medicine suggests. There's no need for a pineal gland to act as a portal between world and self. As science is increasingly making clear, consciousness is fully embodied, and the body is fully conscious: the self only exists embedded in the world.

Descartes anatomical error was one that came with its own license for supremacy. If only thinking things could suffer—and Descartes and his ilk recognized one another as thinking things—then they were able to reserve for themselves the power to adjudicate what kinds of life might suffer authentically. As we've seen, the pain of women and BIPOC people is disbelieved or, when acknowledged, matters less. And by the same token, the suffering of the rest of the web of life has been ignored. That animals might suffer remains controversial.[149] Often the terms of dealing with that suffering is to cast it as a rights issue, expanding the original language and law of colonialism to entities to which it was never intended to stretch. More recently, Indigenous groups and ecological movements have pushed to accord rights to nature. This is something with which we're sympathetic but that misses the deeper medicine. The language of rights depends a lot on the state to recognize the right to have to rights. In this view, rights are a kind of private property guaranteed by a legal contract. We need a new language, one that doesn't require sanction by the state—a language that might dramatically change the relationship between humans and the world around us.

It is possible to imagine urban spaces filled with biodiversity. But without addressing the rhythms of colonial capitalism that, literally, stop us from taking a minute to smell the flowers, we're unlikely to be able to engage with the web of life as we need to. Cities are built to run all day and all night, with workers on shift around the clock, in a social architecture that pollutes with light and noise and loneliness. Human rhythms are severed from those with which humans evolved.[150] Granting rights to animals or to nature can't address this deeper deficit in the cosmology of capitalist colonialism.

Engaging in deep medicine means understanding how every human's internal state synchronizes with the environment around them, and helping that dialogue speak in as many languages as possible. The extermination of these languages was a central part of the colonial project.[151] In North America, the locus of that extinction was the boarding school, to which generations of Indigenous people were kidnapped to be civilized by the state, as we observed in Chapter 5.[152]

The Indigenous ethnobotanist Linda Black Elk says, "For Indigenous people in North America, health has four components: physical, mental, emotional, and spiritual. The genocide of Indigenous people has created lasting intergenerational trauma." A large part of this "soul wound" was created through cutting the ties that bind through language.[153]

Some Indigenous groups are working to heal the connections that were violently severed through these schools and policies of cultural erasure.[154] Maintaining and revitalizing one's native language has positive health effects, specifically in those diseases where inflammation plays a role.[155] Oxytocin is involved in the social process of language learning, knitting together the reciprocal relations of hearing and repeating and understanding semantic relations as taught by experienced speakers.[156] More surprising, like an exposure to nature in youth, exposure to a noncolonized linguistic cosmology may have a medical benefit. First Nations people in Alberta who maintain their language seem to be shielded against diabetes. Even after controlling for socioeconomic factors, the higher the language knowledge among Indigenous groups, the lower their level of diabetes. A strong knowledge of language may reflect better organized community resistance to the damaging effects of colonialism, and its toxic pathways of disease.[157] Language can play a protective role in youth suicide, which is a sign of cultural distress that affects Indigenous people around the world. One study found that groups of Indigenous people where more than 50 percent of the tribe spoke their language had youth suicide rates six times lower than those where less than 50 percent spoke their language.[158] The cultural continuity of language helps Indigenous people "be who we are" and fend off "a sickness of colonization we fight every day."[159]

Tipiziwin Tolman, who teaches the Lakȟóta language to young children, has some ideas on why language plays a protective role in health. Her parents were both forced away from their Lakȟóta-speaking families into boarding schools, where their language was stolen. Her grandfather tried to make the best of a situation he could not fight, telling his daughter that it was important for her to learn how to speak English, what he called "the money language."

But Tolman knew that there are things more powerful than money. "Speaking our own language, it's our superpower," she said. If hormones are the chemical connections braiding together the systems of our body to respond to the world around us, then language is the way human relationships are woven in the world. Tolman puts it like this:

> Without our language, we forgot these integral, ancient connections to our spiritual ancestors. We come from the sun. We come from the moon. We come from this Earth. They are our ancient grandmothers and grandfathers. And without our language to really reinforce this, we have been violently severed from those relationships. When we're not in relationship, then we're not in respect, and we're not being embraced with this love that they have for us.
>
> They still love us. They are still here. I always think about them like forgotten grandmothers and grandfathers who are over in a nursing home. We don't see them or acknowledge them. We don't visit with them. We don't say their names. We don't remember their names in the manner in which we used to. The Moon, the Sun, the Earth. Yes. All

of those ancient grandmothers. "Uŋčí" means grandmother. Like the water, Uŋčí Úŋk. That is the name of the water and everything that comes from the water. Our people used to practice these songs for her. These acknowledgments. And we don't anymore. Most of our people don't even remember her name.

In 2016 a prayer camp formed at Standing Rock where thousands of Lakȟóta people with their comrades—Indigenous people from all over the world as well as settlers—came together to stop the Dakota Access Pipeline from crossing the Mni Sose, or Missouri River. In early August, as the heavy construction machines were digging a trench for the pipeline, two of Tolman's sisters jumped the fence and stood in front of the machines in order to stop them. They succeeded. Construction stopped for several months until the hired private armies arrived.[160] The day after the sisters stopped the machines, they went down to the river. Tolman recounts:

> One of my sisters, she said, "There was a grandmother with us when we got to the river. We could hear crying and the crying was like grief, like how a mom sounds when her child dies." They stopped and looked at each other to see who it was. And then they realized that it was coming from the water.
>
> We took this spiritual happening to our spiritual leaders. And what was told to us in ceremony was that it was our grandmother, the water, Uŋčí Úŋk. And she was crying out of grief and anger and sadness all mixed together, at the state of our people. She said, "Everyone wants to defend the water right now, but nobody even remembers my name. And no one even remembers my songs. And nobody even acknowledges me anymore."
>
> And that was real for us. And so we started reimplementing simple protocol with the water. We'll pray. We'll say her name. We'll bring her name back to our mouths. Uŋčí Úŋk.

Tolman has taught Lakȟóta language in an immersion program for young children on the Standing Rock reservation for over five years. She returns these words back into the mouths of the next generation, and in doing so she awakens ancient relationships so the children are able to name themselves in relation to the world around them and the world that came before. She has noticed that families where the children are speaking their language seem to be doing better than families where no Lakȟóta is spoken. The language connects people to their past.

Watching her own children speak Lakȟóta, Tolman is joined to the future. At a Sun Dance ceremony a few years back, her five-year-old son was receiving a blessing. As he walked toward the sacred tree and touched it, he turned around to his mother and said in his language, "*Iná, waŋná mawášteya.*" Mom, now I am okay.

In the Cheyenne language, the word for *home* is "Eńovó," which means "you are home." Not "your home." "You are home": which could mean falling asleep on the couch at your grandmother's or sitting at the table of your auntie while she cooks or returning to the land your family takes care of or speaking your community's language. "You are home" defines a system of relationships between humans, and between humans and their built environment and the web of life. A sense of well-being comes with a shared language, shared purpose, and common cause, a political community that stretches beyond the concept of nation with its vocabulary of rights. It is a consciousness of balance and happiness that is reflected in the very chemistry of our bodies.

8

NERVOUS SYSTEM

THE WEB OF LIFE

PANDO/PANDO

The Trembling Giant Aspen/Bolivian massacre site

Trembling giant
  bulging under siege
Pando
  /Pando

waving I spread
  banned from streets
perpendicular to leaf blade
Pando/
  Pando

  havoc, natural gas
petiole flattened
  opposition pushing right autonomy
rush, lift, breaking cover, tremble
  on the fourth day of
yellow-white-grayish-yellow
Pando/Pando

hunger strike, assailants
lobbed a green grenade
forced to knees   shirtless
peasantry
tree
Pando
   /Pando

Pando/
   Pando
aspen man spreads uprising
flowering, flower,
spreading root sprout
Pando
   ambush
   where Morales has stayed
biomass   clone cross   giant uprising
deeply rooted Indigenous growth
   prevent, Bolivia from splintering apart
Pando/Pando

   visiting Santa Cruz
one hundred acres
   dynamite blasts
fourteen million pounds
   public humiliation
Pando/Pando

rooted eighty thousand years
   fifty Indigenous mayors rooted
   thirty Andeans killed this week
   paralyzed borders
   Argentina, Brazil, Paraguay
Pando/Pando
clonal colony
   colonial massacre
singular genetic individual
   Morales, an Aymara Indian,
Pando/Pando
   organized opposition, university

student conservatives, forced terrified
Indigenous people, to their knees
forced refugee people to
apologize for coming to Sucre
forced chanted insults to their hero Evo
then conservatives set fire
to blue, black, white Aymara flag
seized hand-woven Aymara ponchos
Aymara people
Pando/Pando

Pando/Pando
rhizome, basal shoot
   shot,   seven dead
shooting—genet/ramet
   peasant farmers

organism overtaking
   not supported by current evidence

Fishlake quaking
   Amazon
   Pando
aspen   life in largest
   singular germination
Pando/Pando
   Pando/Pando
Pando/Pando
   Pando/Pando
Pando/Pando
   Pando/Pando
Pando/Pando

—ALLISON ADELLE HEDGE COKE

No individual or species is privileged in the world of nature:
All eat and are eaten; all become sick and die in their turn.
Humans are part of an interconnected continuum of life.

—LISA KEMMERER[1]

For animals, as well as plants, there have never been individuals. This new paradigm for biology asks new questions and seeks new relationships among the different
living entities on Earth. We are all lichens.

—SCOTT F. GILBERT, JAN SAPP, AND ALFRED TAUBER[2]

Pando is the name of a great forest in Utah and also the name of
the region in Bolivia where, on September 11, 2008, paramilitary
forces killed at least eleven supporters of then-Bolivian president
Evo Morales. The victims had been on their way to a union organizing
meeting when they were ambushed by paramilitary thugs supported
by the local government.[3] Students from a nearby teachers' college
joined the Aymara protesters in an act of solidarity. Three were killed
and mutilated. The anthropologist Bret Gustafson reports that survivors of the massacre were whipped with barbed wire, a method of
assault on Indigenous Bolivians carried over from the early years of
colonization.[4]

The Indigenous poet Allison Adelle Hedge Coke published her
startling poem *Pando/Pando* five years before Leopoldo Fernández,
the regional governor, had joined others in Bolivia's wealthy landowning elite to stage a coup in 2019 against Morales, an Indigenous
Aymara leader and head of the Movement Toward Socialism (MAS)
party.[5] The coup government was supported by the United States,
which had long been involved in backing right-wing regimes in the
region, and in pushing neoliberal economic policies that opened up
land for the extraction of resources needed by the North.[6] Bolivia is
rich in the lithium needed to manufacture all the batteries that keep
our home electronics, including smartphones, and electric cars running. Unsurprisingly, the coup plotters were more aligned with US
interests over the control of these resources than MAS, which had
instituted a law on the rights of Pacha Mama, Mother Earth.[7] Elon

Musk tweeted in support of the undemocratic government, saying "We will coup whoever we want! Deal with it." Morales, responding to the coup, recalled the same colonial history as the murders in Pando did: "My crime, my sin, is to be an Indian."[8]

But in death and in grief, there is the possibility of regeneration. From the killings came the coup, but the coup ended and Morales's party was back in power by 2020, democratically restored in a landslide. In Hedge Coke's poem, the Bolivian region, stained with the blood of its Indigenous people, transforms into Pando the forest. The catalyst for this shift is the language of ramets and rhizomes, the tendrils of life that emerge from the soil.

Pando, named from the Latin for "I spread," is one of the largest and oldest living creatures on Earth. It appears as a forest of quaking aspens, but each tree is just a stem. All forty-seven thousand stems are parts of a single organism, possibly thousands of years old—the world's heaviest being, stretching over forty-three hectares underground.[9]

Pando is a single being but also many. This should sound very familiar by now. We contain multitudes; the border between self and other is as fluid and in motion as life itself. In *Pando/Pando*, we see how a single name can be plural; we hear the shots of those who were killed in Bolivia reverberating through the thousands of trees of a swaying forest in Utah. The poem describes a process of becoming, of the self embedded in the web of life and intersected by history. It is a vision of blood spilled so that others might become.

We began our journey into the immune system with Donna Haraway's observation that "biology is about recognition and misrecognition." Playing with a homonym, *Pando/Pando* juxtaposes two moments of life and death, recognized and misrecognized, above ground and below. In the interplay of two meanings of Pando, we can find the poetry of a new, radical understanding of health.

Reflecting on the poem, Hedge Coke observed, "We are Pando and never the single quaking aspen appearance, presentation, one may (mis)identify as (individual) tree. Poetry behaves like the wonderfully gelatinous Blob, oscillating unicellular intelligence—like a bit of the heart of Sky Woman extending throughout us, our world."[10]

SUBTERRANEAN SOLIDARITY

Life's oscillating intelligence is part of our deep history. In the creation story told by Western science, about 2.4 billion years ago,[11] there was a vast expansion of biodiversity called the Great Oxygenation Event. A proliferation of new life-forms was made possible by the cumulative effect of cyanobacteria floating in the oceans. Through photosynthesis, these bacteria created oxygen, enabling the evolution of new kinds of organisms who could use this molecule as an energy source.[12] Single-cell organisms expanded in size until they hit a limitation of diffusion: any bigger, and the surface-area-to-volume ratio works against getting nutrients into and waste products out of a cell.[13] When they could no longer grow, they started creating mutually beneficial systems of relationships with one another.

An archaeon fused with a bacterium to form the first nucleated cell.[14] A photosynthetic bacterium got incorporated into a nucleated cell to form the first plant cell. That bacterium now exists as the chloroplast in today's plant world.[15] Single-cellular organisms compartmentalized functions, joining together to make multicellular organisms, in which each individual cellular unit works for the benefit of the whole system in autonomous and converging ways. For plants, this evolution led to the biological tools that eventually made it possible for them to cover almost the entire surface of the terrestrial planet. But before that could happen, the hard rock surface of Earth had to be broken down into minerals available for life. And that would not have been possible without fungi.

Although fungi represent only 10 percent of life on Earth, no terrestrial life as we know it would exist without them.[16] Fungi can be found in every ecosystem on the planet—on rocks, in rivers, in the hot desert of the Mojave and the cold deserts of the Arctic, in forests, in tropical jungles, in thermal hot springs—even in the depths, on the ocean floors, which may be one of the largest fungal habitats.[17]

Lichens, the first life-form to emerge on the rocky surface of the Earth, are a composite organism, made up of species from two or more kingdoms, often fungi and bacteria. While fungi usually get their energy from organic material around them, lichens' cyanobacteria get their energy from the sun and share this resource with the fungi who bore into rock, liberating mineral nutrients and creating soil. Today these ancient relationships endure, as lichens cover 10 percent of the planet's surface, literally laying the groundwork for more life.[18]

In 1867 the Swiss botanist Simon Schwendener first suggested that lichens were made up of two different kingdoms within a single life-form. The initial response by the scientific community was ridicule.[19] Modern biology, and the medicine that rests upon it, has been part of an epic misrecognition of self and other. Hence the quote at the beginning of this chapter, from a remarkable scholarly takedown of the biological idea of individualism, by biologists Scott F. Gilbert and Jan Sapp, and physician and philosopher Alfred I. Tauber. The truth is that we are all systems of life that stretch across biological kingdoms and across space and time. Individual organisms are constituted in mutualism and exchange in which the borders between self and other are fluid. That we have failed to appreciate the significance of this web of life reflects on the individualist strain in the human sciences, the sciences borne of modern liberalism. If your biological theory allows you only to look for individuals, then the research technology you'll develop as a result will be very good at investigating individuals. But if your theory is different, the world is cracked open.[20]

Sophisticated ecological systems thinking in Europe and North America dates from the mid-twentieth century. For thousands of years, however, Indigenous forms of knowledge have revealed and attended to the interconnected systems, the complex networks, that make life possible. We've drawn on Indigenous systems thinking and on research in biology, ecology, and political economy to see individuals within systems in a new way: interacting through relationships of power, history, mutualism, and care. Within those networks, the processes of birth and death and regeneration constitute the cycles of life on Earth.

A system approaching a steady state, or a type of homeostasis, is a highly interconnected network in which positive and negative feedback balance and benefit the whole structure. Such a system is stable and resilient to disturbance when the distribution of energy and resources is even and when care of the whole network is prioritized.[21] Colonial capitalism suppresses the equitable distribution of resources, expending great energy—through extraction, border construction, incarceration, and the creation of supremacist cosmologies and institutions—to maintain a structure that prioritizes individuals over communities. Without the networking-capacity benefit of communities, society under colonial capitalism is more vulnerable to the shocks and failures of systems within systems, which we see with pandemics, raging wildfires, and stock market volatility.

At this historic moment, when the web of life is in unprecedented peril, engagement with systems thinking is critical, allowing us to locate medicine, health, and care in new ways. Our diagnostic journey has shown how disease is situated in the spaces around the body, in the exposome, and in the cumulative history of relationships lived through our bodies and minds. We are complex holobionts, with emergent properties that can't be predicted by looking discretely at the parts. There's no greater demonstration of this complexity and relationality than in the emergent behavior of consciousness in our nervous system. Consciousness, understood as an emergent systemic property that confers a remarkable social intelligence and empathy for others, is the opposite of Descartes's dualism.[22] We exist in and are made by our connections to the world. Pando is and becomes Pando.

THE TREE OF LIFE

The science of human biology has been overtaken by the insight that to understand how we function optimally and how we get sick, we must develop a more sophisticated understanding of systems-level interactions. While the last century's frontiers of biology focused on the gene, this century is defined by its fascination with systems, from the gut microbiome to neural networks. Both of these systems impact the biology of the mind, which is not located simply in the brain but is a composite of phenomena that occur throughout the body—an oscillating identity, fully embodied but not restricted to one site.

The nervous system is the fastest system of communication in the body, facilitating the sending and receiving of electrical signals through a network of specialized nerve cells called neurons. Neurons can be bundled together with connective tissue and blood vessels to create nerves, which branch out from the brain and spinal cord (the central nervous system) like a tree, extending the tiniest twigs into every tissue in the body (the peripheral nervous system).[23] While neurons do the bulk of the communication work in the nervous system, there are just as many support cells that protect, insulate, and nourish neurons, called glial cells.[24]

Three main functions of the nervous system include receiving sensory input from sensory receptors (like our eyes), integrating those signals into information by the brain (a tiger), then sending out signals to tell the muscles what to do in response to that integration (run!). But other functions are just as important, like integrating sensations of love into a sense of knowing where we belong and with whom.[25] We experience the world by merging different sensory inputs. The nervous system brings together all the other systems. It is the conductor of the body's orchestra, one that doesn't dominate but unifies the different voices, sets the tempo, listens critically, and shapes the interpretation of the music, keeping all the parts moving together as an integrated whole.

From the instruments of this orchestra emerges the experience of consciousness.[26] Although no individual neuron is capable of consciousness, the network of neurons throughout our body is a system sufficiently complex for new properties to emerge. Consciousness isn't merely an epiphenomenon of our brains—it confers an evolutionary advantage in helping us predict the world around us and, in particular, to anticipate, understand, and learn from other people.[27]

The shape of a neuron matters to its function. Its small finger-like projections called dendrites receive multiple signals, sometimes at the same moment. These signals travel to the cell body, where they are summed up into one singular signal and then sent down the axon. When the signal reaches the terminus, it changes from an electrical impulse to a chemical one through the release of neurotransmitters, such as dopamine or serotonin, into the space between connecting neurons called the synapse. From a systems perspective, a neuron is an information node with many inputs and only one output.[28] A neural network is made up of interconnected neurons, taking in signals both from the world and from our bodies and correlating them with outgoing signals.[29] Over time, the network receives more inputs and sends output signals based on prior learning. This is how we accumulate knowledge based on experience: learning.[30]

Learning is how we nongenetically transmit information that is vital for our survival. And language is a critical aspect of cultural learning and transmission. Language development occurs simultaneously with brain network development, so it's not surprising that childhood is the time when the greatest learning happens.[31] There appears to be a critical window in development beyond which language learning is far less successful. But all hope is not lost for adults. Learning a second language in adulthood, although difficult, can be done and is accompanied by an increase in brain size to handle the new information, the growth proportional to how well you pick up the language and how much effort you put into learning it.[32] The networks that are laid out, used, and reinforced through language learning are a powerful example of a system functioning at higher levels of order than the sum of its individual neurons.

When neurological systems are working well, you're able to engage in fluent conversation, to read, to name and recall, to ponder and imagine and explore and analyze. Colonial capitalism puts pressure on this system, straining these cognitive capacities, particularly in people who are denied the means for survival. Poverty is a cognitive burden.[33] Working in poverty so that you and your family may eat every day takes a neurological toll: poverty is associated with lower attention and lower working memory capacity. Rallying talk from the wealthy to pull oneself up by one's bootstraps rings particularly hollow when one's mental faculties are consumed by the demands of survival. Worse yet, the experience of surviving within the systems of exploitation within colonial capitalism has been individualized. Government policy and medicine are often blind to the ways the nervous system is connected to the world. You are encouraged to develop resilience, a personal habit of being robust to the shocks of a system that you cannot change.[34]

INFLAMMAGING

The erosion of neural networks is seen in the inflammatory brain disease Alzheimer's dementia. In dementia, the self becomes fragmented, not in a pattern of normal aging but through the damage of neuroinflammation. The system starts to break down. And the loss of language is the first place it's often detected. Linguistic markers can predict the likelihood of developing Alzheimer's with remarkable accuracy.[35] People forget the names of objects and of the people with whom they have shared their whole lives, a loss that has profound consequences for the sense of self that is made through these connections.

George Connolly's family knew him as ornery and cantankerous. He had spent his life working blue-collar jobs in San Francisco, from sandblasting ships at the Hunters Point shipyard in his youth to repairing cars as an auto mechanic for several decades. He hated going to doctors, calling them "phonies" when they advised him to get yearly checkups or pursue preventive care measures like tracking his cholesterol level. Even as he aged and was suffering from various ailments, he interacted with the health care system as little as possible. At eighty years old, he lived alone in a small one-bedroom apartment in San Francisco's Richmond District. He had been divorced for forty years but had two adult children who checked in on him. Often when they came by, he would criticize their help: they didn't bring the right groceries, they arrived at the wrong time, they stayed either too briefly or too long. When George walked to the local corner store to get sundries, he would pause every block or so to catch his breath, taking in the foggy air. He had no friends, in spite of having lived in the same area since he was in his twenties.

Adam Connolly worried when his father didn't return his calls for two days; sure enough, when he went to go check up on him, George was on the couch, looking pale and running a fever. George was hospitalized for a urinary tract infection that had spread to his blood, and while he was being treated, his son stayed by his bedside. Adam noticed that George had been unusually withdrawn and quiet, but with antibiotics and fluids, he perked right up. That was when he asked to speak privately to the care team.

"Something's wrong with my dad," he confided. "He's usually really cranky and kind of unbearable. But over the past month or so, he's become really considerate. He's asking me how I'm doing when I go to visit him. He thanks me for the things I bring over, which is totally not like him. Sometimes he seems to be confused as to where he is when he's walking around his own place. He seems totally with it when I talk to him, but this is so out of character for him. Something's off."

When the hospital team investigated, they found that George's cognitive abilities were in fact quite compromised. In casual conversation, he chatted you up with stories of his youth, his old-man charm giving you no reason to suspect that anything was wrong. But when you probed deeper, posing questions that required recollection, spatial analysis, or fixing new memories, he faltered. If you asked him what year it was, he'd confidently reply, "1965," with a look like you were an idiot for asking in the first place. After a referral to memory specialists and the completion of diagnostic tests, it was clear that George had Alzheimer's dementia. This was the reason his personality had changed toward the end of his life.

Dementia is a set of symptoms associated with memory deficits and problems in reasoning skills. It is not a normal part of aging and is caused by damage to cellular communication in the brain, which can lead to cognitive, emotional, and behavioral changes. One of the most precious aspects of elderhood is sharing the hard-earned wisdom of lived experience with younger generations—often in stories of shocking audacity. Such stories tell younger people who they are and where they come from. Our elders are our living historians, serving as vital links between the past, the present, and the future. With dementia, their wisdom is lost.

There are many types of dementia, but Alzheimer's is overwhelmingly the most common. More than 35 million people worldwide suffer from it; death can be expected just three to nine years after diagnosis.[36] Nearly six million people in the United States currently live with Alzheimer's, a number predicted to rise up to 16 million by 2050 due to the growing elderly population. Between 2000 and 2018, deaths from heart disease decreased 7.8 percent, while deaths from Alzheimer's increased 146 percent.[37] The main risk factor is age, but an extensive study of a 115-year-old woman shows that the disease is not a necessary outcome of aging.[38] The brain changes that accompany Alzheimer's are not inevitable.[39]

For decades, researchers have been trying to understand what causes Alzheimer's dementia. One characteristic finding in the brains of Alzheimer's patients is the buildup of two proteins, amyloid-β and tau. Amyloid-β is the main constituent of the plaques that are deposited in the brain and lead to cell death, vascular injury, and the clinical phenomenon of dementia.[40] Tau protein makes neurofibrillary tangles between nerve cells, and its amount is associated with the disease's severity.[41] Where these plaques and tangles show up determines what parts of the brain (and therefore the mind) are impacted. It makes sense for scientists to conclude that preventing or reducing the buildup of these proteins would improve Alzheimer's symptoms. In fact, however, none of the drugs that target buildup have prevented or even halted the progression of symptoms.[42] Indeed, one trial showed that removing the proteins made the symptoms worse.[43]

Researchers then asked more upstream questions about the disease, following clues from the past to understand why the plaques appeared in the first place. Over a million survivors of the 1918 flu pandemic went on to develop Parkinson's disease, another form of dementia, which is characterized by the buildup of the protein α-synuclein.[44] One has to wonder how the brain fog and dementia-like symptoms impacting many Covid survivors today portends increased neurological issues in the future.[45] Alzheimer's amyloid-β and Parkinson's α-synuclein levels both rise with infection. Produced by the brain's innate immune response, they behave as antimicrobials.[46] Genetic analysis has tied almost all the genes involved in the development of Alzheimer's to the immune system.[47] Its plaques are closely associated with a type of immune cell called microglial cells.[48]

Microglial cells are the immune cells residing in the brain, where they serve as the mediators of inflammation, becoming activated in the face of infection, cell damage, or other stress. An activated microglial cell is the nervous system equivalent of an activated macrophage in the body's periphery. In fact, microglial cells are derived from macrophages that migrate during embryonic development and take up permanent residence in the brain, where they differentiate into their mature form.[49] As the brain's macrophages, they are in charge of immune defense and the maintenance of homeostasis. Rudolf Virchow offered us the first images of activated microglial cells more than 150 years ago, in his seminal work, *Cellular Pathology*.[50] He understood them as cells in the brain that aren't nerve cells but rather some sort of filler in the space between neurons.

Microglial cells are not just passive filler. They are in fact like parent cells to neurons, existing in two different states. One is supportive and works to keep the area around neurons clean. In this housekeeping role, they help to repair tissue, to secrete growth factor, and to phagocytose infectious elements, dead neurons, and other debris, even amyloid-β.[51] The other state is pro-inflammatory. They secrete cytokines and free radicals, such as reactive oxygen species and IL-1β, which can injure nearby nerve cells.[52] Astrocytes are another brain cell closely related to microglial cells. They also regulate neuroinflammation.[53] Chronic stress can invoke a senescence-associated secretory phenotype in astrocytes, making them a source of localized inflammation in the brain.[54]

As with macrophages in wound healing, balance is key. Normally, pro-inflammatory activity is self-limited, turning off once homeostasis is achieved. Sustained activation means that an inflammatory stimulus is chronic or the response simply fails to stop. When it continues unabated, it produces the inflammation that is a hallmark of neurodegenerative conditions such as Alzheimer's, Parkinson's, Huntington's, multiple sclerosis, and amyotrophic lateral sclerosis.[55] Understanding what flips a microglial cell from the housekeeping state to the inflammatory state, and keeps it there, will be key to further characterizing the pathophysiology of these diseases. What is no longer in question, in the face of abundant evidence, is that inflammation drives the network breakdown we see in these neurodegenerative diseases.

Consider two experiments with rats and mice. In a laboratory, researchers repeatedly introduced young male rats into cages with older, larger aggressor rats.[56] After a few confrontations, the younger rats, socially defeated, were loaded with stress signals. Their immune systems changed. Stress primed their monocytes, the precursors to macrophages, to throw off more pro-inflammatory signals than before they were socially defeated. Under stress, monocytes travel across the blood-brain barrier, where they can directly impact the brain. In a second experiment, mice were given an electrical shock to the foot; others close to them had higher levels of inflammation-primed cells in their brains.[57] Pain and social defeat, ours and that of others, brings inflammation to the brain.

Here it becomes startlingly clear how our nervous system is connected to the immune system, and how these systems are connected to our experience of the world, to the systems that cause suffering to others. Our reaction to others' pain can inflame our brains. Our consciousness is a tool through which we can understand others, to sympathize and to be moved to care. When the violent ordering of colonial capitalism makes some people suffer, we all do.

JUSTICE IS THE MEDICINE

On December 2, 2015, San Francisco Police Department officers killed twenty-six-year-old Mario Woods in the predominantly Black neighborhood of Bayview, and no cops were held accountable for the murder. His family and other community members fighting for justice asked the doctors of the Do No Harm Coalition to design a research study to answer a critical question: if a police killing is a wound, and justice is the medicine, what happens to our community's health if the medicine is withheld? The findings are obvious. When police murder with impunity, everyone suffers. Preliminary results indicated that killings create widespread PTSD and that lack of justice compounds this effect. As we have seen, trauma and PTSD are potent activators of inflammation. Erica Garner died of a heart attack at the age of twenty-seven, just three years after police killed her father, Eric Garner, showing the toll this violence takes by way of inflammation.[58] A police killing creates concentric circles of death in its wake and erodes a community's health from the inside out.

That the trauma caused by police killings had to be documented by a research study in order to influence policy is another example of how Black testimony doesn't matter. The stories of suffering and violent video recordings should say enough. But one striking takeaway from the Justice Study's findings was this: while Black and brown community members are most impacted by the trauma, white people suffer too.[59] Our consciousness has evolved to recognize the suffering of other beings. Even if we are taught over a lifetime to depersonalize the web of life, and other people, we have evolved over millennia to care about suffering, because we have evolved as social animals. When injustice to one person happens, all who witness it carry the allostatic load.

The Justice Study from the Do No Harm Coalition also found that this load is not distributed equally, as BIPOC carry the heaviest burden. Stress ages the brain in ways that lead to cognitive decline. The impact is dose dependent: the more stressful events you experience, the greater your degree of mental impairment will be. Which is why it's important to remember that lifetimes of stress add up differently for different communities. A stressful event can cause changes in the brain that create a permanent cognitive impairment by literally changing the architecture of neurons and the density of connectivity.[60] A tragedy like losing a child can result in lower scores in tests of memory and executive function. In white people, that cognitive loss is the equivalent to a year of aging. For Black people in the United States, the same stressful event led to the equivalent of aging four years.[61] Black people report up to 84 percent more mean lifetime stressful events than white folks.[62] Cumulative lifetime stress accelerates the aging of the brain, and the rate of acceleration is directly proportional to how damaging the exposome is.[63]

As we have seen, racism is a cognitive load that is experienced throughout the body. It provokes a cascading series of responses, just like what you experience during fight-or-flight: your heartbeat will rise, your breath will quicken, and you'll start to sweat. When you are under stress, your body's sympathetic nervous system will ready you for action. As a result of this involuntary nervous system activity, the electrical resistance across your skin drops.[64] This used to be called the electrogalvanic response, but now it's known as electrodermal response, and it can be measured with some simple electronics. (These are also the responses that polygraphs or lie detectors look for to determine whether you're lying—your body tells the truth through its autonomic actions.[65])

A recent study measured the racism Black and Latinx students experience on a majority-white midwestern U.S. university campus.[66] The researchers provided the students with a wearable device to track skin conductivity, and a journal in which they were to reflect on their experiences with racism in three-hour blocks. This method made it possible in real time to see the intensity of the allostatic load borne by people of color in a white supremacist society. Carried out under the Donald Trump presidency, a time of increasing hate crimes and the racist stigmatization of immigrants, when 70 percent of Black and 56 percent of Latinx students reported racism on campus, the burden was unmistakable.

Over a lifetime, the allostatic load of race and class creates a disproportionately toxic exposome for the brain. Chronic stress and allostatic load affect the whole brain and cause atrophy of neurons in the specific regions responsible for behavior and cognitive function—the hippocampus, the amygdala, and the prefrontal cortex.[67] And this all plays out in the dramatic racial disparities of who will suffer from Alzheimer's. In the United States, a sixty-five-year-old Black person faces a 38 percent likelihood of developing Alzheimer's in the next twenty-five years. For Native Americans, the risk is 35 percent, and 32 percent for Latinx, 25 percent for Pacific Islanders, 30 percent for whites, and 28 percent for Asian-Americans.[68] It's clear that Black people suffer disproportionately from Alzheimer's.[69] Social support systems and income offer some buffer to stress's effects on the brain, but simply put, injustice ages us and makes us more prone to cognitive decline.[70] That inequality is the result of social choices—segregation, domination, and supremacy—made by the few. To change the cognitive outcomes experienced by people of color, those choices must be undone.

THE MIND OUTSIDE YOUR BRAIN

All systems within the body are connected to systems outside. Social and ecological stressors cause depression and cognitive decline through inflammation not just in the brain. Inflammation in other bodily systems—circulatory, digestive, endocrine, and so one—also affect our consciousness and mental states. One study, after adjusting for demographics and cardiovascular risk factors associated with inflammation, found that people in their forties and fifties with higher markers of *systemic* inflammation were more likely to have greater mental impairment over the following twenty years.[71] Systemic inflammation also worsens the progression of cognitive decline in Alzheimer's patients.[72] One means by which systemic inflammation is translated into brain inflammation is a pro-inflammatory cytokine— tumor necrosis factor α (TNF-α)—that is produced by circulating macrophages. Once it is in the central nervous system, TNF-α activates microglial cells along the inflammatory pathway that causes and exacerbates neurodegeneration.[73] There is still much to untangle in the complex mechanics of inflammation, but current research is dramatically changing our understanding of the very nature of the mind-body relationship.

For decades, the brain was viewed as a site that does not develop the same kind of inflammatory response as other parts of the body—it was thought to have "immune privilege."[74] That view suggests a kind of upstairs-downstairs dynamic, in which the brain is somehow cordoned off from the body's other organs, not deigning to interact with whatever lowly processes are happening below.

Recent discoveries, however, contradict this understanding. In fact, the brain is directly tied to and influenced by those processes, and nothing better demonstrates this fact than the gut microbiome.

What we know now about the importance of the forest living inside us gives us a glimpse of how a robust gut microbiome is vital to modulating the brain's functions. For example, some people who receive successful fecal transplants to counter *Clostridium difficile* infection—the hard-to-treat bacterium that can cause life-threatening illness when out of balance in the colon—enjoy not only the relief of their gastrointestinal symptoms but also improved mental health.[75]

Through blood and the microcircuits of neural connections, the brain and the digestive system are intertwined in what is called the *gut-brain-microbiota axis*.[76] The science of gut-brain connections is very young, but what we are learning is already remarkable.[77] The gut produces up to 90 percent the body's serotonin, controlled by signals coming from our microbes.[78] Serotonin, as we saw in Chapter 7, is a hormone and neurotransmitter that creates a sense of well-being, derived from the essential amino acid tryptophan. Like melatonin, for which it serves as a precursor, serotonin is ubiquitous in the animal and plant kingdom. The pathway for making serotonin is the same in humans as it ever was, back when cyanobacteria were floating in the primordial oceans, changing Earth's atmosphere one oxygen molecule at a time. When plant life evolved from single-cell organisms to multicellular complexity, levels of serotonin inside them rose dramatically.[79] Tryptophan is the molecule in plants responsible for harnessing the energy of the sun, and serotonin was beneficial in minimizing UV damage in the face of this energizing event.[80] In humans, sunlight also plays a role in serotonin levels. Seasonal depression in the winter months is caused by low serotonin levels and can be treated with light therapy. When we don't have enough of this hormone, we are prone to depression and other stress-related states, including, at the most extreme, suicidal ideation.[81]

Traditionally, researchers studied the development of the nervous system by focusing on the brain. But over the past few decades, it has become clear that signals from outside the brain are central to this process. Not only is the gut the largest portal between the inside of the body and the world around us, but molecules in our food can directly affect how the brain develops.[82] Recently, a burst of research has demonstrated that gut microbes communicate with the nervous system, in a dialogue crucial for healthy development, behavior, and immune response.[83] Disruptions in that communication are implicated in depression, anxiety, cognitive problems, and autism.[84]

During gestation and the early months of infancy, gut microbes are involved in signaling that shapes the growing nervous system. They play a role in the development of the blood-brain barrier,[85] the uniquely selective lining of blood vessels that tightly regulates the movement of molecules, ions, and cells into and out of the brain. This barrier is critical to homeostasis and keeps the brain safe when the body is exposed to a toxin or experiences wild fluctuations in ions such as sodium.[86] This may be one of the pathways through which the exposures—or lack of them—in youth come to make such a difference in bodies across different social groups as we age.

Gut microbes are also crucial to myelination, the coating of neurons' long fibers with insulation that acts like the covering on an electric wire.[87] Without these microbes, nerve signals don't reach their destination. And this microbial caretaking may be continuous: a study of autoimmune encephalomyelitis, in which the brain and myelin are inflamed, found that polysaccharide A, produced by the gut bacteria *Bacteroides fragilis*, travels to the brain and protects the central nervous system from demyelination and inflammation.[88] Moreover, gut microbes play a critical role in the maturation of microglial cells, which are so central to our discussion of neurodegenerative diseases and inflammation.[89]

Throughout our lives, the gut microbiome shapes and influences the brain and therefore the mind. The feces of people with Alzheimer's dementia contain less microbial biodiversity than those of age-matched, sex-matched elders with no dementia.[90] Our gut micro-biome changes as we age, which may make us more prone to developing cognitive difficulties. After young mice were transfused with feces from old mice with spatial reasoning issues, their microbiomes shifted to match those of the older mice, and they too began to display spatial reasoning issues.[91] It's as if cognitive skills or lack thereof were somehow transplanted by way of the feces. One has to wonder what would happen if the experiment were reversed—would the old mice regain spatial functioning?

Gut dysbiosis is associated with several kinds of mental illness. Depression and anxiety are often explained either as personal failures or as hardwired into the brain. But evidence now shows that social stress, particularly poverty, has inflammatory effects that change our gut, which in turn can reduce microbial diversity and lead to changes in the brain.[92] Your depression and anxiety may be less an intrinsic part of your character than a consequence of experiencing intersecting forces of colonial capitalism. They may be what it feels like to be embedded in the converging systems of our biology and our exposome. The allostatic load of oppression, lived through and recorded within our bodies, reshapes our minds. While all these associations are pointing toward underlying causation, and while large gaps in our understanding remain, the challenge that such discoveries pose to assumptions of mind-body dualism—and even to the very concept of self—is striking.[93]

The idea that the presence or absence of organisms in our gut can directly affect the development and functioning of our brain is expanding the limits of our imagination. Instead of focusing simply on plaques and tangles, for instance, doctors who study neurodegenerative disease are now looking at the whole body and at how systemic and localized inflammation accelerates it. Path-breaking research into the role of tending the "other"—microbes—in taking care of ourselves has fundamentally changed our understanding of health and well-being. These examples of how our health is an effect of systems within systems show how ineffective reductionist frameworks are for understanding the causes of the many inflammatory diseases that are making us sick.

Despite these strides in our comprehension, humans continue to treat one another, and the web of life, as disposable. They continue to treat the mind as separate from both the body and the natural world. The colonial cosmology of infinite growth, infinite greed, and a planet that can infinitely absorb our follies is becoming increasingly hard to sustain. The violence needed to enforce that delusion causes widespread trauma and the deaths of the people and world we love. Yet even as we mourn, we can find hope. Our collective rituals of grief can knit us together, like the oscillating intelligence of the Pando forest, its tens of thousands of trees united under the soil as one being, a multiplicity that itself is overwritten by the memory of killings in Bolivia.

COMPOSTING OUR GRIEF

Funerals of those killed by the state have long been rituals of political community, sites for collective mourning. The British, during their colonization of India in the nineteenth century, moved to restrict women's public lamentations. In 1985 the South African apartheid regime banned funerals for more than one person. In Belgrade, the Women in Black protest the official denial of the Srebrenica massacre.[94] In Buenos Aires's Plaza de Mayo, the mothers of the Argentinian disappeared protest that silence.[95] And in a Houston church, people gathered, even under Covid lockdown, to grieve together the murder of George Floyd.[96] A funeral can be a collective act of diagnosis, telling the story of a killing not simply through biology but through the social and political conditions that precipitated it. Collective mourning allows the bereaved an opportunity to crack grief open and find the hope inside. It is a moment for testimonies of injustice to be witnessed, heard, and held.

Funerals offer us a chance to connect to one another politically through stories that narrate the story of illness, but they are also a reminder of each body's place in the web of life, a lesson in ecology for the living. In some traditions, the body of a dead person is returned to the soil to decompose. In others, it is cremated and scattered in a river, to become sediment and life again. The Zoroastrian religion mandates a sky burial: when a person has died, they are to receive their death rites, and then their body is left in the open as an offering to vultures.[97] In India, as Zoroastrians moved into cities, they built Towers of Silence, open-air temples where bodies could be ritually consumed.

Today the vultures are disappearing, poisoned by humans. Vultures sit at the top of the food chain, feeding on the carcasses of animals that have been exposed to the industrial chemistry of Indian industrial agriculture. Their bodies accumulate the toxins, like DDT, and are now in catastrophic population decline. There aren't enough vultures left to allow Zoroastrian humans to pass into the spirit world.[98]

Zoroastrian traditions share with every other tradition some route for the dead human body to reintegrate back into the web of life. Care for the dead is also care for the living, and a reminder that we came from air, water, dust—and that to there, we will return. Whatever rituals we use to grieve our dead, they all transmute the pain of grief into healing. Vocalizing our grief—storytelling, groaning, wailing, and singing—can be healing, quite literally: when we use our voices, the nervous system works to counter inflammation.

The vagus nerve is the longest in the human body. Starting in the brainstem, it gets its name from the Latin *vagus*, "wandering," and like a vagabond, it travels to and innervates most of our internal organs, influencing how fast the heart beats and when digestive juices are secreted into the intestines.[99] Whereas the sympathetic nervous system makes up part of the stress response, the vagus nerve is a part of the opposing parasympathetic nervous system, which prepares the body to rest and digest. It plays an important role in modulating the immune response, and the cytokines it induces are decidedly anti-inflammatory.[100]

When the vagus nerve is well toned through regular stimulation, it creates greater resilience in the face of stress.[101] The anti-inflammatory state that comes with vagus nerve stimulation is being applied as treatment for inflammatory bowel disease and depression.[102] Excitation of the vagus nerve with electricity can have an immediate impact on stopping inflammatory cytokine production and has been demonstrated to improve survival in experimental models of sepsis.[103] A better way to stimulate the nerve than submitting oneself to electric shocks is through singing or chanting. The vagus nerve courses through the back of the throat and innervates the vocal cords. Chanting may coax it to exert its anti-inflammatory effect.[104] The nerve also innervates the lungs and may explain why contemplative activities that include focus on breathing, such as mediation, lower inflammation.[105] Singing has a range of demonstrable health benefits, from upregulating oxytocin, to improving outcomes with dementia patients, to building social bonds that sustain and enrich our lives.[106] Singing with one another has always been a form of protest against colonialism, a way of transmuting grief over the illness and death that it causes. Settlers have always understood this power, teaching hymns that drown out the voices of the colonized and enforcing the compulsory amnesia of the healing songs of Indigenous peoples.[107]

THE ORIGINAL WORLD WIDE WEB

When Solomon Reese, the Tsimshian Saulteaux man whom we met in Chapter 3, said, "The land is made of our ancestors' bodies reentering the life cycle," he was speaking directly of the alchemy that is the work of the fungal kingdom, turning death back into life as it recycles nutrients through its network. On a cellular level, fungi sit somewhere between plants and animals, sharing characteristics of both groups and serving as a bridge between them. As our bodies are sent to decompose, our mourning songs generate real biological change within the living. Fungi will ultimately transform the dead back into new life.

Today the largest organism on the planet isn't a blue whale. It is an agent of both death and decomposition, and of regeneration and rebirth. A honey fungus in Oregon—"the humongous fungus"—is a parasite more than two thousand years old and hundreds of hectares wide.[108] Known as *Armillaria ostoyae*, it threads through the soil and roots of what is now called the Malheur National Forest, in Paiute territory. It exists as a thick, white, rubbery substance that secretes digestive enzymes, killing trees from the inside, slowly, over decades, rendering them useless to commercial foresting projects.[109] The honey fungus's long-term effect is uncertain: it shortens the lives of trees but is also one of the few organisms able to break them down into the soil from which new trees can emerge.[110] Climate change is complicating the picture, making the conditions for its spread, and the spread of pathogenic fungi in general, more favorable, to the detriment of symbiotic fungi.[111] From this death, too, can come rebirth.

The word *mycorrhiza* comes from the Greek *mycos*, "fungus," and *rhiza*, "root," and denotes a relationship between fungus and the roots of plants.[112] In fact, plant roots coevolved with the fungal elements of the mycorrhizae.[113] When early plant cells emerged from the ocean onto land, they couldn't access the micronutrients present in the rocks. So they partnered with fungi, who break down rock, making minerals such as phosphorus, zinc, and copper available to the plants. In turn, the plants make sugar from the sunlight, 20 percent of which it gives to the fungus. It is a relationship that continues today. Up to 90 percent of modern land-based plants have mycorrhizae, an example of one of the oldest and most enduring symbiotic relationships between kingdoms.[114]

Mycorrhizae operate as a system of care for plants and for the ecosystem where those plants grow. They extend the functional surface area of a plant's root system by sending their threadlike projections deeper into the soil. Through them, the plant can absorb more water and vital nutrients. The mycorrhizae retain water and make it available to the plant, helping it to resist drought.[115] They secrete acids that break down neighboring dead organic matter, enabling their uptake by the host. Mycorrhizae also protect plants from heavy metals by clearing them from soil[116] and can even mop up oil spills, making them star players in bioremediation.[117]

If you plant a tree in soil unfamiliar to it, it may not thrive without some dirt—including the dirt's fungi—from its native territory.[118] That dirt protects the plant from pathogens and other stresses.[119] Only after mycorrhizae were established did plants cover the Earth, evolving traits, such as flowers, fruits, and seeds, that made animal life possible. All these functions boost the host plant's immunity and resilience.[120]

Mycorrhizae connect plants to one another through exquisitely fine white threads, hyphae, and to the larger network of fungi in the soil, known as the mycelial web.[121] As the biologist Merlin Sheldrake writes, "The total length of mycorrhizal hyphae in the top ten centimeters of soil is around half the width of our galaxy."[122] The mycelial web looks like a network of neurons—and indeed plays this role for plants—extending through the dirt, sending molecular messages between plants, like the electrical impulses of the nervous system. These signals can confer greater resistance to disease for the plants.[123] And like neural networks, systems of plants communicate through them and even learn, leading to what the ecologist Suzanne Simard calls "forest wisdom."[124] You can see the mycelial web when you turn over the top inch of healthy soil or a decaying piece of wood. In some forests, this web helps to transfer carbon from one plant to another.[125]

Nutrient exchange may appear to be an altruistic behavior by trees—they seem to be giving away resources for the good of the community. But if we could imagine the consciousness of this network, we might say that the mycelial web functions as a life-form involved in care. Mycelia tend the forest for the mutual benefit of fungi and trees. The mycelial web looks after itself only by taking care of, and in symbiosis with, the world that it inhabits. Flourishing is predicated on generosity toward the life of others.

MUSHROOM MEDICINE

The fungal kingdom is a bridge between plants, animals, and microbes, facilitating a vast network of interkingdom communication, collaboration, and exchange. And the intersections and interactions between these kingdoms open the way for new insight and understanding to emerge. Mushrooms with hallucinogenic properties from the *Psilocybe* and *Amanita* genuses have featured in Indigenous cultures from Mesoamerica to Siberia to North Africa for thousands of years.[126] Debates about how long mushrooms and other mind-altering substances have been used and what role they have actually played in these cultures are challenging to settle. Pictographs and statues can tell us only so much. Like other forms of Indigenous knowledge, living histories of cultures' relationships with these medicines have gone underground after centuries of damage inflicted by colonialism.

Hallucinogenic mushrooms contain psychedelic substances that act upon the central nervous system to produce profoundly altered states of consciousness. While psycho*active* substances like coffee and wine have been used as medicines across cultures for millennia,[127] the use of psychedelic substances, from plants that can produce hallucinations, appears to be more restricted, usually in the context of ritualistic healing. From peyote cactus to medicinal mushrooms to fermented brews, mind-altering substances were part of many traditional societies' medicine practices, where the healer often consumed the substance to gain the power to address an affliction, which was often described in mixed spiritual and physical terminology.[128] One cross-cultural survey from the 1970s looked at

488 different societies and found that 90 percent of them had cultural practices involving altered states of consciousness. Of the cultures that used these practices, those with the highest rates were Indigenous people from North America. Those with the lowest rates of use were societies where monotheism thrives: North Africa, the Middle East, and Europe, including overseas Europeans.[129]

While industrial societies dose themselves on caffeine, nicotine, and alcohol to alter mood and enhance productivity, nonindustrial societies opt for substances that have the capacity to alter consciousness. Some ethnobotanists point to the role that monotheism played in eliminating the Indigenous science of plant medicine in Europe and the Middle East.[130] In a concerning shift, people from European-structured societies are now increasingly seeking out psychedelic experiences, through venues such as Ayahuasca tourism in the Peruvian Amazon. These spiritual tourists, while boosting the economic input of impoverished Indigenous communities, damage the ability of Indigenous shaman to heal within their own communities, continuing a long cycle of colonial plunder.[131]

Psychedelic substances that produce hallucinations—such as N,N-dimethyltryptamine (DMT) from ayahuasca, psilocybin from mushrooms, mescaline from peyote, and synthetic LSD from the fungus ergot[132]—all affect the same receptor in the brain: the $5HT_{2A}$ receptor.[133] This is also where the neurotransmitter serotonin acts.[134] As we have seen, serotonin is an ancient molecule critical for maintaining homeostasis in the brain.[135] Many modern antidepressants work by blocking the clearance of whatever little bit you may have from the active space between nerve cells, so it can continue to stimulate its receptors, producing what we would call a sense of well-being. The $5HT_{2A}$ receptor's activation also has potent anti-inflammatory effects, not just in the brain but all over the body, where serotonin acts as a hormone.[136] This is why both psychedelics and serotonin reuptake inhibitors such as Prozac are useful in treating depression, suicidality, and their accompanying inflammation.[137]

Before we conclude that all we need to make us feel better is more serotonin in our lives, it is important to understand that mood is created through interactions of systems within systems, with other neurotransmitters that also act as hormones, such as dopamine and adrenaline, and the dance between the immune, endocrine, and nervous systems.[138] Those interactions are influenced by the exposome. Nonetheless, a molecular focus on the $5HT_{2A}$ receptor is, in close up, very revealing of systems thinking that has until recently been anathema to colonial cosmology.

The feeling of being an "I" is an effect of these systems within systems. Psychedelics that activate the $5HT_{2A}$ receptor expand that "I" by changing the way networks interact in the brain. LSD frees brain activity from its anatomical constraints, loosening the association between brain structure and its functional connectivity. With psychedelics, systems of neural networks that are usually segregated into subnetworks become more integrated globally, and this highly integrated state is correlated with the subjective sense of the ego dissolving.[139] What was small and localized becomes infinite and decentralized, extending that "I" into the space beyond our own perceived anatomy. Psilocybin has a similar effect of ego dissolution.[140]

These substances are also known as empathogens because they cultivate a deep sense of empathy for beings outside ourselves—it's easier for us to care for others when our own ego is a little more dissolved. Psychedelics can correct our vision. If colonial capitalist cosmology sees *things* where *persons* once were, empathogens enable us to see the personhood once more. We cannot properly care for others, whether fellow humans or other animals or forests or mountains, unless we can see them. In the right context, with the correct guidance, psychedelics can return to us the capacity for which consciousness may have evolved in social creatures like ourselves: to recognize and empathize with other beings, making it possible for us to thrive.

Psychedelics offer potent medicine in these times of reconnection, as we heal from all the ways colonialism has damaged our relationships to each other and to the world. Today's standard treatments for PTSD are mostly ineffective and limited, but psychedelic medicines are opening new horizons.[141] Ironically, many medical studies demonstrating the healing effects of these medicines have been focused on military personnel, those who have been conscripted to inflict trauma on other people. US combat veterans with PTSD, after a three-day psychedelic clinic program in Mexico, had significant lasting improvements in suicidal ideation, depression, anxiety, and PTSD symptoms. Most of the participants ranked their experience as in the top five of meaningful, psychologically insightful, and spiritually significant moments of their lives.[142] A small study found that therapy with MDMA (another $5HT_{2A}$-activating substance) ameliorated PTSD symptoms in 76 percent of participants with chronic PTSD, with improvements lasting one year out.[143]

Psychedelic medicines also show promise for the treatment of depression and anxiety by fostering feelings of reconnection.[144] Patients at the end of life, who need help managing understandable anxiety around death, are also finding benefit, as the medicines promote more meaningful time with their families.[145] One dose of psilocybin was enough to lower anxiety and depression in cancer patients experiencing psychological distress.[146] Following up with the surviving patients of that study four years later, the beneficial effects from that one dose persisted, as a majority of the participants rated the experience as one of the most meaningful of their lives.[147] These medicines may even help with healing the connections injured by colonial medicine, through healing the wounded perpetrators—the physician. Using a combination of psychedelics and therapy, Dr. Mellody Hayes experienced relief from physician burnout and "deep relational healing."[148] Small studies show that psychedelics simultaneously lower symptoms of depression and reduce signs of chronic inflammation.[149]

Western uses of psychedelics have been highly individualistic: in quests for personal transformation, recreation, or increasing creative productivity through micro-dosing. While self-care is important, expanding that sense of self is urgent, as we teeter on the edge of global systems failure, through economic shocks, climate shocks, and pandemics. We must develop a greater understanding of the social use of these medicines, which is how the Indigenous cultures who have stewarded these medicines and practices have kept them alive.[150] It is through communities of care and communities of medicine that we must work to heal this wound that is too great for any one of us to heal alone.

SYSTEMS OF CARE

Earth, human societies, our bodies, and our minds are interconnected systems, and they all are in desperate need of care. We are now living in a catastrophe wrought by five centuries of extractive and individualist cosmology. Under colonial capitalism, this want of care becomes an opportunity for profit. Consider the sites of the earliest and most horrific concentrations of death under Covid: nursing homes.[151] In Europe, in the early stages of the outbreak, more than 50 percent of deaths were linked to long-term-care facilities. In Quebec, nearly 90 percent of deaths were in nursing homes.[152] Under late capitalism, the care of elders is a fix—in the vein of a prison system—to warehouse a low-income population, exploiting carers from communities where neoliberalism has devastated other forms of employment.[153] Treating elders and their carers in this way is lucrative. The global long-term-care industry was a trillion-dollar business in 2019.

Herein lies the tension. Evolution predisposes us for care. The planet, our own bodies, and our consciousness are wired for the care of others. But capitalist economic and social systems teach us to restrict the set of beings whom we're prepared to recognize as people, and to suppress the urge to care, unless money might be made from it. They misdirect our attention and obfuscate our capacity to recognize one another, and the care we need.

Humans have broken the world. The air that renders neurological disease more likely has to be cleaned.[154] Industrial agriculture has massively degraded the land, and it will take a profound shift in priorities to reverse the killing of the flora, fauna, and fungi beneath our feet.[155] In the United States, as elsewhere in the world, waterways are being polluted by agriculture and fossil fuels, and the defenders of that water are being attacked.[156] The leader of the Poor People's Campaign, Rev. William Barber, points out that "as many as five and a half million people in this nation can buy unleaded gas, but can't get unleaded water from their faucets at home."[157]

But grand visions of "care and repair," to use Naomi Klein's term, can move us beyond the failures of contemporary capitalism. Ideas like a Green New Deal are international calls to care for humans and the planet.[158] Rebuilding schools, hospitals, clinics and day cares, bridges, and transmission lines for a zero-carbon future are all important works of repair. In a sustainable future, clean air and water for every human, health care and education for all, safe and sustainable housing for everyone, an end to hunger, and even fifteen thousand kilometers of zero-carbon travel per person per year are possible.[159]

The Green New Deal, at least as it stands in the United States, is a promissory note that is already insufficient.[160] It doesn't begin to recognize that for justice to prevail outside the country, consumption within the country must be limited—people in the United States must live more simply so that others might simply live.[161] As the plant breeder Stan Cox has written, the idea of permanent economic growth allows us to escape the demands of ecology and pretend that business as usual, just "slapping solar panels on top of Walmart," is all that's needed to address the climate catastrophe.[162] But a zero-carbon economy is entirely compatible with colonial capitalism, as the Bolivian coup, and Elon Musk's support for it, suggests.

The US Green New Deal doesn't call for an end to fossil fuel consumption. For communities that have been on the front lines of fighting extraction and pollution, that's more than an oversight—it's consonant with history.[163] In the original New Deal between 1933 and 1941, the back-and-forth of strikes and struggles made compromises. Among those who were compromised: immigrants, workers, Black people, women, the infirm, the poor, and Indigenous people.

Women's rights were not guaranteed at the federal level but were left for individual states to decide; as Ruth Wilson Gilmore puts it, "men received automatically what women had to apply for individually."[164] While native-born workers enjoyed workplace protections, immigrant laborers endured "a decade of betrayal," interrupted by the largely women- and communist-led 1938 San Antonio pecan shellers' strike, which won victories against employers and the Immigration and Naturalization Service.[165] Landowning farmers did well, but tenant farmers, particularly in the South, were ineligible for direct subsidy because they were renters. Indeed, the Southern Tenants and Farmers Union called the New Deal "that economic monstrosity and bastard child of a decadent capitalism and a youthful fascism."[166]

This history is not lost on a new generation of climate activists, which is why Indigenous-led groups like the Red Nation have responded by calling for a Red Deal.[167] Like the Movement for Black Lives does, the Red Deal calls for the abolition of colonial institutions that sunder communities. And acknowledging the intersecting systems in which we are embedded, the collective behind the Red Deal demands a return to kinship with the web of life.

Under a more expansive cosmology, the ideas of "care" and "repair" shift from being investments in health care and public works programs to something far deeper. The "repair" in "care and repair" is about recognizing our need to make reparation to one another. In that process, it is the communities most offended against—whose exposomes have put them at greatest risk of harm—who can and must lead: BIPOC communities in the United States; Black, Asian, and minority ethnic communities in the UK; Indigenous peoples worldwide; those in the Global South who fell under European empires; and those vassaled to the needs of US, Chinese, Indian, Japanese, South African, and Brazilian capital. Following the lead of the Movement for Black Lives, the Red Deal sees change emerging through mass movement building rather than benevolent policy tweaks.

Decolonizing care means expanding the community with whom and for whom care is given and taken. Feminists have recognized that the duties of care have invariably fallen on women's shoulders. *Care Revolution*, written by the social scientist Gabriele Winker, is a book for an international movement to democratize care on the basis of need, to make the resources available so that we can all care for one another and, through that, ourselves.[168] Childcare, eldercare, care for the disabled, teaching, fostering, educating, healing, feeding, and tending—all these are low-carbon professions degraded by colonial capitalism and often delegated to women. But caretaking is central to the deep medicine we need to reduce the inflammation coursing through our air, water, soil, and blood. Extending that care beyond humans to all beings through the web of life is a lesson in medicine from civilizations that predate colonial capitalism.

A pan-species care revolution cannot happen, however, without a reckoning. The decolonizing project isn't a one-off reparations payment from oppressor to oppressed, from white to Black, from bourgeoisie to the working class, from men to women, from settler to Indigenous. Reparation is certainly part of the process of healing, but it cannot be dispensed through a single payment. Reparative care requires a transformation in the way we hold, exchange, and interact with one another and the web of life.

Unlearning capitalist cosmology cannot be done alone, as a project of individual therapy. It is not about an individual decision to "be kind" or to "be antiracist." Rather, it's about the solidarity of political communities, of networks of people, engaged in systemic change. A decolonial idea of care extends not just to other humans but to all relations in the web of life. We can learn new songs, but not while the old ones are being sung. Such learning is always social. To achieve that will require a vision of comprehensive abolition. Ruth Wilson Gilmore explains that "abolition is about presence, not absence. It's about building life-affirming institutions." As we together compost our grief and transmute death into life, we liberate the resources necessary to transform our world through the creation of a culture of care.

Health is not the static condition of an independent organism but a state of dynamic interaction of systems within systems, synchronized and harmonized in ways that support the thriving of the entire whole. Health is not something we can attain as individuals, for ourselves, hermetically sealed off from the world around us. An injury to one is an injury to all.

We can be healthy only when the entire community is also healthy, meaning all beings: plants, animals, water, people, soil, and air, the ancestors, and those not yet born. And this is achievable only through social, economic, political, ecological, and cosmological spheres working in an integrated fashion for the benefit of all, where resources are distributed in ways that support vitality for all, not just for a privileged few. This vision is not wishful thinking but is already in our midst. Indigenous knowledge systems and the people for whom this understanding is not about theoretical possibilities but part of their lived truths can show us how it's done—once they're protected and uplifted as the leaders in this movement, and once we understand that our own place in this work is to follow their lead.

As we move to correct our course, we are equipped with everything we need to transform our world into one that heals. The immune system, and its interconnections to the nervous and other systems, is our own internal tuning device, reflecting back to us how close we are to health. If we can train our ears to listen to what our bodies are telling us, we will know what needs to be done. And when we are on the right path, it will be clear. We will no longer be inflamed.

9

DEEP MEDICINE

MAKING THE BODY WHOLE

Decolonization, which sets out to change the order of the world, is, obviously, a program of complete disorder. But it cannot come as a result of magical practices, nor of a natural shock, nor of a friendly understanding. Decolonization, as we know, is a historical process: that is to say that it cannot be understood, it cannot become intelligible nor clear to itself except in the exact measure that we can discern the movements which give it historical form and content. Decolonization is the meeting of two forces, opposed to each other by their very nature, which in fact owe their originality to that sort of substantification which results from and is nourished by the situation in the colonies. Their first encounter was marked by violence and their existence together—that is to say the exploitation of the native by the settler—was carried on by dint of a great array of bayonets and cannons. The settler and the native are old acquaintances. In fact, the settler is right when he speaks of knowing "them" well. For it is the settler who has brought the native into existence and who perpetuates his existence. The settler owes the fact of his very existence, that is to say, his property, to the colonial system.

—FRANTZ FANON[1]

There is a speech convention called "double wampum" that once served the ceremonial purpose of allowing multiple speakers to address multiple audiences. . . . I realize that the double wampum format tends to be confusing to westerners, to whom the monologue is construed as natural, while multilogue is dismissed as disorder. Linearity is not, however, an immutable law of discourse, but a learned, cultural preference. Stepping beyond it is not hazardous to one's health. If the reader just lies down for an hour or so, the dizzy feeling will pass. She will then be able to cope with this book, her equanimity restored with the realization that the work *is* organized, after all.

—BARBARA A. MANN[2]

The coalition emerges out of your recognition that it's fucked up for you, in the same way that we've already recognized that it's fucked up for us. I don't need your help. I just need you to recognize that this shit is killing you, too, however much more softly, you stupid motherfucker, you know?

—FRED MOTEN[3]

Deep medicine brings together several kinds of stories, each showing how illness is written on the body through histories and relationships. Rather than taking things apart to know (dia-gnosis), deep medicine puts the pieces back together to understand and to heal what's been divided. It never separates a person or a community away from the web of relationships that confer sickness or health. It is from that place of understanding that healing actions become possible.

We began this book with the story of Shelia McCarley, a woman whose suffering was so protracted that she ultimately surrendered to her body's inflammatory attack on itself. By the time she arrived at the hospital in San Francisco, she had already been in the offices and hospitals of several highly trained physicians. All had taken her medical history according to standard procedure, but it was always a selective act; what counted as "history of present illness" was what medicine had already decided was relevant. Colonial medicine can't admit to a diagnosis for which colonialism itself is responsible. Dissected from her exposome, her official diagnosis couldn't possibly explain why she was so sick and why she wasn't getting better.

The first time anyone asked McCarley about her childhood exposures to industrial chemicals, she'd already been in and out of the ICU many times over and was just days away from her death. Her exposome included growing up in the Tennessee Valley Authority's industrial effluent, drinking water pulled from that ground. The Tennessee River and its toxins flowed through her, and they may well have been responsible for her death.[4] But because her doctors didn't ask the right question—what burdens her body had carried over a lifetime—we'll never know for sure.

What we do know is that she died, her immune system reacting to her exposome and her illness trapped within the oppressive bounds of colonial medicine's narratives.

MODERN MEDICINE IS A PRISON, ABOLITION IS THE CURE

When Covid put us all under lockdown, capitalism magnified the crisis. The SARS-CoV-2 virus that causes Covid thrives in places of incarceration. By the end of 2020, one in five prisoners in the United

States were infected, and thousands were dead.[5] The virus ravaged the Navajo nation, Diné Bikéyah, where Indigenous people have been hemmed into reservations on their own ancestral lands, at times with no access to running water.[6] It jumped species in places where bats have become enclosed as city limits expanded and felled forests.[7] The virus moved through millions of caged Danish mink, kept in captivity to harvest their skins for coats and fake eyelashes. The state's solution, as usual, was extermination: 17 million mink were slaughtered and buried.[8] Lacking facilities to incinerate so many corpses, farmers buried them in shallow graves. When their bodies decomposed, they bloated and were pushed above ground, threatening to pollute the groundwater.[9]

Covid spread where elders are warehoused, in nursing homes where aging has become a condition to be managed rather than honored. In a San Francisco group shelter for the unhoused, 67 percent of residents and 17 percent of staff tested positive, while thirty thousand hotel rooms that would have afforded safe quarters through the pandemic sat empty.[10] In Singapore, over 50 percent of low-wage workers got infected. While the rest of the economy opened up, they were confined to dormitories.[11]

As the world anxiously awaited a vaccine to address the Covid pandemic, the virus kept mutating, developing new maneuvers to continue expanding its reach. Deep medicine recognizes that the virus runs rampant through spaces of incarceration, spaces that have been created through systems of domination that colonialism has entrenched. Those institutions must be liberated, through the transformation of our relationships—social, economic, ecological, and interpersonal. While we can keep engineering vaccines for the next pandemic, endless shots of mRNA may not be as effective as ensuring these viruses can't get a foothold in the first place. To prevent the next coronavirus, we must transform the very exposome that colonialism creates.

• • •

Now that we've diagnosed the link between Covid and the institutions of incarceration, we have treatment options. Vaccines, mask-
ing, and social distancing are important in the short term. In the long
term, however, what we prescribe is fugitivity. In his book *Stolen
Life* (from the second volume in the *consent not to be a single being*
trilogy), the Black antischolar Fred Moten explains that fugitivity "is
a desire for and a spirit of escape and transgression of the proper
and the proposed. It's a desire for the outside, for a playing or being
outside, an outlaw edge proper to the now always already improper
voice or instrument."[12]

Fugitivity requires direct action to evade the structures and logic
that have come with liberal settler colonialism.[13] It calls for escaping
the bounds of the state and its colonial institutions, from the hospital
and the university to the prison and the military, and weaving political communities dedicated to healing together. Only then can we
birth a new world.

This is why abolition is one of deep medicine's central prescriptions. In her book *Are Prisons Obsolete?*, Angela Davis offers an object for meditation: "Imagine a constellation of alternative strategies
and institutions, with the ultimate aim of removing the prison from
the social and ideological landscapes of our society."[14] This idea may
seem fanciful today, but that's because a tremendous amount of resources and violence has been expended to suppress movements
that have proposed such alternatives.

Prison abolitionists like Angela Davis were fortified in their commitment to prison abolition through incarceration. In prison, writing *If They Come in the Morning* with a range of Black scholars, she
invited readers to imagine what it might be like to live in a world
without the prison-industrial complex.[15] Activist-thinkers, incarcerated and in movements like Critical Resistance, used the language
of abolition as a marker for the unfinished work of the Thirteenth
Amendment, abolishing slavery in the United States, and the incipi-
ent fascism that maintains it.[16] The work of abolition remains incom-
plete. Racial capitalism fights back, in part by spreading the myth

that prison abolition is just about opening the doors to prison and walking away.

Abolition isn't a negative rejection but a positive embrace of a better way of doing things. Abolishing prisons doesn't mean letting violence go unfettered but rather establishing systems of justice that hold the entire community accountable for the traumas that induce such violence. Abolishing the military industrial complex doesn't mean leaving American citizens vulnerable but rather decreasing the rates of trauma and subsequent inflammation being perpetrated on brown and Black people around the world.[17] Abolishing the modern private corporation doesn't mean ending coordinated enterprise but rather holding it accountable to the people it serves. Abolishing private health care doesn't mean casting individuals out into the world alone but rather opening the possibility of new institutions of healing that know to relieve suffering where it hurts to most. Abolishing means holding life precious.[18]

If the imaginative work of creating new worlds feels difficult and overwhelming to you, that's because it is. The world we live in makes such ideas feel wrong, abnormal, deviant, and sick. Colonialism wants you to feel powerless and alone. A paper cut feels bad because of inflammation, but the way we feel about ourselves and our world has less to do with biology than with the colonial cosmology that shapes our lives. How, then, do we mend what the cultural theorist Raymond Williams called the "structures of feeling" that tilt against a better future?[19]

The language of abolition in the United States is tightly woven with that of freedom from slavery. Harriet Tubman spoke of the work of abolition like this: "I had crossed the line of which I had so long been dreaming. I was free, but there was no one to welcome me to the land of freedom, I was a stranger in a strange land, and my home after all was down in the old cabin quarter, with the old folks and my brothers and sisters. But to this solemn resolution I came; I was free, and they should be free also; I would make a home for them."[20]

We began this book faulting the limits of diagnosis, of medicine's narrative. Michel Foucault understood that modern medicine meant controlling the land according to colonialism's mandates: "doctors were, along with the military, the first managers of collective space."[21] To be fugitive from colonialism's carceral enclosures, then, is to move to the edge of the life you know. It is at that border, that ecotone, that a new exchange of life can happen. Abolition is a place-making activity, with a geography that reaches into the soil and across trade routes, into the air and onto the internet. It is also a collective action, an act of reweaving ourselves back into symbiosis with one another and with our place.

Only then might we begin to plant and tend a home for freedom, as Tubman suggested. Abolition is an activity of making a home *with others*—not an individual prescription but a social one.

BEYOND THE SELF FOR DEEP MEDICINE

The first written documentation of meditation comes from India in 1500 BCE, in the texts of the Vedanta philosophical tradition. Before that, wall art in the Indus Valley, dating to between 5000 and 3500 BCE, depicted people sitting in meditative postures with their eyes half closed.[22] In the Vedas, *dhyāna* is described as the training of the mind. The Sanskrit root of the word is *dhi*, which can be translated as "imaginative vision." Meditation is common to many of the world's spiritual traditions and offers people a sense of oneness or unity, altering the perception of a separate and individual identity.

It's also now a multimillion-dollar industry, with apps, celebrity promoters, and leaderboards. Once associated with hippie enclaves such as Marin in Northern California, wellness culture has made its way into the mainstream. Corporations use meditation apps to help managers focus[23] and to wring productivity from workers in jobs they despise.[24] The executive Pierre Wack brought incense and meditation practices to Royal Dutch/Shell offices. Tapping into meditation's capacity to open up the imagination helped the company develop techniques of scenario planning that anticipated the 1973 oil shock.[25] The global holistic health industry is itself big business, expected to be worth almost $300 billion by 2027. But in servicing the very real pathologies and anxieties experienced by individuals navigating the modern world, the industry compounds the diseases it purports to treat.

The modern individual has been made through centuries of disconnection—from the world around us, from others, and even from our own bodies. While wellness trends can help us to reconnect on some level, they incorrectly focus on the power of an individual to improve their own health while ignoring—or worse, defusing— another power: our ability to collectively dismantle the hierarchies that cause these disconnections and consequently a large share of the illnesses that we face.

Holistic medicine would be a good thing if it did what it promises. But absent an analysis of power and a historical perspective on colonial cosmology, it is shallow. Holistic physicians extol the importance of the gut and soil microbiomes while insisting that white supremacy is "outside their field." They celebrate regenerative agriculture without contending with land theft or the ongoing genocide of Indigenous people. They counsel immune self-defense without worrying about police violence. Blind to power, holism in medicine has its limits—because to practice it fully would be to indict the invariably white physician in sandals peddling Indigenous knowledge and the wisdom of the East.

Truly holistic health must contend with the elements that continue to make all people unwell, locating the disease-causing entities in social structures and the grave misunderstandings that created them. Systems that position humans as supreme over the entire web of life, settler over Indigenous, a singular religion over all other worldviews, male over female and nonbinary understandings of gender, white over every other shade of skin—these must be dismantled and composted. We must reimagine our wellness collectively, not simply as individuals or communities but in relation to all the entities that support the possibility of healthy lives. These relationships, precisely because they are vital for health, are worthy of our care.

The problem is when inclusion becomes enclosure—when the radically transformative projects, theories, and futures led by Indigenous and poor people are sterilized by liberalism, and when the language and other signifiers of revolution are co-opted and incorporated into some giant soup of civil rights struggles.[26] (Think tolerance and broken window policing.) For those living in settler societies, the work of being in solidarity specifically with Indigenous-led movements is particularly critical. The collapse of ecological, social, and bodily health is an outcome of over six hundred years of cosmological warfare.

Forging new forms of solidarity is not easy. It requires abandoning colonial ties and creating new relations with other fugitives.[27] Reconnecting relations that colonialism sundered is simultaneously a personal and political project. Colonialism reproduces itself through a hegemony that has been widely internalized. Transcending it won't require just therapy, or antiracist book clubs, or some individual process of self-scrutiny. It will involve a collective journey to new forms of exchange and relations. In their paper "Decolonization Is Not a Metaphor," the Indigenous scholar Eve Tuck and the decolonial thinker Wayne Yang argue that "solidarity is an uneasy, reserved, unsettled matter that neither reconciles present grievances nor forecloses future conflicts."[28] But it is a critical step in centering an epistemology and praxis of care.

DOUBLE WAMPUM

"Physician, heal thyself" is an old retort, and we, the authors, do not pretend that we aren't on others' lands. As the Tuscarora writer Alicia Elliott says of Indigenous people, "We're here, in diaspora on our own lands. We're watching as the same exploitive process that pushed our people out centuries ago continues to push out others today—an updated version with different copyrights attached."[29]

Decolonization in medicine, and anywhere else, is hard.[30] We know that, too. Hearing individual stories, and the outlines of power in those stories, is an essential part of that practice. As we near the end of our journey in this book, we thought we might move from the mode of duet, in which we have written this book, to our solo voices, just for a moment. Here we try to understand our experiences of diaspora through conversation with each other.

RAJ I learned growing up in Britain that I was part of a diaspora, but I'm not quite sure which one. I was born in the UK, but my parents were born in British colonies, my father in Fiji, my mother in Kenya, and their ancestors a few generations back in south Asia. My great-grandparents left their families, following the trail of British theft, pulled by the opportunities of the colonial metropole, pushed by the still-rippling shock waves that the British Empire created when it brought Indians over to its footholds in Africa and the Pacific. I left Britain for similar reasons—drawn by the chance of being able to study across a range of disciplines and pushed by the racism. There was nothing unusual in being stopped and frisked, of walking home in fear of being assaulted in the waves of "Paki bashing," being spat at and told to "go back home." But it was clear that home wasn't India. I don't share the chauvinisms, Islamophobia, sexism, contempt for untouchables, or Hindu nationalism of my family there. I am, in that way, proudly a Bad Indian. Wherever there seems to be an identity, there seems to be an identity politics police ready to point out my inadequacies at just the moment I'm ready to point out theirs.

So I now live in Texas, the only US state that fought for slavery twice, once as part of the Confederacy, and once against Mexico. I live on land that's a palimpsest of Alabama-Coushatta, Caddo, Carrizo/Comecrudo, Coahuiltecan, Comanche, Kickapoo, Lipan Apache, Tonkawa, and Ysleta del Sur Pueblo territory.[31] I have no idea how to relate to it. If I were in the UK, the question would be different: I'd ask how all this wealth accrued through the theft of land elsewhere, through the exploitation of workers here and abroad, through the creation of diasporas throughout the empire. I'd know better how to navigate questions about land and money. I'd know who to accuse, but I wouldn't be thinking as hard about the theft of land as I do here.

I turned to a friend and comrade to help me understand this feeling of being orphaned from place, because she herself had gone through it. Kandace Vallejo's family "was from Texas before Texas was Texas." Their experiences with colonialism, Spanish and American and Mexican, have attenuated her connection to them to the extent that it doesn't make sense for her to identify with any specific Indigenous nation. When I asked her how I ought to relate to the ground beneath my feet, as someone who doesn't intend to colonize or gentrify or obliterate a history but does so anyway, she said:

> I believe that wherever we go, the earth is our home. I recognize that that's a dangerous statement in this stage of late capitalist colonization, because it can be misinterpreted. But on my travels, I pack a little altar prayer-space kit. Whenever I arrive, I burn some of the medicines that I carry with me. I recognize the four directions, because wherever I am at, the four directions are also there. I honor and am grateful to the caretakers of that particular land and to the people whose land I am on, whether or not I know their names, and I ask for their blessing and their permission and commit to being a respectful person, like I'm walking on your land. And I do my best to uphold those laws. That's actually not just something that only people of Indigenous descent can do.

She encouraged me to cultivate a humility and curiosity about connection in time and space, reminding me that humans share 70 percent of our genes with worms,[32] and to be a sensualist in my connection with the web of life. But she also reminded me that this can't be a solo project, that it has to involve community. She leads Youth Rise Texas, a group dedicated to helping young people who have been harmed by family separation policies, deportations, and the criminal justice system—youths who've had the sweep of the border pass over them. She's a border medic. Her spiritual work is also communal, as part of the Native American church.

The symbol of that church is a teepee. It's odd, because no one in the southern United States ever used one. "We're all revivalists," she explained. The church recycled a colonial representation of Indigeneity into a new vision. She reminded me that I've seen this before, in the international peasant movement La Via Campesina. Every one of its meetings begins with burning incense and pointing to the four directions, in an entirely manufactured and nonetheless moving ceremony called *La mistica*. It makes me remember that traditions can and should be invented. I just worry about the people who authorize themselves to say "You're doing it wrong." You've had more engagement with traditions of diaspora and Indigenous nations within the United States than I have, though, Rupa. How do you wrestle with the tension of being a settler here?

RUPA To be in diaspora, to me, is to be in a state of becoming, to hold many possible futures. It is a state of being in relationship, simultaneously, to the ancestors of this land and to my own ancestors—to the past, present, and future, the way seeds are. For my life right now, that means working in close connection with our Indigenous friends to help them achieve their stated goal of getting their land back. It is being in ceremony with them when invited. It is creating ceremonies with my family, through poetic acts that can bring together our mixed lineages into a language that can transmit love of our community, honor for the caretakers of this place, and recognition of the land, air, seeds, and water that sustain us. This is my home. But this is not my homeland.

I was born in occupied Ramaytush Ohlone territory, in what is now called Mountain View, California. My parents were immigrants from northern India who left their homelands to follow economic opportunity. My father moved first to New Mexico, where he studied electrical engineering. He fell in love with the fluidity of culture there—the mixture of Pueblo people, Mexicans, and folks from around the world. He saw how settler colonialism in North America was different from the extractive colonialism he experienced growing up amid the intense wealth disparities that still characterize postcolonial India. He used to tell me that the disparities of India were not the past of a backward nation; they were the future of places like the United States. My mother was a classically trained musician, a Beatles fanatic, and up for adventure in faraway places when she married my father at nineteen years old. They moved to California and had my brothers and me there.

Our family vacations when I was young consisted of us driving around the western United States, going to the beautiful national parks. When we drove through an Indian reservation, my father would often remark, "Look at what they did to these people here. Look at how they took their land. Look at the way they forced them to live." Traveling through New Mexico, at any pit stop, my father insisted that I learn to talk with the people. The conversations my eight-year-old self engaged in with Indigenous people, and the distress I could feel from my father when he spoke of these injustices, were the seeds of my own inquiry into why things are the way they are on this land.

Growing up in the United States, I was frequently told as a child to "go back to where you came from!" But I never felt at home in India, where I was mocked for my Americanized Hindi accent, and my tomboy attitudes didn't sit well with the entrenched patriarchy. Where I did feel at home was in the oak trees in the hills above our house, where, as you walk through a canyon, grassland savanna gives way to bay groves, which transform into families of redwoods towering over banana slugs and fern-lined winding creeks. When I walked in these places, I could sense a presence here that felt out of step with the strip malls, the freeways, and the manufactured quality of Silicon Valley. It was a presence I recognized from my time spent in India. It felt ancient.

I didn't learn about this presence in the fourth grade when we were taught about the California missions and the arrival of the Spanish in this land. The teachers didn't talk about the genocide of California native people. They didn't talk about the way the Indigenous people here had songs for every act of daily life, from harvesting acorns to building boats out of tule reeds. They didn't teach us about the diversity of cultures here. I spent my young adulthood moved by this sense of presence, trying to understand it and my relationship to it. It wasn't until I started spending more time in wilder places, in solitude with my guitar, writing music, reading more, and reaching out to Indigenous people here, that I began to learn, through friendship and through a deep desire to understand. I felt a similar presence sleeping on the ground at the prayer camp at Standing Rock, in Lakȟóta territory, when I was called there by California native activists to assist with medical response as the state acted with increasing violence toward the Indigenous people trying to stop a petroleum pipeline from crossing their source of drinking water. Connecting to this presence wherever I am feels like a vital part of being diaspora. It can start with something as seemingly trivial as taking off my shoes and walking on the Earth. "To let her know you're here," as my husband says.

My grandfather passed in this land. He was cremated here and his ashes taken back to India. My father was also cremated here. My two sons were born here. My husband is a farmer, growing our food in this land. I am a physician, practicing medicine in this land. One day I asked my friend Gregg Castro, who is a culture bearer for the Ramaytush Ohlone tribe, if I could have his blessing and permission to practice my medicine in his homelands. To my surprise, the question, asked so plainly, made me cry and made his eyes well up with tears. It was a moment of tender historical correction, where humility and acknowledgment took center stage. There's a quiet and important power in this simple request for permission. It is the power of learning to be a good guest in someone else's homelands. I'm still learning. And it's something many more of us will need to learn. As more and more people are forced into migrations by climate catastrophes, many more will become part of other diasporas.

RAJ "Can I do X here?" is a powerful question, and one that I've not thought to ask of my practices in Texas. It's such an obvious way of being a good guest, yet to ask the question is to disrupt one of the deepest tenets of the Texas way: if you own it, you need ask no one.

I'm struck in our dialogue by the importance of biography and inheritance. They are ways to emplace ourselves because we don't have a story to tell about our connection to land and people here. Those stories can get bundled up in ways that, for me, are worrying. I'm thinking of the nationalism that I see across the political spectrum, of flags being waved as signs of collective biography and *patria*. Part of the deep medicine of writing this book with you has been learning how to build a relation to self/place/history that doesn't involve nationalism. I don't care for the deep green nationalists, and there are many, waving flags to England's Green and Pleasant Lands, or the ethnonationalists here in Texas who see the climate catastrophe as reason to kill immigrants coming for "our stuff."

In our discussion, we've landed again and again on the social fissures that colonial capitalism has wrought. As we experience the paroxysms of late capitalism, nationalisms become the last redoubt of those pining for the certainties of childhood that never were. I'm thinking here of the National Fronts in France and England, the Hindu fanatics of the Rashtriya Swayamsevak Sangh in India, the white nationalists in Bolivia and the United States. For me the question of nation gets dissolved by queering boundaries, as we mentioned in our look at the Movement for Black Lives and border medicine, by belonging to several nations simultaneously. I'd like to wear nation like language, speaking many and being able to move through them to see how they might combine and learn, expanding and sharing grammars and words that can't be thought of in other ways. I've heard this called "two-eyed seeing," and I think we'll find our way through the fog of national certainties only by seeing with as many subaltern eyes as possible.[33]

National ambiguity is the curse and gift of diaspora. We can't just don nationhoods like hoodies. We've both had experiences in the remains of British colonialism and now find ourselves in the bellies of ongoing colonial struggle. That said, there's no pretending that we have no "move to innocence" to make here, as Eve Tuck and Wayne Yang put it in their important essay.[34] Our experience of colonialism doesn't render us immune to complicity in the colonial project. You've been on the front lines of that in Standing Rock. What lessons did you learn there that might help us navigate this question of collective identity and decolonization?

RUPA How do we understand our identities when colonial institutions have created so much of them and reinforced them on a daily basis? You have to learn to stop caring for other people and the world around you. You see it when middle-class parents teach their kids not to wonder at the unhoused people on the streets.

This "violent act of looking away," as my friend Lisa "Tiny" Gray-Garcia, who used to be unhoused, says, is part of re-creating this system today, as people walk past those who are in tent encampments on the streets of major cities without stopping to ask, "Are you okay? How can I help?" I believe that every act of looking away is a tacit agreement that things should continue as they are, and that that agreement further cuts us off from our own humanity. Whether by the violence of conquest or the violence of seduction by power, in the end we are all cut off from our relationships in this system.

Identity is central to this issue, because the identity that feels the most whole is the most fluid, whether we are speaking collectively or even as individuals. My understandings have come from the spaces of intersection of identities, as a physician/artist, as a doctor who has been disempowered when I have been sick as a patient, as a settler on colonized land from ancestral lands that have also been colonized, as an activist who has accompanied families who have lost loved ones to police violence, as a person with a lived immigrant experience in white supremacist nations, as a partner to an incredible farmer who is in love with the soil, and as a mother who has been awed by the commonplace but also surreal experience of harboring two heartbeats in one body. All these experiences become networks of my own understanding of who I am and where I am, and it is in the transitional spaces, neither here nor there, that I feel the possibility of new futures, for my sense of who I am and for a collective identity.

When I went to Standing Rock, I saw a glimpse of another way of being in community, which allowed us to reconnect to that pluripotency that has been broken by colonialism. I went out there with a crew of health workers from the newly formed Do No Harm Coalition. We had provided medical accompaniment to people protesting police killings of Black, brown, and Indigenous people in the San Francisco Bay Area. When the police (and, now we know, the hired mercenaries from TigerSwan)[35] in Dakȟóta/Lakȟóta territory became increasingly violent toward the Indigenous people protecting their water by stopping the construction of the Dakota Access Pipeline, we were called to come help.

I will never forget the drive down to the camp, passing signs on neighboring ranchers' properties that said things like "WILL SHOOT INDIANS GOING TO STANDING ROCK." It was as if time were standing still, and we were back in the era of colonial conquest. I had already known this conceptually, but it was there that I really understood in every cell of my body that colonialism is an ongoing project that reproduces itself across generations. It never stopped. For the system to continue, its power relations must be re-created every day, and that re-creation occurs because individuals are coerced, voluntarily agree, or simply cannot imagine how not to participate in the rules set out before us.

When we turned the corner into the camp and stopped at the checkpoint, a group of young Indigenous men approached the car. They were the *akicita*, the security team. The seemingly youngest wore a red baseball cap with the words "MAKE AMERICA NATIVE AGAIN."

They inspected what we were bringing in (medical supplies and our tents) and reminded us of the rules: no firearms, no drugs, no alcohol.

As I moved through the camp, meeting various uŋčí (grandmothers) and learning the medical lay of the land, I was also receiving a rundown of the ancient relationships and a blunt schooling on my need to abandon my settler arrogance. There was the Očhéthi Šakówiŋ, the Seven Council Fires, which brought together Lakȟóta, Dakȟóta, and Nakȟóta people. I learned that at camp, I was sleeping with my ear close to the ground in Dakȟóta Lakȟóta homelands. The different tribes, including the Mandan, would gather at those banks of the Mni Sose river for ceremony, trading, and gathering food and medicine since the beginning of time. The Lakȟóta are made up of seven bands, who were gathered there in camp: Húŋkpapȟa, Oglála, Sičáŋǧu, Itázipčho, Sihásapa, Oóhenuŋpa, and Mnikȟóžu. These groups have kept one fire alive together. The concept of nationhood was important, as evidenced in their customs and songs. However, what transcended nationhood was the fire, metaphoric and literal, because so many things in Lakȟóta culture are simultaneously metaphoric and literal. Here it was the common cause, the common value of care and the community that was created among Indigenous people from all corners of the globe who ended up spending time at Standing Rock. There was no money exchanged in this camp, which had about two thousand people when I first arrived and twelve thousand people at its height a few months later. There were several camp kitchens, and no one ever went without food. A massive tent was set up for clothing, and as the winter months arrived, donations came in and people got what they needed for themselves or their families. A school was set up to educate the children in the camp. Structures were built for solar power and composting toilets. Teepees were set up throughout the camp, which stood proudly while the first big windstorm battered and flattened modern camping tents. There was singing with drumming, almost all the time deep into the night.

As we drove down the main path, with flags from Indigenous nations around the world lining both sides, I felt as if I had slipped into another reality. When I arrived, a main medic space had been set up, and with time a whole healing village emerged, staffed by practitioners of every imaginable persuasion. A whole team from National Nurses United was there, assisting throughout the encampment. I was impressed by the readiness of these nurses, some of whom I worked with on the hospital floors back at home. They translated their clinical experiences directly into treating mass casualties from police violence there and to digging out people in tents who had been buried in snow from the blizzards.

There were frontline medics who were agile and well trained to do rapid decontamination from chemical weapons and treatment of mass occurrences of hypothermia when law enforcement sprayed the people with water in subzero conditions at night. Those medics did a lot of the first response in the medic tent, triaging and treating minor injuries, and major ones too. Indigenous midwives monitored a birth in camp and tended to reproductive and women's health issues. Herbalists kept a respiratory-health tea available at all times and prepared concoctions as needed from an incredible apothecary on site. There were guided walks on the plains to learn to identify and forage native medicines. There were acupuncturists, massage therapists, trauma-informed psychotherapists, traditional healers, and physicians such as myself who had to learn a whole other way of working, in which our views, values, and perspectives were not centered in the health care experience.

The Indigenous people who came to the healing village reported never experiencing anything like this. They had had access to only Indian Health Services or the racist clinical environments in the local hospitals. They had never had a say in what kind of wellness modality would work best for what ailed them. Under the leadership of the Oglala Lakȟóta physician Sara Jumping Eagle and ethnobotanist Linda Black Elk, the medic response was dynamic and fluid, evolving to match both what was happening in the camp socially and politically and the impact events might have on the people's bodies, minds, and spirits. It was highly responsive care. It worked so well that people who weren't staying in camp would drive up to have their medical needs taken care of.

This model of a healing village was something the *uŋčí* saw great value in. They didn't want it to go away when the camp dissolved. They asked some of us to create something like this as a lasting tribute to the community. So we are building, under the leadership of the Lakȟóta health workers Tasha Peltier and Alayna Eagleshield, the Mni Wiconi Clinic and Farm—because as Lakȟóta elder Candace Ducheanaux said, "You cannot decolonize medicine without decolonizing our foods." The *uŋčí* saw something in the camp with their imaginative vision, something that did not yet exist but that should exist, to heal those things that were fractured and that continue to be reinjured by colonialism.

RAJ I've seen and felt these moments, at the World Trade Organization protest in Seattle in 1999 and at some of the Occupy encampments, at meetings of Abahlali baseMjondolo, in the favelas in Rio—where the infrastructure of change isn't just logistical but the living example of the better world. In it, time feels different—it's "movement time," filled with tenderness, tending, and joy. Even amid mourning and grief, without any misty romanticism, there is laughter. And what that signifies, above all, is what happens when people come together in a community that is moved by care.

RUPA Yes, I agree. I also believe there's something in these places that is generative, and joyful, because of this fluid community of care. I can compare it only to the feeling I get when I write a song that I know is going to move other people, because the song feels deeply life-affirming. The feeling is one of encountering the space between what is known, this world as it is, and what is not yet known, the imagined future. And in that space there is intense creativity, which is alive with experimentation. What if we were to relate to one another differently? At Standing Rock, in the autonomously organized Indigenous territories in Chiapas, in the anarchist collective Nosotros in Exarchia,

Athens, in the community center in Gulbai Tekra, Ahmedabad, I feel this fertile presence of the imagination, which is what makes our lives a living artform. And in all those projects, the central ethic at play was one of care: for one another, for the environment, for the foods, for the space they held and for the future. All these elements they create around them go back and impact the body. They are changing their exposomes, retooling language, bringing back stories, symbols, and relationships that ultimately change both the nature of time and the chemistry inside their own bodies. They are building new worlds around them that their bodies will harmonize with and that harmony sounds like good health.

A CULTURE OF CARE

We become inflamed when we are in abusive relationships with our soils, our rivers, our microbial passengers, our animal and plant relatives, our air, and each other. An anti-imperial people's Green New Deal offers a path to healing, through care and repair. But there has to be a shift in grammar. The verb *care about*—as in "I care about the suffering of Indigenous people"—can simply re-create colonial paternalism. "Caring about" along axes of oppression and charity allows supremacies to re-create themselves surreptitiously. Part of colonialism's sleight of hand is its normalization of the capitalist political, economic, and ecological framework in which care is practiced. The economic system that allocates care as a good, on the basis of ability to pay, turns something inherently relational into something to be consumed like a hamburger. Covid has shown how well different communities care for one another. Some countries in Asia have already been through SARS. Taiwan, Singapore, and South Korea learned their lessons well. Within India in Dharavi and Kerala, histories of investment in care, and the faith in one another that this produces, helped keep the disease under control and help communities care for the long-term sick.

So rather than "care about," we follow Tronto's suggestion to "care with."[36] The English word *care* has its origins in the Gothic *karôn*, "to lament, to grieve."[37] We don't underestimate the work of grief and emotional labor ahead. To center care in our world is to reframe liberal questions of property—"Who gets what?"—into questions of work: "Who does what?" In a properly decolonizing approach, "Who does what?" must be answered alongside "Who has had what done to them?" To create a decolonizing ethic of care, to imagine futures in which the injuries of colonialism can be healed, care priorities must be decided by those who have been the most impacted by six hundred years of carelessness.

Care cannot simply be a rearranging of civil society to spread material wealth. Although the rich white men of the ecomodernist movement prophesy plenty for everyone tomorrow, the weight of evidence suggests that capitalism has broken the planet, with the richest having done far more damage than they're on track ever to clean up. Reparation and redistribution from Global North to Global South is a sine qua non of any future. And in the driving seat must be those whose existence has been in a position of peril. The agenda cannot be set by the Global North, by the medical establishment, by the non-Indigenous, by whiteness. Any attempts to direct the care work from those positions of superiority leave it privy to the degrading mentality that has brought us to this moment. Because of its pervasiveness and its historicity, none of us are immune. The directives must come from underneath. All power, then, to the carers.

Carers have been doing the work of decolonization around the world. In the nursing profession, there is a growing debate about the need to recognize the damage that settler colonialism has caused.[38] Decolonizing nursing involves the difficult, collective work of examining culpability—individual and social—for past injustices, to repair and prevent them in the future. Concrete actions of solidarity, from organizational critique of the health care system to radical listening for new knowledge, are both new to the field of nursing, and ancient wisdom. In Maori, it's *"Ka mua, Ka muri"*;[39] in Hawai'i, it's *"Ka Wā Ma Mua, Ka Wā Ma Hope."*[40] In English, it's "walking backwards into the future." In every case, the goal is the end of settler society.

Deep medicine requires new cosmologies, ones that can braid our lives with the planet and the web of life around us. The anatomy of justice stretches from the hospital to the forest, from the ocean to the school, from the prison to the sky. The process of decolonizing must be deeply unsettling and highly creative. It will transform us all. As Frantz Fanon observed, "Decolonization never takes place unnoticed, for it influences individuals and modifies them fundamentally."[41] It requires engaging with material things, as in restoring sovereignty over land, water, and seeds and securing the ability to protect them again. It requires resources to build anew. It requires the recognition that there will be honest mistakes, and dishonest ones.[42] And it requires the kinds of analysis and imagination that dissolve fixed identities, so we can find our way back to aspects of our humanness that center care—for one another, for the Earth, for our own bodies and minds as an assemblage of organisms and systems, for all the plant and animal relatives around us, for the water. Settler ideologies have circumscribed the imagination. Perhaps the most important thing in this work is to exercise it, to escape, so that those borders and limits can be erased and people can begin to see the way forward. This is not a hearkening back to a time gone by but an active envisioning of a future.

"To decolonize" in Lakȟóta is *KhiLakȟóta*: *Khi* means "return to our own" and *Lakȟóta* "the people/the humans." To Tipiziwin Tolman, the *Lakȟóta* language revitalist, this translates to "a return to ourselves, our true selves." And that is the radical promise of decolonizing. It is to become humble once more in the face of life's greater intelligence. It is to create a community of care that can heal what has been broken, in which we can all take part, with fire in our hearts, to cool our veins, our minds, our communities, and our planet, with recognition of how dependent we are on water, wind, earth, fire, and the entire web of life. It is to become human again.

NOTES

INTRODUCTION

1. Quoted by Frantz Fanon, *Black Skin, White Masks*. Translated by Charles Lam Markmann (London: Pluto Press, 1952), p. 9.
2. Michel Foucault, *Discipline and Punish: The Birth of the Prison*. Translated by Alan Sheridan (New York: Vintage Books, 1979), 25–26.
3. Sandro Galea and Salma M. Abdalla, "Covid-19 Pandemic, Unemployment, and Civil Unrest: Underlying Deep Racial and Socioeconomic Divides," *JAMA* 324, no. 3 (2020), doi.org/10.1001/jama.2020.11132.
4. Jeremy Hess et al., "Petroleum and Health Care: Evaluating and Managing Health Care's Vulnerability to Petroleum Supply Shifts," *American Journal of Public Health* 101, no. 9 (2011), doi.org/10.2105/AJPH.2011.300233.
5. Jordi Bascompte, "Disentangling the Web of Life," *Science* 325, no. 5939 (2009), doi.org/10.1126/science.1170749; Moreno Di Marco et al., "Changes in Human Footprint Drive Changes in Species Extinction Risk," *Nature Communications* 9, no. 1 (2018), doi.org/10.1038/s41467-018-07049-5.
6. Chelsea Brentzel, "3M Admits to Illegal Chemical Release in Tennessee River," *News19* (Decatur, AL), June 14, 2019, whnt.com/news/decatur/3m-admits-to-illegal-chemical-release-in-tennessee-river/; Mayra Quirindongo et al., *Lost and Found: Missing Mercury from Chemical Plants Pollutes Air and Water* (New York: Natural Resources Defense Council, 2006).
7. K. R. Miner et al., "Deposition of PFAS 'Forever Chemicals' on Mt. Everest," *Science of the Total Environment* 759 (2021), doi.org/10.1016/j.scitotenv.2020.144421.
8. Elizabeth R. Daly et al., "Per- and Polyfluoroalkyl Substance (PFAS) Exposure Assessment in a Community Exposed to Contaminated Drinking Water, New Hampshire, 2015," *International Journal of Hygiene and Environmental Health* 221, no. 3 (2018), doi.org/10.1016/j.ijheh.2018.02.007.
9. Annie Sneed, "Forever Chemicals Are Widespread in U.S. Drinking Water," *Scientific American*, January 21, 2021, tinyurl.com/kdr3opl8.
10. Sharon Lerner, "3M Knew About the Dangers of PFOA and PFOS Decades Ago, Internal Documents Show," *The Intercept*, July 31, 2018, theintercept.com/2018/07/31/3m-pfas-minnesota-pfoa-pfos/; Brentzel, "3M Admits to Illegal Chemical Release."
11. Carolin Fleischmann et al., "Assessment of Global Incidence and Mortality of Hospital-Treated Sepsis. Current Estimates and Limitations," *American Jour-*

nal of Respiratory and Critical Care Medicine 193, no. 3 (2016), doi.org/10.1164 /rccm.201504-0781oc.

12. Kristina E. Rudd et al., "Global, Regional, and National Sepsis Incidence and Mortality, 1990–2017: Analysis for the Global Burden of Disease Study," *The Lancet* 395, no. 10219 (2020), doi.org/10.1016/S0140-6736(19)32989-7.

13. J. Karavitis and E. J. Kovacs, "Macrophage Phagocytosis: Effects of Environmental Pollutants, Alcohol, Cigarette Smoke, and Other External Factors," *Journal of Leukocyte Biology* 90, no. 6 (2011), doi.org/10.1189/jlb.0311114; Vijay Kumar, "Macrophages: The Potent Immunoregulatory Innate Immune Cells" (IntechOpen, 2019), doi.org/10.5772/intechopen.88013.

14. A. Prüss-Ustün et al., *Preventing Disease through Healthy Environments: A Global Assessment of the Burden of Disease from Environmental Risks* (Geneva: World Health Organization, 2016), tinyurl.com/dabo23d2.

15. Julian Cribb, *Surviving the 21st Century: Humanity's Ten Great Challenges and How We Can Overcome Them* (Switzerland: Springer, 2016), link.springer.com/10.1007 /978-3-319-41270-2; Roberto Binetti, Francesca Marina Costamagna, and Ida Marcello, "Exponential Growth of New Chemicals and Evolution of Information Relevant to Risk Control," *Annali-istituto superiore di sanità* 44, no. 1 (2008).

16. Zhe Xu et al., "Pathological Findings of Covid-19 Associated with Acute Respiratory Distress Syndrome," *Lancet Respiratory Medicine* (2020), doi.org /10.1016/S2213-2600(20)30076-X.

17. Oxford English Dictionary, "Diagnosis, N.," *Oxford English Dictionary* (Oxford University Press).

18. Covid exploded in places where workers are incarcerated, in the meat-packing plants, in the fulfillment centers, and in the fields where farmworkers grow our food. Leah Douglas, "Mapping Covid-19 Outbreaks in the Food System," *Food and Environment Reporting Network*, April 22, 2020, thefern.org /2020/04/mapping-covid-19-in-meat-and-food-processing-plants/.

19. Jack Nicas, "A Pastor, a School Bus and a Trip Through a Scorched Oregon Town," *The New York Times*, September 15, 2020, tinyurl.com/1asgb899.

20. We use the term *Latinx* recognizing that it is a placeholder term, one that fails to capture the complex and different histories of Indigenous communities, and those of African and European origin in South America. It isn't freighted with the heteronormativity of *Latino* or the binarism of *Latin@*. But we fully imagine that this is a term that will date quickly. We look forward to its replacement.

21. Lindsay Schnell, "'Like Smoking Multiple Packs a Day': Hazardous Air Quality Worries West Coast Parents," *USA Today*, September 20, 2020, tinyurl.com /2og3xuxl.

22. Zachary S. Wettstein et al., "Cardiovascular and Cerebrovascular Emergency Department Visits Associated with Wildfire Smoke Exposure in California in 2015," *Journal of the American Heart Association* 7, no. 8 (2018), doi.org/10 .1161/jaha.117.007492.

23. Silvia Comunian et al., "Air Pollution and Covid-19: The Role of Particulate Matter in the Spread and Increase of Covid-19's Morbidity and Mortality," *International Journal of Environmental Research and Public Health* 17, no. 12 (2020), doi.org/10.3390/ijerph17124487; Wettstein et al., "Cardiovascular and Cerebrovascular Emergency Department Visits."

24. Whaley, for instance, writes on why it makes sense to see the "western expansion" as a particularly vicious moment in the bloody history of US coloni-

zation. Gray H. Whaley, "Oregon, Illahee, and the Empire Republic: A Case Study of American Colonialism, 1843–1858," *Western Historical Quarterly* 36, no. 2 (2005), doi.org/10.2307/25443145.

25. Aníbal Quijano, "Coloniality and Modernity/Rationality," *Cultural Studies* 21, no. 2–3 (2007), doi.org/10.1080/09502380601164353.

26. Michel Foucault, *The Birth of the Clinic: An Archaeology of Medical Perception*, trans. A. M. Sheridan (New York: Vintage, 1975), 174.

27. David Abram, *Becoming Animal: An Earthly Cosmology* (New York: Pantheon, 2010).

28. Global Witness, *Enemies of the State: How Governments and Business Silence Land and Environmental Defenders* (London: Global Witness, 2019), www .globalwitness.org/en/campaigns/environmental-activists/enemies-state/.

29. Tony Barta, "Sorry, and Not Sorry, in Australia: How the Apology to the Stolen Generations Buried a History of Genocide," *Journal of Genocide Research* 10, no. 2 (2008), doi.org/10.1080/14623520802065438.

30. Mark Gibney, *The Age of Apology: Facing Up to the Past* (Philadelphia: University of Pennsylvania Press, 2008).

31. US Government, "Indian Entities Recognized by and Eligible to Receive Services from the United States Bureau of Indian Affairs," *Federal Register* 84, no. 22 (2019); Alexa Koenig and Jonathan Stein, "Federalism and the State Recognition of Native American Tribes: A Survey of State-Recognized Tribes and State Recognition Processes across the United States," *Santa Clara Law Review* 48 (2008).

32. The "under God" part was added in 1953.

33. Karina Czyzewski, "Colonialism as a Broader Social Determinant of Health," *International Indigenous Policy Journal* 2, no. 1 (2011); Ian Anderson et al., "Indigenous and Tribal Peoples' Health (*The Lancet*–Lowitja Institute Global Collaboration): A Population Study," *The Lancet* 388, no. 10040 (2016), doi.org /10.1016/S0140-6736(16)00345-7.

34. L. Dwyer-Lindgren et al., "Inequalities in Life Expectancy Among US Counties, 1980 to 2014: Temporal Trends and Key Drivers," *JAMA Internal Medicine* 177, no. 7 (2017), doi.org/10.1001/jamainternmed.2017.0918.

35. We come to this mindful that *settler colonialism* is a distinct form of control. We use this term in preference to *imperialism* because, particularly for the US reader, it's easy to forget that the United States is a colonial project, and that the practices of empire are still enforced in the settler colony in which we write. Edward Said observes a more traditional distinction between imperialism and colonialism: "'Imperialism' means the practice, the theory, and the attitudes of a dominating metropolitan centre ruling a distant territory; 'colonialism,' which is almost always a consequence of imperialism, is the implanting of settlements on distant territory." Edward W. Said, *Culture and Imperialism* (New York: Knopf, 1993), 9. See also Edward Cavanagh and Lorenzo Veracini, eds., *The Routledge Handbook of the History of Settler Colonialism* (London: Routledge, 2017); and Ronald J. Horvath, "A Definition of Colonialism," *Current Anthropology* 13, no. 1 (1972), doi.org/10.1086/201248.

36. Raj Patel and Jason W. Moore, *A History of the World in Seven Cheap Things: A Guide to Capitalism, Nature, and the Future of the Planet* (Berkeley: University of California Press, 2017); Tink Tinker and Mark Freeland, "Thief, Slave Trader, Murderer: Christopher Columbus and Caribbean Population Decline," *Wičazo Ša Review* 23, no. 1 (2008), jstor.org/stable/30131245.

37. Lee Raye, "The Early Extinction Date of the Beaver (Castor Fiber) in Britain," *Historical Biology* 27, no. 8 (2015), doi.org/10.1080/08912963.2014.927871.

38. To be accurate, the fiber at the base of the fur was ground up and used in hat making. James L. Clayton, "The Growth and Economic Significance of the American Fur Trade, 1790–1890," *Minnesota History* 40, no. 4 (1966): 211, jstor.org/stable/20177863.

39. Robert J. Naiman, Carol A. Johnston, and James C. Kelley, "Alteration of North American Streams by Beaver," *BioScience* 38, no. 11 (1988), doi.org/10.2307/1310784.

40. Ibid.

41. Erica Neeganagwedgin, "'Chattling the Indigenous Other': A Historical Examination of the Enslavement of Aboriginal Peoples in Canada," *AlterNative: An International Journal of Indigenous Peoples* 8, no. 1 (2012), doi.org/10.1177/117718011200800102. The entanglements of Indigenous and settler men and women were also, it's worth noting, opportunities for Indigenous women to engage in forms of resistance that have remained largely outside the mainstream histories of colonialism. Sylvia Van Kirk, *Many Tender Ties: Women in Fur-Trade Society, 1670–1870* (Norman: University of Oklahoma Press, 1983).

42. Catherine Meyers, "Tuberculosis Followed the Fur Trade," *Science*, April 4, 2011, www.sciencemag.org/news/2011/04/tuberculosis-followed-fur-trade.

43. P. Collen and R. J. Gibson, "The General Ecology of Beavers (Castor Spp.), as Related to Their Influence on Stream Ecosystems and Riparian Habitats, and the Subsequent Effects on Fish—a Review," *Reviews in Fish Biology and Fisheries* 10, no. 4 (2000): 450, doi.org/10.1023/a:1012262217012.

44. Michael M. Pollock et al., "The Importance of Beaver Ponds to Coho Salmon Production in the Stillaguamish River Basin, Washington, USA," *North American Journal of Fisheries Management* 24, no. 3 (2004), doi.org/10.1577/M03-156.1.

45. Spencer B. Beebe et al., *Salmon Nation: People. Place. Welcome Home* (2019), 3, medium.com/@salmonnation/salmon-nation-a-place-and-an-idea-1f18e4776362.

46. Ibid.

47. Adam Hochschild, *King Leopold's Ghost: A Story of Greed, Terror, and Heroism in Colonial Africa* (Boston: Houghton Mifflin, 1998), 198.

48. Corey J. A. Bradshaw, "Little Left to Lose: Deforestation and Forest Degradation in Australia Since European Colonization," *Journal of Plant Ecology* 5, no. 1 (2012), doi.org/10.1093/jpe/rtr038.

49. By 1494, Columbus was explaining to Ferdinand and Isabella, in the medical language of the day, that Spanish sailors weren't able to thrive in the Western Hemisphere because the food and climate were not conducive to the maintenance of healthy European bodies. Rebecca Earle, "'If You Eat Their Food . . .': Diets and Bodies in Early Colonial Spanish America," *American Historical Review* 115, no. 3 (2010), doi.org/10.1086/ahr.115.3.688.

50. The acrobatics of Descartes's arguments are the stuff of undergraduate philosophy, but we encourage readers to begin at the Third Meditation and then consider its consequences. René Descartes, *Meditations on First Philosophy: With Selections from the Objections and Replies*, trans. Michael Moriarty (Oxford: Oxford University Press, 2008); Kay Anderson, "Mind over Matter? On Decentring the Human in Human Geography," *Cultural Geographies* 21, no. 1 (2013), doi.org/10.1177/1474474013513409.

51. This, at least, is what was possible for Steven Pinker to write in 2018 in a popular celebration of the Enlightenment. The same forces that unleashed the Enlightenment, and its medicine, also made possible the sixth extinction, austerity economics, opioid addiction, and the climate catastrophe. You can't celebrate one without acknowledging them all.

52. Howard K. Koh, Anand K. Parekh, and John J. Park, "Confronting the Rise and Fall of US Life Expectancy," *JAMA* 322, no. 20 (2019), doi.org/10.1001 /jama.2019.17303; Laura Parry, Nick Steel, and John Ford, "Slowing of Life Expectancy in the UK: Global Burden of Disease Study 2016," *The Lancet* 392 (2018), doi.org/10.1016/S0140-6736(18)32906-4.

53. Theresa Andrasfay and Noreen Goldman, "Reductions in 2020 US Life Expectancy Due to Covid-19 and the Disproportionate Impact on the Black and Latino Populations," *Proceedings of the National Academy of Sciences of the United States of America* 118, no. 5 (2021), doi.org/10.1073/pnas.2014746118.

54. Lorraine C. Boyd, *Pregnancy-Associated Mortality Report, 2006–2010* (New York City Department of Health and Mental Hygiene, 2010).

55. UN Food and Agricultural Organization, *The State of Food Insecurity and Nutrition in the World: Safeguarding against Economic Slowdowns and Downturns* (Rome: FAO, 2019). This, note, despite figures that themselves had been gerrymandered to fit a narrative that all was well in world hunger. Frances Moore Lappé et al., "How We Count Hunger Matters," *Ethics and International Affairs* 27, no. 03 (2013), doi.org/doi:10.1017/S0892679413000191.

56. Ian Bailey, "Edward Jenner (1749–1823): Naturalist, Scientist, Country Doctor, Benefactor to Mankind," *Journal of Medical Biography* 4, no. 2 (1996).

57. Stefan Riedel, "Edward Jenner and the History of Smallpox and Vaccination," *Baylor University Medical Center Proceedings* 18, no. 1 (2005), doi.org/10.1080 /08998280.2005.11928028.

58. Jennifer Meyer, Vasileios Margaritis, and Aaron Mendelsohn, "Consequences of Community Water Fluoridation Cessation for Medicaid-Eligible Children and Adolescents in Juneau, Alaska," *BMC Oral Health* 18, no. 1 (2018), doi.org /10.1186/s12903-018-0684-2.

59. Stephen Peckham, "Slaying Sacred Cows: Is It Time to Pull the Plug on Water Fluoridation?," *Critical Public Health* 22, no. 2 (2012), doi.org/10.1080 /09581596.2011.596818.

60. Anna L. Choi et al., "Developmental Fluoride Neurotoxicity: A Systematic Review and Meta-Analysis," *Environmental Health Perspectives* 120, no. 10 (2012), doi.org/10.1289/ehp.1104912.

61. TRUDP105. *NPR/PBS Newshour/Marist Poll National Tables March 13th through March 14th, 2020* (2020), maristpoll.marist.edu/wp-content/uploads/2020/03 /NPR_PBS-NewsHour_Marist-Poll_USA-NOS-and-Tables_2003151338.pdf.

62. Noni E. Macdonald, "Vaccine Hesitancy: Definition, Scope and Determinants," *Vaccine* 33, no. 34 (2015), doi.org/10.1016/j.vaccine.2015.04.036; World Health Organization, "Ten Threats to Global Health in 2019" (2019), www.who.int /news-room/spotlight/ten-threats-to-global-health-in-2019.

63. Alexandre De Figueiredo et al., "Mapping Global Trends in Vaccine Confidence and Investigating Barriers to Vaccine Uptake: A Large-Scale Retrospective Temporal Modelling Study," *The Lancet* 396, no. 10255 (2020), doi .org/10.1016/s0140-6736(20)31558-0; Jeremy K. Ward et al., "Vaccine Hesitancy and Coercion: All Eyes on France," *Nature Immunology* 20, no. 10

(2019), doi.org/10.1038/s41590-019-0488-9; Kim Willsher, "Vaccine Scepticism in France Reflects 'Dissatisfaction with Political Class,'" *The Guardian*, January 11, 2021, tinyurl.com/10tc14qr; AFP-Tokyo, "Fraught History Haunts Japan Covid-19 Vaccine Roll-Out," *Deccan Herald*, January 8, 2021, tinyurl.com/1eoorei3.

64. Naomi Klein, *The Shock Doctrine: The Rise of Disaster Capitalism* (New York: Metropolitan Books, 2007).

65. Lauren Bunch, "A Tale of Two Crises: Addressing Covid-19 Vaccine Hesitancy as Promoting Racial Justice," *HEC Forum* (2021), link.springer.com/article/10 .1007%2Fs10730-021-09440-0.

66. Refusal is the opposite of recognition, as Audra Simpson puts it. Audra Simpson, *Mohawk Interruptus: Political Life Across the Borders of Settler States* (Durham, NC: Duke University Press, 2014).

67. Yehonatan Turner and Irith Hadas-Halpern, "The Effects of Including a Patient's Photograph to the Radiographic Examination," Radiological Society of North America 2008 Scientific Assembly and Annual Meeting (Chicago, 2008), archive.rsna.org/2008/6008880.html.

68. Yehudit Hasin, Marcus Seldin, and Aldons Lusis, "Multi-Omics Approaches to Disease," *Genome Biology* 18, no. 1 (2017), doi.org/10.1186/s13059-017-1215-1.

69. Katherine Byrns, "Angela Davis Speaks About Justice and Equality," *Colgate Maroon-News*, 2009, thecolgatemaroonnews.com/10555/news/angela-davis -speaks-about-justice-and-equality/.

70. James Tully, "Life Sustains Life 2. The Ways of Re-Engagement with the Living Earth." In *Nature and Value*, edited by Akeel Bilgrami (New York: Columbia University Press, 2020).

71. Ibid.

72. William B. Karesh et al., "Ecology of Zoonoses: Natural and Unnatural Histories," *The Lancet* 380, no. 9857 (2012), doi.org/10.1016/s0140-6736(12)61678-x.

73. Rob Wallace, *Big Farms Make Big Flu: Dispatches on Infectious Disease, Agribusiness and the Nature of Science* (New York: Monthly Review Press, 2016).

74. James Gorman, "The Coronavirus Kills Mink, So They Too May Get a Vaccine," *The New York Times,* January 25, 2021, tinyurl.com/32o9qj3m.

75. D. L. Martin, "Health Conditions before Columbus: Paleopathology of Native North Americans," *Western Journal of Medicine* 176, no. 1 (2002), doi.org/10 .1136/ewjm.176.1.65; Mohammed Al-Hariri, "Sweet Bones: The Pathogenesis of Bone Alteration in Diabetes," *Journal of Diabetes Research* 2016 (2016), doi .org/10.1155/2016/6969040.

76. Nancy Macdonald, "Bella Bella, B.C.: The Town That Solved Suicide," *Maclean's*, September 22, 2016, www.macleans.ca/news/bella-bella-the-town-that-solved -suicide/.

77. Michael J. Chandler and Christopher Lalonde, "Cultural Continuity as a Hedge against Suicide in Canada's First Nations," *Transcultural Psychiatry* 35, no. 2 (1998), doi.org/10.1177/136346159803500202.

1. IMMUNE SYSTEM

1. Donna Haraway, "The Biopolitics of Postmodern Bodies: Determinations of Self in Immune System Discourse," in *Feminist Theory and the Body: A Reader*, ed. Janet Price and Margrit Shildrick (Edinburgh: Edinburgh University Press, 1999), 211.

2. Nanna Mik-Meyer, "The Social Negotiation of Illness: Doctors' Role as Clinical or Political in Diagnosing Patients with Medically Unexplained Symptoms," *Social Theory and Health* 13, no. 1 (2015), doi.org/10.1057/sth.2014.15.

3. Malcolm X, "The Ballot or the Bullet," speech delivered at King Solomon Baptist Church, Detroit, 1964.

4. David Furman et al., "Chronic Inflammation in the Etiology of Disease across the Life Span," *Nature Medicine* 25, no. 12 (2019), doi.org/10.1038/s41591-019-0675-0.

5. Melody G. Duvall and Bruce D. Levy, "DHA- and EPA-Derived Resolvins, Protectins, and Maresins in Airway Inflammation," *European Journal of Pharmacology* 785 (2016), doi.org/10.1016/j.ejphar.2015.11.001.

6. A. Liston and S. L. Masters, "Homeostasis-Altering Molecular Processes as Mechanisms of Inflammasome Activation," *Nature Reviews Immunology* 17, no. 3 (2017), doi.org/10.1038/nri.2016.151.

7. Nicola R. Sproston and Jason J. Ashworth, "Role of C-Reactive Protein at Sites of Inflammation and Infection," *Frontiers in Immunology* 9 (2018), doi.org/10.3389/fimmu.2018.00754.

8. Liston and Masters, "Homeostasis-Altering Molecular Processes."

9. Ibid.

10. M. Bonafe, J. Sabbatinelli, and F. Olivieri, "Exploiting the Telomere Machinery to Put the Brakes on Inflamm-Aging," *Ageing Research Reviews* 59 (2020), doi.org/10.1016/j.arr.2020.101027; Jingwen Zhang et al., "Ageing and the Telomere Connection: An Intimate Relationship with Inflammation," *Ageing Research Reviews* 25 (2016), doi.org/10.1016/j.arr.2015.11.006.

11. Naoko Ohtani, "Deciphering the Mechanism for Induction of Senescence-Associated Secretory Phenotype (SASP) and Its Role in Ageing and Cancer Development," *Journal of Biochemistry* 166, no. 4 (2019), doi.org/10.1093/jb/mvz055; Francis Rodier et al., "Persistent DNA Damage Signalling Triggers Senescence-Associated Inflammatory Cytokine Secretion," *Nature Cell Biology* 11, no. 8 (2009), doi.org/10.1038/ncb1909.

12. Tamara Tchkonia et al., "Cellular Senescence and the Senescent Secretory Phenotype: Therapeutic Opportunities," *Journal of Clinical Investigation* 123, no. 3 (2013), doi.org/10.1172/jci64098; Y. Zhu et al., "Cellular Senescence and the Senescent Secretory Phenotype in Age-Related Chronic Diseases," *Current Opinions in Clinical Nutrition and Metabolic Care* 17, no. 4 (2014), doi.org/10.1097/MCO.0000000000000065; Wen-Juan Wang, Guang-Yan Cai, and Xiang-Mei Chen, "Cellular Senescence, Senescence-Associated Secretory Phenotype, and Chronic Kidney Disease," *Oncotarget* 8, no. 38 (2017), doi.org/10.18632/oncotarget.17327; Manish Kumar, Werner Seeger, and Robert Voswinckel, "Senescence-Associated Secretory Phenotype and Its Possible Role in Chronic Obstructive Pulmonary Disease," *American Journal of Respiratory Cell and Molecular Biology* 51, no. 3 (2014), doi.org/10.1165/rcmb.2013-0382ps; Frej Fyhrquist, Outi Saijonmaa, and Timo Strandberg, "The Roles of Senescence and Telomere Shortening in Cardiovascular Disease," *Nature Reviews Cardiology* 10, no. 5 (2013), doi.org/10.1038/nrcardio.2013.30; Rekha Bhat et al., "Astrocyte Senescence as a Component of Alzheimer's Disease," *PLOS One* 7, no. 9 (2012), doi.org/10.1371/journal.pone.0045069; Antero Salminen et al., "Astrocytes in the Aging Brain Express Characteristics of Senescence-Associated Secretory Phenotype," *European*

Journal of Neuroscience 34, no. 1 (2011), doi.org/10.1111/j.1460-9568.2011 .07738.x.

13. Arne N. Akbar and Derek W. Gilroy, "Aging Immunity May Exacerbate Covid-19," *Science* 369, no. 6501 (2020), doi.org/10.1126/science.abb0762; Jamil Nehme et al., "Cellular Senescence as a Potential Mediator of Covid-19 Severity in the Elderly," *Aging Cell* 19, no. 10 (2020), doi.org/10.1111/acel.13237.

14. Cornelia M. Weyand, Zhen Yang, and Jörg J. Goronzy, "T-Cell Aging in Rheumatoid Arthritis," *Current Opinion in Rheumatology* 26, no. 1 (2014), doi.org/10 .1097/bor.0000000000000011.

15. Ohtani, "Deciphering the Mechanism for Induction"; Rodier et al., "Persistent DNA Damage"; J. Mu et al., "Interspecies Communication Between Plant and Mouse Gut Host Cells Through Edible Plant Derived Exosome-Like Nanoparticles," *Molecular Nutrition and Food Research* 58, no. 7 (2014), doi.org/10.1002/mnfr.201300729. Some of the causes of premature senescence that trigger the onset of the senescence-associated secretory phenotype include telomere erosion, damaged DNA, epigenetic changes, and mitochondrial dysfunction. Akbar and Gilroy, "Aging Immunity May Exacerbate Covid-19."

16. Tchkonia et al., "Cellular Senescence and the Senescent Secretory Phenotype"; Zhu et al., "Cellular Senescence and the Senescent Secretory Phenotype in Age-Related Chronic Diseases"; P. Brodin et al., "Variation in the Human Immune System Is Largely Driven by Non-Heritable Influences," *Cell* 160, no. 1–2 (2015), doi.org/10.1016/j.cell.2014.12.020.

17. Gwyneira Isaac et al., "Native American Perspectives on Health and Traditional Ecological Knowledge," *Environmental Health Perspectives* 126, no. 12 (2018), doi.org/10.1289/ehp1944; M. M. Niedzwiecki et al., "The Exposome: Molecules to Populations," *Annual Review of Pharmacology and Toxicology* 59 (2019), doi.org/10.1146/annurev-pharmtox-010818-021315.

18. Ohtani, "Deciphering the Mechanism for Induction"; Rodier et al., "Persistent DNA Damage"; Zhu et al., "Cellular Senescence and the Senescent Secretory Phenotype in Age-Related Chronic Diseases."

19. Jose C. Clemente, Julia Manasson, and Jose U. Scher, "The Role of the Gut Microbiome in Systemic Inflammatory Disease," *BMJ* (2018), doi.org/10.1136 /bmj.j5145.

20. C. Fiuza-Luces et al., "Exercise Benefits in Cardiovascular Disease: Beyond Attenuation of Traditional Risk Factors," *Nature Reviews Cardiology* 15, no. 12 (2018), doi.org/10.1038/s41569-018-0065-1.

21. P. Carrera-Bastos, "The Western Diet and Lifestyle and Diseases of Civilization," *Research Reports in Clinical Cardiology*, no. 2 (2011), doi.org/10.2147 /RRCC.S16919.

22. Carrera-Bastos, "Western Diet and Lifestyle."

23. T. W. McDade et al., "Analysis of Variability of High Sensitivity C-Reactive Protein in Lowland Ecuador Reveals No Evidence of Chronic Low-Grade Inflammation," *American Journal of Human Biology* 24, no. 5 (2012), doi.org/10 .1002/ajhb.22296.

24. David A. Raichlen et al., "Physical Activity Patterns and Biomarkers of Cardiovascular Disease Risk in Hunter-Gatherers," *American Journal of Human Biology* 29, no. 2 (2017), doi.org/10.1002/ajhb.22919.

25. Hillard Kaplan et al., "Coronary Atherosclerosis in Indigenous South Amer-

ican Tsimane: A Cross-Sectional Cohort Study," *The Lancet* 389, no. 10080 (2017), doi.org/10.1016/s0140-6736(17)30752-3.

26. Nancy Agmon-Levin et al., "Antitreponemal Antibodies Leading to Autoantibody Production and Protection from Atherosclerosis in Kitavans from Papua New Guinea," *Annals of the New York Academy of Sciences* 1173, no. 1 (2009), doi.org/10.1111/j.1749-6632.2009.04671.x.

27. David M. Keohane et al., "Microbiome and Health Implications for Ethnic Minorities after Enforced Lifestyle Changes," *Nature Medicine* 26 (2020), doi.org/10.1038/s41591-020-0963-8.

28. T. W. McDade, "Early Environments and the Ecology of Inflammation," *Proceedings of the National Academy of Sciences of the United States of America* 109, suppl. 2 (2012), doi.org/10.1073/pnas.1202244109.

29. Saman Khalatbari-Soltani et al., "Importance of Collecting Data on Socioeconomic Determinants from the Early Stage of the Covid-19 Outbreak Onwards," *Journal of Epidemiology and Community Health* (2020), doi.org/10.1136/jech-2020-214297.

30. Yu Shi et al., "Host Susceptibility to Severe Covid-19 and Establishment of a Host Risk Score: Findings of 487 Cases Outside Wuhan," *Critical Care* 24, no. 1 (2020), doi.org/10.1186/s13054-020-2833-7.

31. C. E. Rose et al., "Coronavirus Disease Among Workers in Food Processing, Food Manufacturing, and Agriculture Workplaces," *Emerging Infectious Diseases* 27, no. 1 (2021), doi.org/10.3201/eid2701.203821.

32. Marie C. Lewis et al., "Direct Experimental Evidence That Early-Life Farm Environment Influences Regulation of Immune Responses," *Pediatric Allergy and Immunology* 23, no. 3 (2012), doi.org/10.1111/j.1399-3038.2011.01258.x.

33. M. Hatori et al., "Global Rise of Potential Health Hazards Caused by Blue Light-Induced Circadian Disruption in Modern Aging Societies," *NPJ Aging and Mechanisms of Disease* 3, no. 9 (2017), doi.org/10.1038/s41514-017-0010-2.

34. Russel J. Reiter et al., "Melatonin as an Antioxidant: Under Promises but over Delivers," *Journal of Pineal Research* 61, no. 3 (2016), doi.org/10.1111/jpi.12360; Gaia Favero, "Melatonin as an Anti-Inflammatory Agent Modulating Inflammasome Activation," *International Journal of Endocrinology* (2017), doi.org/10.1155/2017/1835195; Yong Zhang et al., "Melatonin Alleviates Acute Lung Injury Through Inhibiting the NLRP3 Inflammasome," *Journal of Pineal Research* 60, no. 4 (2016), doi.org/10.1111/jpi.12322.

35. R. Leproult, U. Holmback, and E. Van Cauter, "Circadian Misalignment Augments Markers of Insulin Resistance and Inflammation, Independently of Sleep Loss," *Diabetes* 63, no. 6 (2014), doi.org/10.2337/db13-1546.

36. Tarani Chandola, Eric Brunner, and Michael Marmot, "Chronic Stress at Work and the Metabolic Syndrome: Prospective Study," *BMJ* 332, no. 7540 (2006), doi.org/10.1136/bmj.38693.435301.80.

37. S. Cohen et al., "Chronic Stress, Glucocorticoid Receptor Resistance, Inflammation, and Disease Risk," *Proceedings of the National Academy of Sciences of the United States of America* 109, no. 16 (2012), doi.org/10.1073/pnas.1118355109.

38. H. Renz et al., "An Exposome Perspective: Early-Life Events and Immune Development in a Changing World," *Journal of Allergy and Clinical Immunology* 140, no. 1 (2017), doi.org/10.1016/j.jaci.2017.05.015.

39. Caroline Isaksson, "Urbanization, Oxidative Stress and Inflammation: A

Question of Evolving, Acclimatizing or Coping with Urban Environmental Stress," *Functional Ecology* 29, no. 7 (2015), doi.org/10.1111/1365-2435.12477.

40. J. R. Swiston et al., "Wood Smoke Exposure Induces a Pulmonary and Systemic Inflammatory Response in Firefighters," *European Respiratory Journal* 32, no. 1 (2008), doi.org/10.1183/09031936.00097707.

41. A. J. Bartlett and Justin Clemens, *Alain Badiou: Key Concepts* (Durham, NC: Acumen, 2010), 9.

42. Ed Cohen, *A Body Worth Defending: Immunity, Biopolitics, and the Apotheosis of the Modern Body* (Durham, N.C.: Duke University Press, 2009), 41–45.

43. Steven I. Hajdu, "Rudolph Virchow, Pathologist, Armed Revolutionist, Politician, and Anthropologist," *Annals of Clinical and Laboratory Science* 35, no. 2 (2005): 204.

44. Friedrich Engels, *The Condition of the Working Class in England in 1844,* trans. Florence Kelley Wischnewetzky (New York: John W. Lovell Co., 1887).

45. Ibid., 64.

46. Ibid., 334.

47. Theodore M. Brown and Elizabeth Fee, "Rudolf Carl Virchow," *American Journal of Public Health* 96, no. 12 (2006), doi.org/10.2105/ajph.2005.078436.

48. Rex Taylor and Annelie Rieger, "Medicine as Social Science: Rudolf Virchow on the Typhus Epidemic in Upper Silesia," *International Journal of Health Services* 15, no. 4 (1985): 548.

49. Michael Titford, "Rudolf Virchow: Cellular Pathologist," *Laboratory Medicine* 41, no. 5 (2010), doi.org/10.1309/LM3GYQTY79CPYLBI.

50. Taylor and Rieger, "Medicine as Social Science."

51. Ibid., 550.

52. Ibid., 551.

53. George A. Silver, "Virchow, the Heroic Model in Medicine: Health Policy by Accolade," *American Journal of Public Health* 77, no. 1 (1987): 83, doi.org/10 .2105/ajph.77.1.82; Kazimierz Popiołek, "1848 in Silesia," *Slavonic and East European Review* 26, no. 7 (1948), www.jstor.org/stable/4203953.

54. Silver, "Virchow, the Heroic Model," 84.

55. "Weekly Commercial Times, Banker's Gazette and Railway Monitor," *Economist* 4, no. 163 (1846): 1315, books.google.com/books?id=kEdUAAAAcAAJ. The historian Jim Handy, who points us to the original quote, has a fine analysis, and notes with Michael Kirkpatric and Carla Fehr the similarities between *The Economist*'s rhetoric in Ireland and India. Jim Handy, "'Almost Idiotic Wretchedness': A Long History of Blaming Peasants," *Journal of Peasant Studies* 36, no. 2 (2009/04/01 2009), doi.org/10.1080/03066150902928306; Jim Handy and Michael D. Kirkpatrick, "'A Terrible Necessity': *The Economist* on India," *Canadian Journal of History* 51, no. 2 (2016), doi.org/10.3138/cjh.ach.51.2.02; Jim Handy and Carla Fehr, "'The Free Exercise of Self-Love': *The Economist* on Ireland," *Studies in Political Economy* 94, no. 1 (2014), doi.org/10.1080/19187033.2014.11674955.

56. "The Effect of the Government Feeding the Irish," *The Economist* 4, no. 155 (1846): 1050.

57. Hermann Beck, "State and Society in Pre-March Prussia: The Weavers' Uprising, the Bureaucracy, and the Association for the Welfare of Workers," *Central European History* 25, no. 3 (1992), jstor.org/stable/4546275.

58. Richard Grove, "The Influence of El Niño on World Crises in the Nineteenth Century," in *El Niño in World History*, ed. Richard Grove and George Adam-

son (London: Palgrave Macmillan UK, 2018); Cormac Ó Gráda and Andrés Eiríksson, *Ireland's Great Famine: Interdisciplinary Perspectives* (Dublin: University College Dublin Press, 2006).

59. Phelim P. Boyle and Cormac O. Grada, "Fertility Trends, Excess Mortality, and the Great Irish Famine," *Demography* 23, no. 4 (1986), doi.org/10.2307/2061350.

60. Helge Berger and Mark Spoerer, "Economic Crises and the European Revolutions of 1848," *Journal of Economic History* 61, no. 2 (2001), www.jstor.org /stable/2698022.

61. Izet Masic, "The Most Influential Scientists in the Development of Public Health (2): Rudolf Ludwig Virchow (1821–1902)," *Materia Socio Medica* 31, no. 2 (2019), doi.org/10.5455/msm.2019.31.151-152.

62. Howard Waitzkin, "The Social Origins of Illness: A Neglected History," 11, no. 1 (1981), doi.org/10.2190/5cdv-p4fe-y6hn-jacd.

63. Silver, "Virchow, the Heroic Model in Medicine: Health Policy by Accolade."

64. Jonathan Marks, "Why Be against Darwin? Creationism, Racism, and the Roots of Anthropology," *American Journal of Physical Anthropology* 149, no. S55 (2012), doi.org/10.1002/ajpa.22163.

65. Andrew Zimmerman, "Anti-Semitism as Skill: Rudolf Virchow's Schulstatistik and the Racial Composition of Germany," *Central European History* 32, no. 04 (1999), doi.org/10.1017/s0008938900021762.

66. Charles Darwin, *The Origin of Species by Means of Natural Selection* (New York: D. Appleton, 1898), 305, books.google.com/books?id = zt8yAQAAMAAJ.

67. Élie Metchnikoff, *Souvenirs: Recueil d'articles autobiographique*, trans. L. Piatagorski (Moscow: En Langues Étrangères, 1959), 97 in Cohen, *A Body Worth Defending: Immunity, Biopolitics, and the Apotheosis of the Modern Body*, 1.

68. Élie Metchnikoff, *Lectures on Comparative Pathology of Inflammation* (London: Kegan Paul, Trench, Trübner, 1893), 63, books.google.com/books?id = KjszAQAAMAAJ.

69. Ibid., 13.

70. Ibid.

71. Ibid., 1; Darwin. *Origin of Species.*

72. Metchnikoff, *Lectures on Comparative Pathology of Inflammation*, 3.

73. Ibid., lecture 2.

74. Ibid., 39.

75. Plants have a sophisticated innate immune system, but Metchnikoff was not alive to this. Hence his relatively brusque treatment of inflammation in plants, which he thought "would thus be only an irritation of the tissues (tumefaction, growth) *plus* a vascular congestion." In fact, plants have a robust innate immune response that becomes activated by pathogen-associated molecular patterns (PAMPs) expressed on a pathogen. Jonathan D. G. Jones and Jeffery L. Dangl, "The Plant Immune System," *Nature* 444, no. 7117 (2006), doi.org/10.1038/nature05286.

76. Natalya Yutin et al., "The Origins of Phagocytosis and Eukaryogenesis," *Biology Direct* 4 (2009), doi.org/10.1186/1745-6150-4-9. But cf. Katsumi Ueda et al., "Phagocytosis in Plant Protoplasts," *Cell Structure and Function* 3, no. 1 (1978). Plants *are* able to engulf and devour—just at the root, where Metchnikoff wasn't looking. We'll return to this in our penultimate chapter, in the discussion of the mycelial web.

77. Metchnikoff, *Lectures on Comparative Pathology of Inflammation*, 58.

78. Metchnikoff, *Lectures on Comparative Pathology of Inflammation*, 109–10.
79. Daniel M. Davis, *The Beautiful Cure: The Revolution in Immunology and What It Means for Your Health* (Chicago: The University of Chicago Press, 2018).
80. Akiko Iwasaki and Ruslan Medzhitov, "Control of Adaptive Immunity by the Innate Immune System," *Nature Immunology* 16, no. 4 (2015), doi.org/10.1038/ni.3123.
81. A. O'Garra, "Cytokines Induce the Development of Functionally Heterogeneous T Helper Cell Subsets," *Immunity* 8, no. 3 (1998), doi.org/10.1016/s1074-7613(00)80533-6.
82. Francesco Annunziato, Chiara Romagnani, and Sergio Romagnani, "The 3 Major Types of Innate and Adaptive Cell-Mediated Effector Immunity," *Journal of Allergy and Clinical Immunology* 135, no. 3 (2015), doi.org/10.1016/j.jaci.2014.11.001.
83. Ibid.
84. M. M. Stein et al., "Innate Immunity and Asthma Risk in Amish and Hutterite Farm Children," *New England Journal of Medicine* 375, no. 5 (2016), doi.org/10.1056/NEJMoa1508749.
85. Paurene Duramad et al., "Early Environmental Exposures and Intracellular Th1/Th2 Cytokine Profiles in 24-Month Old Children Living in an Agricultural Area," *Environmental Health Perspectives* 114, no. 2 (2006), doi.org/10.1289/ehp.9306.
86. Sergio Romagnani, "The Th1/Th2 Paradigm," *Immunology Today* 18, no. 6 (1997), doi.org/10.1016/s0167-5699(97)80019-9; Annunziato, Romagnani, and Romagnani, "3 Major Types of Effector Immunity."
87. Graham A. W. Rook, Christopher A. Lowry, and Charles L. Raison, "Microbial 'Old Friends,' Immunoregulation and Stress Resilience," *Evolution, Medicine, and Public Health* 2013, no. 1 (2013), doi.org/10.1093/emph/eot004.
88. Jérôme Hadjadj et al., "Impaired Type I Interferon Activity and Inflammatory Responses in Severe Covid-19 Patients," *Science* 369, no. 6504 (2020), doi.org/10.1126/science.abc6027.
89. Finlay McNab et al., "Type I Interferons in Infectious Disease," *Nature Reviews Immunology* 15, no. 2 (2015), doi.org/10.1038/nri3787.
90. Alfons Billiau, "Anti-Inflammatory Properties of Type I Interferons," *Antiviral Research* 71, no. 2–3 (2006), doi.org/10.1016/j.antiviral.2006.03.006.
91. Amit K. Maiti, "The African-American Population with a Low Allele Frequency of SNP rs1990760 (T allele) in IFIH1 Predicts Less IFN-Beta Expression and Potential Vulnerability to Covid-19 Infection," *Immunogenetics* 72, no. 6–7 (2020), doi.org/10.1007/s00251-020-01174-6.
92. N. D. Powell et al., "Social Stress Up-Regulates Inflammatory Gene Expression in the Leukocyte Transcriptome via Beta-Adrenergic Induction of Myelopoiesis," *Proceedings of the National Academy of Sciences of the United States of America* 110, no. 41 (2013), doi.org/10.1073/pnas.1310655110; S. W. Cole et al., "Transcriptional Modulation of the Developing Immune System by Early Life Social Adversity," *Proceedings of the National Academy of Sciences of the United States of America* 109, no. 50 (2012), doi.org/10.1073/pnas.1218253109.
93. Nehme et al., "Cellular Senescence as a Potential Mediator."
94. Naoko Ohtani, "Deciphering the Mechanism for Induction of Senescence-Associated Secretory Phenotype (SASP) and Its Role in Ageing and Cancer

Development," *Journal of Biochemistry* 166, no. 4 (2019), doi.org/10.1093/jb /mvz055; Francis Rodier et al., "Persistent DNA Damage Signalling Triggers Senescence-Associated Inflammatory Cytokine Secretion," *Nature Cell Biology* 11, no. 8 (2009), doi.org/10.1038/ncb1909.

95. Andrasfay and Goldman, "Reductions in 2020 US Life Expectancy"; Jarvis T. Chen and Nancy Krieger, "Revealing the Unequal Burden of COVID-19 by Income, Race/Ethnicity, and Household Crowding: US County Versus Zip Code Analysis," *Journal of Public Health Management and Practice* 27 (2021), doi.org/10.1097/PHH.0000000000001263.

96. Alfred I. Tauber, *Immunity: The Evolution of an Idea* (New York: Oxford University Press, 2017), 28.

97. Vijay Prashad, *The Darker Nations: A People's History of the Third World* (New York: New Press, 2007).

98. Warwick Anderson and Ian R. Mackay, "Fashioning the Immunological Self: The Biological Individuality of F. Macfarlane Burnet," *Journal of the History of Biology* 47, no. 1 (2014), www.jstor.org/stable/43863733.

99. Hyung Wook Park, "Germs, Hosts, and the Origin of Frank Macfarlane Burnet's Concept of 'Self' and 'Tolerance,' 1936–1949," *Journal of the History of Medicine and Allied Sciences* 61, no. 4 (2006), www.jstor.org/stable/24632317.

100. Wendy Brown, *Regulating Aversion: Tolerance in the Age of Identity and Empire* (Princeton, N.J.: Princeton University Press, 2006), 151.

101. Brown, *Regulating Aversion*, 151; emphasis in original.

102. Claudia Dreifus, "A Conversation with Polly Matzinger; Blazing an Unconventional Trail to a New Theory of Immunity," *The New York Times*, June 16, 1998, tinyurl.com/bqb2clzv.

103. Sarah Richardson, "The End of the Self," *Discover*, April 1, 1996, www .discovermagazine.com/health/the-end-of-the-self.

104. Dreifus, "Conversation with Polly Matzinger."

105. Polly Matzinger and Galadriel Mirkwood, "In a Fully H-2 Incompatible Chimera, T Cells of Donor Origin Can Respond to Minor Histocompatibility Antigens in Association with Either Donor or Host H-2 Type," *Journal of Experimental Medicine* 148, no. 1 (1978).

106. Polly Matzinger, "Tolerance, Danger, and the Extended Family," *Annual Review of Immunology* 12, no. 1 (1994): 922.

107. Ibid., 921.

108. Polly Matzinger, "The Danger Model: A Renewed Sense of Self," *Science* 296, no. 5566 (2002): 301, doi.org/10.1126/science.1071059.

109. Dreifus, "Conversation with Polly Matzinger."

110. Bernard E. Harcourt, *Illusion of Order: The False Promise of Broken Windows Policing* (Cambridge, MA: Harvard University Press, 2001).

111. Matzinger, "Danger Model," 301.

112. Stefania Gallucci and Polly Matzinger, "Danger Signals: SOS to the Immune System," *Current Opinion in Immunology* 13, no. 1 (2001), doi.org/10.1016 /s0952-7915(00)00191-6.

113. David Enard et al., "Viruses Are a Dominant Driver of Protein Adaptation in Mammals," *eLife* 5 (2016), doi.org/10.7554/elife.12469.

114. Sha Mi et al., "Syncytin Is a Captive Retroviral Envelope Protein Involved in Human Placental Morphogenesis," *Nature* 403, no. 6771 (2000), doi.org/10 .1038/35001608.

115. Harold F. Dvorak, "Tumors: Wounds That Do Not Heal," *New England Journal of Medicine* 315, no. 26 (1986), doi.org/10.1056/NEJM198612253152606.

116. Maria B. Witte and Adrian Barbul, "General Principles of Wound Healing," *Surgical Clinics of North America* 77, no. 3 (1997), doi.org/10.1016/s0039-6109(05)70566-1.

117. Ibid.

118. M. B. Witte and A. Barbul, "Role of Nitric Oxide in Wound Repair," *American Journal of Surgery* 183, no. 4 (2002), doi.org/10.1016/s0002-9610(02)00815-2.

119. Witte and Barbul, "General Principles of Wound Healing"; L. M. Coussens and Z. Werb, "Inflammation and Cancer," *Nature* 420, no. 6917 (2002), doi.org/10.1038/nature01322.

120. David L. Steed, "The Role of Growth Factors in Wound Healing," *Surgical Clinics of North America* 77, no. 3 (1997), doi.org/10.1016/s0039-6109(05)70569-7.

121. Coussens and Werb, "Inflammation and Cancer."

122. Witte and Barbul, "General Principles of Wound Healing."

123. S. M. Levenson et al., "The Healing of Rat Skin Wounds," *Annals of Surgery* 161 (1965), doi.org/10.1097/00000658-196502000-00019.

124. Witte and Barbul, "General Principles of Wound Healing."

125. F. Balkwill and A. Mantovani, "Inflammation and Cancer: Back to Virchow?," *The Lancet* 357, no. 9255 (2001), doi.org/10.1016/S0140-6736(00)04046-0.

126. Coussens and Werb, "Inflammation and Cancer."

127. Dvorak, "Tumors: Wounds That Do Not Heal."

128. Matthew D. Vesely et al., "Natural Innate and Adaptive Immunity to Cancer," *Annual Review of Immunology* 29, no. 1 (2011), doi.org/10.1146/annurev-immunol-031210-101324.

129. Jean-Philippe Coppé et al., "The Senescence-Associated Secretory Phenotype: The Dark Side of Tumor Suppression," *Annual Review of Pathology: Mechanisms of Disease* 5, no. 1 (2010), doi.org/10.1146/annurev-pathol-121808-102144.

130. Jeremy B. Swann and Mark J. Smyth, "Immune Surveillance of Tumors," *Journal of Clinical Investigation* 117, no. 5 (2007), doi.org/10.1172/jci31405.

131. Coussens and Werb, "Inflammation and Cancer."

132. Ibid.; G. Deng, "Tumor-Infiltrating Regulatory T Cells: Origins and Features," *American Journal of Clinical and Experimental Immunology* 7, no. 5 (2018), www.ncbi.nlm.nih.gov/pubmed/30498624.

133. Coussens and Werb, "Inflammation and Cancer."

134. E. V. Tsianos, "Risk of Cancer in Inflammatory Bowel Disease (IBD)," *European Journal of Internal Medicine* 11, no. 2 (2000), doi.org/10.1016/s0953-6205(00)00061-3.

135. R. F. Souza, "From Reflux Esophagitis to Esophageal Adenocarcinoma," *Digestive Diseases* 34, no. 5 (2016), doi.org/10.1159/000445225.

136. A. Mantovani et al., "Cancer-Related Inflammation," *Nature* 454, no. 7203 (2008), doi.org/10.1038/nature07205.

137. H. Kuper, H. O. Adami, and D. Trichopoulos, "Infections as a Major Preventable Cause of Human Cancer," *Journal of Internal Medicine* 249, no. S741 (2001), doi.org/10.1046/j.1365-2796.2001.00742.x.

138. Ibid.

139. E. Mirzaie-Kashani et al., "Detection of Human Papillomavirus in Chronic Cervicitis, Cervical Adenocarcinoma, Intraepithelial Neoplasia and Squamus

Cell Carcinoma," *Jundishapur Journal of Microbiology* 7, no. 5 (2014), doi.org /10.5812/jjm.9930.

140. P. Pisani et al., "Cancer and Infection: Estimates of the Attributable Fraction in 1990," *Cancer Epidemiology, Biomarkers, and Prevention* 6, no. 6 (1997), www.ncbi.nlm.nih.gov/pubmed/9184771.

141. Kuper, Adami, and Trichopoulos, "Infections as Major Preventable Cause"; C. H. Wong and K. Goh, "Chronic Hepatitis B Infection and Liver Cancer," *Biomedical Imaging and Intervention Journal of* 2, no. 3 (2006), doi.org/10.2349/biij.2.3.e7.

142. P. B. Ernst and B. D. Gold, "The Disease Spectrum of *Helicobacter pylori*: The Immunopathogenesis of Gastroduodenal Ulcer and Gastric Cancer," *Annual Review of Microbiology* 54 (2000), doi.org/10.1146/annurev.micro.54.1.615.

143. H. Maeda and T. Akaike, "Nitric Oxide and Oxygen Radicals in Infection, Inflammation, and Cancer," *Biochemistry* (Moscow) 63, no. 7 (1998), www.ncbi .nlm.nih.gov/pubmed/9721338.

144. The tumor-suppressor gene P53 encodes a protein involved in regulating the cell life cycle, including apoptosis. It performs a crucial quality-control function in all our cell lines. When it senses cellular stress and injury, it stops cell division. If the harm can't be corrected, P53 can send the cell down the path to self-destruction. Without this gene, we lose a critical checkpoint, allowing cells with damaged DNA to grow uninhibited.

145. Kuper, Adami, and Trichopoulos, "Infections as a Major Preventable Cause of Human Cancer."

146. K. L. Rock and H. Kono, "The Inflammatory Response to Cell Death," *Annual Review of Pathology: Mechanisms of Disease* 3 (2008), doi.org/10.1146/annurev .pathmechdis.3.121806.151456.

147. Coussens and Werb, "Inflammation and Cancer"; Mantovani et al., "Cancer-Related Inflammation."

148. Mantovani et al., "Cancer-Related Inflammation."

149. Rashid Hanif et al., "Effects of Nonsteroidal Anti-Inflammatory Drugs on Proliferation and on Induction of Apoptosis in Colon Cancer Cells by a Prostaglandin-Independent Pathway," *Biochemical Pharmacology* 52, no. 2 (1996), doi.org/10.1016/0006-2952(96)00181-5.

150. Mantovani et al., "Cancer-Related Inflammation," 436.

151. Ibid.

152. T. Hagemann et al., "'Re-Educating' Tumor-Associated Macrophages by Targeting NF-κB," *Journal of Experimental Medicine* 205, no. 6 (2008), doi.org/10 .1084/jem.20080108.

153. Mantovani et al., "Cancer-Related Inflammation."

154. E. F. McCarthy, "The Toxins of William B. Coley and the Treatment of Bone and Soft-Tissue Sarcomas," *Iowa Orthopedic Journal* 26 (2006).

155. Ibid.

156. William Coley, "The Treatment of Malignant Tumors by Repeated Inoculations of Erysipelas: With a Report of Ten Original Cases," *American Journal of the Medical Sciences* 105 (1893).

157. E. Richard Brown, *Rockefeller Medicine Men: Medicine and Capitalism in America* (Berkeley: University of California Press, 1979). The investment paid off as modern medicine now relies on petroleum to transport patients, staff, supplies and to make medical supplies and drugs. Jeremy Hess et al., "Petroleum and Health Care: Evaluating and Managing Health Care's Vulnerability to

Petroleum Supply Shifts," *American Journal of Public Health* 101, no. 9 (2011), doi.org/10.2105/AJPH.2011.300233.

158. B. J. Johnston and E. T. Novales, "Clinical Effect of Coley's Toxin. II. A Seven-Year Study," *Cancer Chemotherapy Reports* 21 (1962), www.ncbi.nlm.nih.gov /pubmed/14452138.

159. H. C. Nauts and J. R. McLaren, "Coley Toxins—The First Century," *Advances in Experimental Medicine and Biology* 267 (1990), doi.org/10.1007/978-1-4684 -5766-7_52.

160. H. W. Herr and A. Morales, "History of Bacillus Calmette-Guerin and Bladder Cancer: An Immunotherapy Success Story," *Journal of Urology* 179, no. 1 (2008), doi.org/10.1016/j.juro.2007.08.122.

161. Ibid.

162. Diwakar Davar et al., "High-Dose Interleukin-2 (HD IL-2) for Advanced Melanoma: A Single Center Experience from the University of Pittsburgh Cancer Institute," *Journal for ImmunoTherapy of Cancer* 5, no. 1 (2017), doi.org/10.1186 /s40425-017-0279-5.

163. Daniel W. Cramer et al., "Mumps and Ovarian Cancer: Modern Interpretation of an Historic Association," *Cancer Causes and Control* 21, no. 8 (2010), doi.org /10.1007/s10552-010-9546-1.

164. Rae Myers et al., "Oncolytic Activities of Approved Mumps and Measles Vaccines for Therapy of Ovarian Cancer," *Cancer Gene Therapy* 12, no. 7 (2005), doi.org/10.1038/sj.cgt.7700823.

165. S. J. Russell and K. W. Peng, "Measles Virus for Cancer Therapy," *Current Topics in Microbiology and Immunology* 330 (2009), doi.org/10.1007/978-3-540 -70617-5_11; Stephen J. Russell et al., "Oncolytic Measles Virotherapy and Opposition to Measles Vaccination," *Mayo Clinic Proceedings* 94, no. 9 (2019), doi.org/10.1016/j.mayocp.2019.05.006.

166. Mel Greaves, "A Causal Mechanism for Childhood Acute Lymphoblastic Leukaemia," *Nature Reviews Cancer* 18, no. 8 (2018), doi.org/10.1038/s41568-018 -0015-6.

167. P. Correa and M. B. Piazuelo, "*Helicobacter pylori* Infection and Gastric Adenocarcinoma," *US Gastroenterology and Hepatology Review* 7, no. 1 (2011), www .ncbi.nlm.nih.gov/pubmed/21857882; Meira Epplein et al., "Race, African Ancestry, and *Helicobacter pylori* Infection in a Low-Income United States Population," *Cancer Epidemiology Biomarkers and Prevention* 20, no. 5 (2011), doi.org /10.1158/1055-9965.epi-10-1258.

168. Correa and Piazuelo, "*Helicobacter pylori* Infection."

169. David E. Elliott, Robert W. Summers, and Joel V. Weinstock, "Helminths as Governors of Immune-Mediated Inflammation," *International Journal for Parasitology* 37, no. 5 (2007), doi.org/10.1016/j.ijpara.2006.12.009.

170. Centers for Disease Control and Prevention, *Cancer Incidence Among African Americans, United States, 2007–2016*, USCS Data Brief, no. 15 (Atlanta, GA: Centers for Disease Control and Prevention, 2020).

171. Correa and Piazuelo, "*Helicobacter pylori* Infection."

172. S. Lederer, "'Porto Ricochet': Joking About Germs, Cancer, and Race Extermination in the 1930s," *American Literary History* 14, no. 4 (2002), www.jstor .org/stable/3568022.

173. Eric T. Rosenthal, "The Rhoads Not Given," *Oncology Times* 25, no. 17 (2003), doi.org/10.1097/01.cot.0000290560.69715.bf.

174. Ibid.; Lederer, "'Porto Ricochet.'"
175. "Cancer Fighter, Cornelius P. Rhoads," *Time*, June 27, 1949.
176. Susan L. Smith, "War! What Is It Good For? Mustard Gas Medicine," *Canadian Medical Association Journal* 189, no. 8 (2017), doi.org/10.1503/cmaj.161032.
177. Matthew Tontonoz, "Beyond Magic Bullets: Helen Coley Nauts and the Battle for Immunotherapy," *Cancer Research Institute*, April 1, 2015, tinyurl.com /by4vdoli.
178. J. Couzin-Frankel, "Cancer Immunotherapy," *Science* 342, no. 6165 (2013), doi .org/10.1126/science.342.6165.1432.
179. Filipe Martins et al., "Adverse Effects of Immune-Checkpoint Inhibitors: Epidemiology, Management and Surveillance," *Nature Reviews Clinical Oncology* 16, no. 9 (2019), doi.org/10.1038/s41571-019-0218-0.
180. Antoni Ribas and Jedd D. Wolchok, "Cancer Immunotherapy Using Checkpoint Blockade," *Science* 359, no. 6382 (2018), doi.org/10.1126/science.aar4060.
181. Ibid.
182. Ibid.; Couzin-Frankel, "Cancer Immunotherapy"; Jedd D. Wolchok et al., "Overall Survival with Combined Nivolumab and Ipilimumab in Advanced Melanoma," *New England Journal of Medicine* 377, no. 14 (2017), doi.org/10.1056 /nejmoa1709684; F. S. Hodi et al., "Nivolumab Plus Ipilimumab or Nivolumab Alone Versus Ipilimumab Alone in Advanced Melanoma (Checkmate 067): 4-Year Outcomes of a Multicentre, Randomised, Phase 3 Trial," *Lancet Oncology* 19, no. 11 (2018), doi.org/10.1016/S1470-2045(18)30700-9; D. F. McDermott et al., "Quality-Adjusted Survival of Nivolumab Plus Ipilimumab or Nivolumab Alone Versus Ipilimumab Alone Among Treatment-Naive Patients with Advanced Melanoma: A Quality-Adjusted Time Without Symptoms or Toxicity (Q-Twist) Analysis," *Quality of Life Research* 28, no. 1 (2019), doi.org/10.1007 /s11136-018-1984-3.
183. Ribas and Wolchok, "Cancer Immunotherapy Using Checkpoint Blockade"; Martins et al., "Adverse Effects of Immune-Checkpoint Inhibitors."
184. Ribas and Wolchok, "Cancer Immunotherapy Using Checkpoint Blockade."
185. Martins et al., "Adverse Effects of Immune-Checkpoint Inhibitors."
186. Ibid.; McDermott et al., "Quality-Adjusted Survival of Nivolumab."
187. A. Andrews, "Treating with Checkpoint Inhibitors—Figure $1 Million per Patient," *American Health and Drug Benefits* 8, spec. issue (2015), www.ncbi.nlm .nih.gov/pubmed/26380599.
188. Freddie Bray et al., "Global Cancer Statistics 2018: Globocan Estimates of Incidence and Mortality Worldwide for 36 Cancers in 185 Countries," *CA: A Cancer Journal for Clinicians* 68, no. 6 (2018), doi.org/10.3322/caac.21492; Wenpeng You and Maciej Henneberg, "Cancer Incidence Increasing Globally: The Role of Relaxed Natural Selection," *Evolutionary Applications* 11, no. 2 (2018), doi.org /10.1111/eva.12523.
189. Bray et al., "Global Cancer Statistics 2018"; J. Ferlay et al., "Estimating the Global Cancer Incidence and Mortality in 2018: Globocan Sources and Methods," *International Journal of Cancer* 144, no. 8 (2019), doi.org/10.1002/ijc .31937.
190. T. Luzzati, A. Parenti, and T. Rughi, "Economic Growth and Cancer Incidence," *Ecological Economics* 146 (2018), doi.org/10.1016/j.ecolecon.2017.11.031.
191. A. Kapoor, "A Train Offers Hope to Punjab's Patients with Cancer but It Isn't Enough," *BMJ* 349 (2014), doi.org/10.1136/bmj.g4484.

192. David Pimentel, "Green Revolution Agriculture and Chemical Hazards," *Science of the Total Environment* 188 (1996), doi.org/10.1016/0048-9697(96)05280-1.

193. Gary M. Williams, Robert Kroes, and Ian C. Munro, "Safety Evaluation and Risk Assessment of the Herbicide Roundup and Its Active Ingredient, Glyphosate, for Humans," *Regulatory Toxicology and Pharmacology* 31, no. 2 (2000), doi .org/10.1006/rtph.1999.1371. Carey Gillam's work has been vital. See, e.g., Carey Gillam, *Whitewash: The Story of a Weed Killer, Cancer, and the Corruption of Science* (Washington, DC: Island Press, 2017), and Carey Gillam, *The Monsanto Papers: Deadly Secrets, Corporate Corruption, and One Man's Search for Justice* (Washington, DC: Island Press, 2021).

194. Rebecca L. Siegel, Kimberly D. Miller, and Ahmedin Jemal, "Colorectal Cancer Mortality Rates in Adults Aged 20 to 54 Years in the United States, 1970–2014," *JAMA* 318, no. 6 (2017), doi.org/10.1001/jama.2017.7630; Rebecca L. Siegel et al., "Colorectal Cancer Incidence Patterns in the United States, 1974–2013," *JNCI: Journal of the National Cancer Institute* 109, no. 8 (2017), doi.org/10.1093/jnci/djw322.

195. Charles M. Benbrook, "Trends in Glyphosate Herbicide Use in the United States and Globally," *Environmental Sciences Europe* 28, no. 1 (2016), doi.org /10.1186/s12302-016-0070-0.

196. IARC Working Group on the Evaluation of Carcinogenic Risks to Humans, "Some Organophosphate Insecticides and Herbicides," *IARC Monographs on the Evaluation of Carcinogenic Risks to Humans* 112 (Lyon, 2015).

197. S. Thongprakaisang et al., "Glyphosate Induces Human Breast Cancer Cells Growth Via Estrogen Receptors," *Food and Chemical Toxicology* 59 (2013), doi .org/10.1016/j.fct.2013.05.057.

198. Wisanti Laohaudomchok et al., "Pesticide Use in Thailand: Current Situation, Health Risks, and Gaps in Research and Policy," *Human and Ecological Risk Assessment: An International Journal* (2020), doi.org/10.1080/10807039.2020 .1808777.

199. Virginia A. Rauh et al., "Impact of Prenatal Chlorpyrifos Exposure on Neurodevelopment in the First 3 Years of Life Among Inner-City Children," *Pediatrics* 118, no. 6 (2006), doi.org/10.1542/peds.2006-0338.

200. Agence France Presse, "Thailand to Ban Glyphosate and Other High-Profile Pesticides," *France 24*, October 22, 2019, tinyurl.com/p7xj4yev.

201. One of the law firms representing plaintiffs in cases against Monsanto keeps a running list of places where glyphosate is banned. "Where Is Glyphosate Banned?" *Baum Hedlund*, December 2020, tinyurl.com/hcg79elx.

202. D. Kubsad et al., "Assessment of Glyphosate Induced Epigenetic Transgenerational Inheritance of Pathologies and Sperm Epimutations: Generational Toxicology," *Scientific Reports* 9, no. 1 (2019), doi.org/10.1038/s41598-019-42860-0.

203. Michael K. Skinner, Mohan Manikkam, and Carlos Guerrero-Bosagna, "Epigenetic Transgenerational Actions of Environmental Factors in Disease Etiology," *Trends in Endocrinology and Metabolism* 21, no. 4 (2010), doi.org/10.1016 /j.tem.2009.12.007; Michael K. Skinner, "Environmental Stress and Epigenetic Transgenerational Inheritance," *BMC Medicine* 12, no. 1 (2014), doi.org/10 .1186/s12916-014-0153-y.

204. Erika Hayasaki, "Identical Twins Hint at How Environments Change Gene Expression," *The Atlantic*, May 15, 2018, tinyurl.com/1irqlske.

205. Luiz Carlos Caires-Júnior et al., "Discordant Congenital Zika Syndrome Twins

Show Differential in Vitro Viral Susceptibility of Neural Progenitor Cells," *Nature Communications* 9, no. 1 (2018), doi.org/10.1038/s41467-017-02790-9.

206. R. Holliday and J. E. Pugh, "DNA Modification Mechanisms and Gene Activity During Development," *Science* 187, no. 4173 (1975), www.ncbi.nlm.nih.gov/pubmed/1111098; Kubsad et al., "Assessment of Glyphosate Induced Epigenetic."

207. Lisa D. Moore, Thuc Le, and Guoping Fan, "DNA Methylation and Its Basic Function," *Neuropsychopharmacology* 38, no. 1 (2013), doi.org/10.1038/npp.2012.112; Adrian Ruiz-Hernandez et al., "Environmental Chemicals and DNA Methylation in Adults: A Systematic Review of the Epidemiologic Evidence," *Clinical Epigenetics* 7, no. 1 (2015), doi.org/10.1186/s13148-015-0055-7.

208. Ruiz-Hernandez et al., "Environmental Chemicals and DNA Methylation."

209. Kubsad et al., "Assessment of Glyphosate Induced Epigenetic."

210. Stephanie J. Waterman, "Home-Going as a Strategy for Success Among Haudenosaunee College and University Students," *Journal of Student Affairs Research and Practice* 49, no. 2 (2012), doi.org/10.1515/jsarp-2012-6378.

211. Axel Adams, Matthew Friesen, and Roy Gerona, "Biomonitoring of Glyphosate Across the United States in Urine and Tap Water Using High-Fidelity LC-MS," Asia Pacific Association of Medical Toxicology, Perth, Australia, 2015, www.apamt.org/wp-content/uploads/2017/06/Poster_Presentation_34.pdf.

212. Paul J. Mills et al., "Excretion of the Herbicide Glyphosate in Older Adults Between 1993 and 2016," *JAMA* 318, no. 16 (2017), doi.org/10.1001/jama.2017.11726.

213. John Fagan et al., "Organic Diet Intervention Significantly Reduces Urinary Glyphosate Levels in U.S. Children and Adults," *Environmental Research* 189 (2020), doi.org/10.1016/j.envres.2020.109898.

214. Chelsea M. Rochman and Timothy Hoellein, "The Global Odyssey of Plastic Pollution," *Science* 368, no. 6496 (2020), doi.org/10.1126/science.abc4428; Philip J. Landrigan et al., "The *Lancet* Commission on Pollution and Health," *The Lancet* 391, no. 10119 (2018), doi.org/10.1016/s0140-6736(17)32345-0.

215. Aubrey K. Hubbard et al., "Trends in International Incidence of Pediatric Cancers in Children Under 5 Years of Age: 1988–2012," *JNCI Cancer Spectrum* 3, no. 1 (2019), doi.org/10.1093/jncics/pkz007.

216. Sumit Gupta et al., "Low Socioeconomic Status Is Associated with Worse Survival in Children with Cancer: A Systematic Review," *PLOS One* 9, no. 2 (2014), doi.org/10.1371/journal.pone.0089482.

217. Debra J. Salazar et al., "Race, Income, and Environmental Inequality in the U.S. States, 1990–2014," *Social Science Quarterly* 100, no. 3 (2019), doi.org/10.1111/ssqu.12608.

218. Tony Castanha, *The Myth of Indigenous Caribbean Extinction: Continuity and Reclamation in Borikén (Puerto Rico)* (New York: Palgrave Macmillan, 2011).

219. J. C. Martinez-Cruzado et al., "Mitochondrial DNA Analysis Reveals Substantial Native American Ancestry in Puerto Rico," *Human Biology* 73, no. 4 (2001), www.jstor.org/stable/41466825?seq = 1.

220. Christina Duffy Burnett and Burke Marshall, "Between the Foreign and the Domestic: The Doctrine of Territorial Incorporation, Invented and Reinvented," in *Foreign in a Domestic Sense: Puerto Rico, American Expansion, and the Constitution*, ed. Christina Duffy Burnett and Burke Marshall (Durham,

NC: Duke University Press, 2001); Lisa Maria Perez, "Citizenship Denied: The 'Insular Cases' and the Fourteenth Amendment," *Virginia Law Review* 94, no. 4 (2008): 1039.

221. Naomi Klein, *The Battle for Paradise: Puerto Rico Takes on the Disaster Capitalists* (Chicago: Haymarket Books, 2018).

222. Maricruz Rivera-Hernandez et al., "Quality of Care for White and Hispanic Medicare Advantage Enrollees in the United States and Puerto Rico," *JAMA Internal Medicine* 176, no. 6 (2016), doi.org/10.1001/jamainternmed.2016.0267.

223. Nishant Kishore et al., "Mortality in Puerto Rico After Hurricane Maria," *New England Journal of Medicine* 379, no. 2 (2018), doi.org/10.1056/nejmsa1803972.

224. Tamar Adler, "The Young Farmers Behind Puerto Rico's Food Revolution," *Vogue*, June 20, 2018, tinyurl.com/yjmogsfm.

225. Joy E. Lin et al., "Associations of Childhood Adversity and Adulthood Trauma with C-Reactive Protein: A Cross-Sectional Population-Based Study," *Brain, Behavior, and Immunity* 53 (2016), doi.org/10.1016/j.bbi.2015.11.015; Aoife O'Donovan et al., "Lifetime Exposure to Traumatic Psychological Stress Is Associated with Elevated Inflammation in the Heart and Soul Study," *Brain, Behavior, and Immunity* 26, no. 4 (2012), doi.org/10.1016/j.bbi.2012.02.003; Aoife O'Donovan and Thomas C. Neylan, "Associations of Trauma and Posttraumatic Stress Disorder with Inflammation and Endothelial Function: On Timing, Specificity, and Mechanisms," *Biological Psychiatry* 82, no. 12 (2017), doi.org/10.1016/j.biopsych.2017.10.002.

226. S. Entringer et al., "Stress Exposure in Intrauterine Life Is Associated with Shorter Telomere Length in Young Adulthood," *Proceedings of the National Academy of Sciences of the United States of America* 108, no. 33 (2011), doi.org/10.1073/pnas.1107759108.

227. Aoife O'Donovan et al., "Childhood Trauma Associated with Short Leukocyte Telomere Length in Posttraumatic Stress Disorder," *Biological Psychiatry* 70, no. 5 (2011), doi.org/10.1016/j.biopsych.2011.01.035.

228. Frank Edwards, Hedwig Lee, and Michael Esposito, "Risk of Being Killed by Police Use of Force in the United States by Age, Race-Ethnicity, and Sex," *Proceedings of the National Academy of Sciences of the United States of America* 116, no. 34 (2019), doi.org/10.1073/pnas.1821204116.

229. Michael J. McFarland et al., "Perceived Unfair Treatment by Police, Race, and Telomere Length: A Nashville Community-Based Sample of Black and White Men," *Journal of Health and Social Behavior* 59, no. 4 (2018), doi.org/10.1177/0022146518811144.

230. O'Donovan et al., "Childhood Trauma Associated."

231. Vesna Gorenjak et al., "Telomere Length Determinants in Childhood," *Clinical Chemistry and Laboratory Medicine* 58, no. 2 (2020), doi.org/10.1515/cclm-2019-0235.

232. Calvin B. Harley, A. Bruce Futcher, and Carol W. Greider, "Telomeres Shorten During Ageing of Human Fibroblasts," *Nature* 345, no. 6274 (1990), doi.org/10.1038/345458a0; R. C. Allsopp et al., "Telomere Shortening Is Associated with Cell Division in Vitro and in Vivo," *Experimental Cell Research* 220, no. 1 (1995), doi.org/10.1006/excr.1995.1306.

233. Utz Herbig et al., "Telomere Shortening Triggers Senescence of Human Cells Through a Pathway Involving ATM, p53, and p21[CIP1], but Not P16[INK4a]," *Molecular Cell* 14, no. 4 (2004), doi.org/10.1016/s1097-2765(04)00256-4.

234. Janet Lindsey et al., "In Vivo Loss of Telomeric Repeats with Age in Humans," *Mutation Research/DNAging* 256, no. 1 (1991), doi.org/10.1016/0921 -8734(91)90032-7.

235. E. Epel, "How 'Reversible' Is Telomeric Aging?," *Cancer Prevention Research* 5, no. 10 (2012), doi.org/10.1158/1940-6207.capr-12-0370.

236. Gorenjak et al., "Telomere Length Determinants in Childhood."

237. Manish Kumar, Werner Seeger, and Robert Voswinckel, "Senescence-Associated Secretory Phenotype and Its Possible Role in Chronic Obstructive Pulmonary Disease," *American Journal of Respiratory Cell and Molecular Biology* 51, no. 3 (2014), doi.org/10.1165/rcmb.2013-0382ps; Katri Savolainen et al., "Associations Between Early Life Stress, Self-Reported Traumatic Experiences Across the Lifespan and Leukocyte Telomere Length in Elderly Adults," *Biological Psychology* 97 (2014), doi.org/10.1016/j.biopsycho.2014.02 .002; Masahiro Irie et al., "Relationships Between Perceived Workload, Stress and Oxidative DNA Damage," *International Archives of Occupational and Environmental Health* 74, no. 2 (2001), doi.org/10.1007/s004200000209; Masahiro Irie et al., "Depressive State Relates to Female Oxidative DNA Damage Via Neutrophil Activation," *Biochemical and Biophysical Research Communications* 311, no. 4 (2003), doi.org/10.1016/j.bbrc.2003.10.105; Xiao Zhang et al., "Republished: Environmental and Occupational Exposure to Chemicals and Telomere Length in Human Studies," *Postgraduate Medical Journal* 89, no. 1058 (2013), doi.org/10.1136/postgradmedj-2012-101350rep; E. S. Epel et al., "Accelerated Telomere Shortening in Response to Life Stress," *Proceedings of the National Academy of Sciences of the United States of America* 101, no. 49 (2004), doi.org/10.1073/pnas.0407162101.

238. Entringer et al., "Stress Exposure in Intrauterine Life."

239. McFarland et al., "Perceived Unfair Treatment by Police."

240. O'Donovan et al., "Childhood Trauma Associated"; Lawrence H. Price et al., "Telomeres and Early-Life Stress: An Overview," *Biological Psychiatry* 73, no. 1 (2013), doi.org/10.1016/j.biopsych.2012.06.025.

241. Youli Yao et al., "Ancestral Exposure to Stress Epigenetically Programs Preterm Birth Risk and Adverse Maternal and Newborn Outcomes," *BMC Medicine* 12, no. 1 (2014), doi.org/10.1186/s12916-014-0121-6.

242. Epel, "How 'Reversible' Is Telomeric Aging?"; Elissa Epel et al., "Can Meditation Slow Rate of Cellular Aging? Cognitive Stress, Mindfulness, and Telomeres," *Annals of the New York Academy of Sciences* 1172, no. 1 (2009), doi.org /10.1111/j.1749-6632.2009.04414.x.

243. N. P. Kellermann, "Epigenetic Transmission of Holocaust Trauma: Can Nightmares Be Inherited?," *Israel Journal of Psychiatry and Related Sciences* 50, no. 1 (2013), www.ncbi.nlm.nih.gov/pubmed/24029109.

244. María J. Molina et al., "Prevalence of Systemic Lupus Erythematosus and Associated Comorbidities in Puerto Rico," *JCR: Journal of Clinical Rheumatology* 13, no. 4 (2007), doi.org/10.1097/rhu.0b013e318124a8af.

245. M. Molokhia and P. McKeigue, "Systemic Lupus Erythematosus: Genes Versus Environment in High Risk Populations," *Lupus* 15, no. 11 (2006), doi.org /10.1177/.

246. Arndt Manzel et al., "Role of 'Western Diet' in Inflammatory Autoimmune Diseases," *Current Allergy and Asthma Reports* 14, no. 1 (2013), doi.org/10.1007 /s11882-013-0404-6.

247. Julia Baudry et al., "Association of Frequency of Organic Food Consumption with Cancer Risk," *JAMA Internal Medicine* 178, no. 12 (2018), doi.org/10.1001/jamainternmed.2018.4357; Elena C. Hemler, Jorge E. Chavarro, and Frank B. Hu, "Organic Foods for Cancer Prevention—Worth the Investment?," *JAMA Internal Medicine* 178, no. 12 (2018), doi.org/10.1001/jamainternmed.2018.4363.

248. Kenneth Dorshkind, Encarnacion Montecino-Rodriguez, and Robert A. J. Signer, "The Ageing Immune System: Is It Ever Too Old to Become Young Again?," *Nature Reviews Immunology* 9, no. 1 (2009), doi.org/10.1038/nri2471; Julie A. Mattison et al., "Caloric Restriction Improves Health and Survival of Rhesus Monkeys," *Nature Communications* 8, no. 1 (2017), doi.org/10.1038/ncomms14063.

249. *The State of Food Security and Nutrition in the World 2020: Transforming Food Systems for Affordable Healthy Diets* (Rome: FAO, 2020), xvi, doi.org/10.4060/ca9692en.

250. Sylvia Cremer, Sophie A. O. Armitage, and Paul Schmid-Hempel, "Social Immunity," *Current Biology* 17, no. 16 (2007), doi.org/10.1016/j.cub.2007.06.008. See also S. C. Cotter and R. M. Kilner, "Personal Immunity Versus Social Immunity," *Behavioral Ecology* 21, no. 4 (2010), doi.org/10.1093/beheco/arq070.

251. Akhil Gupta, *Red Tape: Bureaucracy, Structural Violence, and Poverty in India* (Durham, NC: Duke University Press, 2012).

252. World Bank, *Promoting Green Urban Development in African Cities: Ethekwini, South Africa Urban Environmental Profile* (Washington, DC: World Bank, 2016); Tara Saharan et al., "Comparing Governance and Bargaining of Livelihoods in Informal Settlements in Chennai and Ethekwini," *Cities* (2019), doi.org/10.1016/j.cities.2019.02.017.

253. Monika Kuffer et al., "Do We Underestimate the Global Slum Population?" paper presented at the Joint Urban Remote Sensing Event, Vannes, Frances, 2019, doi.org/10.1109/jurse.2019.8809066.

254. Jamie Bartram and Sandy Cairncross, "Hygiene, Sanitation, and Water: Forgotten Foundations of Health," *PLOS Medicine* 7, no. 11 (2010), doi.org/10.1371/journal.pmed.1000367.

255. Human Rights Watch, *"They Have Robbed Me of My Life" Xenophobic Violence Against Non-Nationals in South Africa* (New York: Human Rights Watch, 2020). There is a police force of a kind in the shack communities—local safety committees make sure that in cases of assault or theft, "the offender can be asked to restore to the victim whatever may be fair to the victim. The offender can also be expelled from the settlement," says Zikode. In the most serious cases, of rape and murder, the state police are called in.

256. Kerry Ryan Chance, *Living Politics in South Africa's Urban Shacklands* (Chicago: University of Chicago Press, 2018); Richard Pithouse, "Burning Message to the State in the Fire of Poor's Rebellion," *Business Day* (Johannesburg), July 23, 2009; Richard Pithouse and Mark Butler, *Lessons from Ethekwini: Pariahs Hold Their Ground Against a State That Is Both Criminal and Democratic* (Pietermaritzburg: Association for Rural Advancement, 2007), abahlali.org/node/984; S'bu Zikode, "The Greatest Threat to Future Stability in Our Country Is the Greatest Strength of the Abahlali baseMjondolo Movement (SA) (Shackdwellers)," *Journal of Asian and African Studies* 43, no. 1 (2008), doi.org/10.1177/0021909607085642.

257. One way of understanding this space is as an "undercommons," a term coined

by Fred Moten and Stefano Harmey. See Stefano Harmey and Fred Moten, *The Undercommons: Fugitive Planning and Black Study* (New York: Minor Compositions, 2013). It is an understanding shared with the Tohono O'odham Nation, whose land is cleaved by the US-Mexico border and who lack the words for *border* and *citizen*. Fernanda Santos, "Border Wall Would Cleave Tribe, and Its Connection to Ancestral Land," *The New York Times*, February 20, 2017, tinyurl.com/1whcxlqi.

258. Donna Haraway, "Situated Knowledges: The Science Question in Feminism and the Privilege of Partial Perspective," *Feminist Studies* 14, no. 3 (1988): 586, doi.org/10.2307/3178066. See also Lisa Weasel, "Dismantling the Self/Other Dichotomy in Science: Towards a Feminist Model of the Immune System," *Hypatia* 16, no. 1 (2001), doi.org/10.1111/j.1527-2001.2001.tb01047.x.

2. CIRCULATORY SYSTEM

1. Shigehisa Kuriyama, *The Expressiveness of the Body and the Divergence of Greek and Chinese Medicine* (New York: Zone Books, 1999), 50.

2. Bureau of Ethnology, *Annual Report of the Bureau of Ethnology to the Secretary of the Smithsonian Institution* (Washington, DC: US Government Printing Office, 1896), 721, books.google.com/books?id=jJ1CAQAAMAAJ.

3. M. N. Jackson, "'Heart Attack' Symptoms and Decision-Making: The Case of Older Rural Women," *Rural Remote Health* (2014), www.ncbi.nlm.nih.gov/pubmed/24793837.

4. Kerstin Dudas et al., "Trends in Out-of-Hospital Deaths Due to Coronary Heart Disease in Sweden (1991 to 2006)," *Circulation* 123, no. 1 (2011), doi.org/10.1161/circulationaha.110.964999.

5. Laxmi S. Mehta et al., "Acute Myocardial Infarction in Women," *Circulation* 133, no. 9 (2016), doi.org/10.1161/cir.0000000000000351.

6. D. Mozaffarian et al., "Heart Disease and Stroke Statistics—2015 Update: A Report from the American Heart Association," *Circulation* 131, no. 4 (2015), doi.org/10.1161/CIR.0000000000000152.

7. Brad N. Greenwood, Seth Carnahan, and Laura Huang, "Patient-Physician Gender Concordance and Increased Mortality Among Female Heart Attack Patients," *Proceedings of the National Academy of Sciences of the United States of America* 115, no. 34 (2018), doi.org/10.1073/pnas.1800097115.

8. Yusuke Tsugawa et al., "Comparison of Hospital Mortality and Readmission Rates for Medicare Patients Treated by Male vs Female Physicians," *JAMA Internal Medicine* 177, no. 2 (2017), doi.org/10.1001/jamainternmed.2016.7875.

9. Debra L. Roter, Judith A. Hall, and Yutaka Aoki, "Physician Gender Effects in Medical Communication," *JAMA* 288, no. 6 (2002), doi.org/10.1001/jama.288.6.756; Magnus Baumhäkel, Ulrike Müller, and Michael Böhm, "Influence of Gender of Physicians and Patients on Guideline-Recommended Treatment of Chronic Heart Failure in a Cross-Sectional Study," *European Journal of Heart Failure* 11, no. 3 (2009), doi.org/10.1093/eurjhf/hfn041.

10. Jennifer P. Stevens et al., "Comparison of Hospital Resource Use and Outcomes Among Hospitalists, Primary Care Physicians, and Other Generalists," *JAMA Internal Medicine* (2017), doi.org/10.1001/jamainternmed.2017.5824.

11. Leslie Kane, *Medscape Physician Compensation Report* (2019), www.medscape.com/slideshow/2019-compensation-overview-6011286#3.

12. Sarah Jaffe, *Work Won't Love You Back: How Devotion to Our Jobs Keeps Us*

Exploited, Exhausted, and Alone (New York: Hachette Books, 2021); Christina Maslach, Wilmar B. Schaufeli, and Michael P. Leiter, "Job Burnout," *Annual Review of Psychology* 52, no. 1 (2001), doi.org/10.1146/annurev.psych.52.1.397; Nathalie Embriaco et al., "Burnout Syndrome Among Critical Care Healthcare Workers," *Current Opinion in Critical Care* 13, no. 5 (2007), doi.org/10.1097/MCC.0b013e3282efd28a.

13. Judith Johnson et al., "Mental Healthcare Staff Well-Being and Burnout: A Narrative Review of Trends, Causes, Implications, and Recommendations for Future Interventions," *International Journal of Mental Health Nursing* 27, no. 1 (2018), doi.org/10.1111/inm.12416; Takahiro Matsuo et al., "Prevalence of Health Care Worker Burnout During the Coronavirus Disease 2019 (Covid-19) Pandemic in Japan," *JAMA Network Open* 3, no. 8 (2020), doi.org/10.1001/jamanetworkopen.2020.17271.

14. InCrowd, *2019 Physician Burnout Survey* (2019), incrowdnow.com/syndicated-reports/physician-burnout-2019.

15. Mark W. Friedberg et al., "Factors Affecting Physician Professional Satisfaction and Their Implications for Patient Care, Health Systems, and Health Policy," *RAND Health Quarterly* 3, no. 4 (2014), pubmed.ncbi.nlm.nih.gov/28083306/.

16. Tait D. Shanafelt et al., "Relationship Between Clerical Burden and Characteristics of the Electronic Environment with Physician Burnout and Professional Satisfaction," *Mayo Clinic Proceedings* 91, no. 7 (2016), doi.org/10.1016/j.mayocp.2016.05.007.

17. Jari J. Hakanen, Arnold B Bakker, and Markku Jokisaari, "A 35-Year Follow-up Study on Burnout Among Finnish Employees," *Journal of Occupational Health Psychology* 16, no. 3 (2011), tinyurl.com/1k2bekcf.

18. Kea Tijdens, Daniel H. De Vries, and Stephanie Steinmetz, "Health Workforce Remuneration: Comparing Wage Levels, Ranking, and Dispersion of 16 Occupational Groups in 20 Countries," *Human Resources for Health* 11, no. 1 (2013), doi.org/10.1186/1478-4491-11-11; Sigrid Dräger, Mario R. Dal Poz, and David B. Evans, "Health Workers Wages: An Overview from Selected Countries," Geneva: World Health Organization, 2006), tinyurl.com/1tp1ly6b.

19. Thomas Hobbes, *Leviathan* (reprint New York: Oxford University Press, 1996). See also Christoffer Basse Eriksen, "Circulation of Blood and Money in *Leviathan*—Hobbes on the Economy of the Body," in *History of Economic Rationalities: Economic Reasoning as Knowledge and Practice Authority*, ed. Jakob Bek-Thomsen et al. (Cham: Springer International, 2017).

20. Hobbes, *Leviathan*, 167. Marx knew that money doesn't do anything if it stays still—it has to move, and exchange, to create value. Karl Marx, *Capital: A Critique of Political Economy*, trans. Ben Fowkes (Harmondsworth: Penguin Books 1978).

21. Hobbes, *Leviathan*, 220. Indeed, as Karen Feldman notes, "Hobbes's worries as to the dangers that metaphor poses to the stability of the commonwealth thereby converge with his worries about the dangers of conscience to the principle of public author." Karen S. Feldman, "Conscience and the Concealments of Metaphor in Hobbes's 'Leviathan,'" *Philosophy and Rhetoric* 34, no. 1 (2001): 21, www.jstor.org/stable/40238078; Eugene F. Miller, "Metaphor and Political Knowledge," *American Political Science Review* 73, no. 1 (1979), doi.org/10.2307/1954738.

22. Raj Patel and Jason W. Moore, *A History of the World in Seven Cheap Things: A*

Guide to Capitalism, Nature, and the Future of the Planet (Berkeley: University of California Press, 2017), 78–79.

23. Dennis O. Flynn and Arturo Giráldez, "Born with a 'Silver Spoon': The Origin of World Trade in 1571," *Journal of World History* 6, no. 2 (1995), www.jstor .org/stable/20078638. Note that 30 percent of that silver ended up, via British traders, in China.

24. Nicholas A. Robins, *Mercury, Mining, and Empire: The Human and Ecological Cost of Colonial Silver Mining in the Andes* (Bloomington: Indiana University Press, 2011).

25. Ibid., 27; Nicole Hagan et al., "Estimating Historical Atmospheric Mercury Concentrations from Silver Mining and Their Legacies in Present-Day Surface Soil in Potosí, Bolivia," *Atmospheric Environment* 45, no. 40 (2011), doi.org /doi.org/10.1016/j.atmosenv.2010.10.009

26. Robins, *Mercury, Mining, and Empire*.

27. Robin A. Bernhoft, "Mercury Toxicity and Treatment: A Review of the Literature," *Journal of Environmental and Public Health* 2012 (2012), doi.org/10.1155 /2012/460508.

28. Patel and Moore, *History of the World in Seven Cheap Things*.

29. Raquel Gil Montero, "Free and Unfree Labour in the Colonial Andes in the Sixteenth and Seventeenth Centuries," *International Review of Social History* 56, no. S19 (2011).

30. Robins, *Mercury, Mining, and Empire*, 168.

31. David Graeber, *Debt: The First 5,000 Years* (New York: Melville House, 2011).

32. Robins, *Mercury, Mining, and Empire*, 139.

33. As one scholar has noted, "No one existed as an authentic 'primitive,' until s/he was colonized, bounded and deprived of practical political relations to 'mainstream' society and to the world." Prathama Banerjee, "Debt, Time and Extravagance: Money and the Making of 'Primitives' in Colonial Bengal," *Indian Economic and Social History Review* 37, no. 4 (2000): 425, doi.org/10 .1177/001946460003700402, cited in Tania Murray Li, "Indigeneity, Capitalism, and the Management of Dispossession," *Current Anthropology* 51, no. 3 (2010): 389, doi.org/10.1086/651942.

34. Charles F. Walker, *Smoldering Ashes: Cuzco and the Creation of Republican Peru, 1780–1840* (Durham, NC: Duke University Press, 1999).

35. Melissa Dell, "The Persistent Effects of Peru's Mining Mita," *Econometrica* 78, no. 6 (2010), doi.org/10.3982/ecta8121.

36. Naomi Klein, *The Shock Doctrine: The Rise of Disaster Capitalism* (New York: Metropolitan Books, 2007); Graeber, *Debt*. Today Indigenous communities are incited to pay off debt by selling culture and tourism. Bunten Alexis Celeste, "More Like Ourselves: Indigenous Capitalism Through Tourism," *American Indian Quarterly* 34, no. 3 (2010), doi.org/10.5250/amerindiquar.34.3.285.

37. Galeano also observes, however, that in Uruguay the military "don't burn books: now they sell them to paper factories, which shred and convert them into pulp for return to the consumer market. It isn't true that Marx is not available to the public. True, not in the form of books, but in the form of paper napkins." Eduardo Galeano, *Open Veins of Latin America: Five Centuries of the Pillage of a Continent* (New York: Monthly Review Press, 1997), 307.

38. US Department of Agriculture, "Farms and Land in Farms: 2019 Summary" (2020), www.nass.usda.gov/Publications/Todays_Reports/reports/fnlo0220.pdf;

US Department of Agriculture, "Tailored Report—Report: Farm Business Income Statement, Subject: Farm Operator Households, Filter 1: Economic Class > Less Than $100,000, Region: All Survey States," in *Economic Research Service and National Agricultural Statistics Service (NASS), Agricultural Resource Management Survey (ARMS)* (Kansas City, MO: US Department of Agriculture, 2021).

39. Garrett Graddy-Lovelace, "U.S. Farm Policy as Fraught Populism: Tracing the Scalar Tensions of Nationalist Agricultural Governance," *Annals of the American Association of Geographers* 109, no. 2 (2019), doi.org/10.1080/24694452.2018.1551722.

40. Vishav Bharti, "Indebtedness and Suicides: Field Notes on Agricultural Labourers of Punjab," *Economic and Political Weekly* 46, no. 14 (2011), tinyurl.com/vd8zxl1r; Francisco J. Limon et al., "Latino Farmworkers and Under-Detection of Depression: A Review of the Literature," *Hispanic Journal of Behavioral Sciences* 40, no. 2 (2018), doi.org/10.1177/0739986318762457; Wendy Ringgenberg et al., "Trends and Characteristics of Occupational Suicide and Homicide in Farmers and Agriculture Workers, 1992–2010," *Journal of Rural Health* 34, no. 3 (2018), doi.org/10.1111/jrh.12245; Marc B. Schenker, "A Global Perspective of Migration and Occupational Health," *American Journal of Industrial Medicine* 53, no. 4 (2010), doi.org/10.1002/ajim.20834; Raj Patel, *Stuffed and Starved: Markets, Power and the Hidden Battle for the World Food System* (London: Portobello Books, 2007).

41. Howard Meltzer et al., "The Relationship Between Personal Debt and Specific Common Mental Disorders," *European Journal of Public Health* 23, no. 1 (2012), doi.org/10.1093/eurpub/cks021.

42. Thomas Richardson, Peter Elliott, and Ronald Roberts, "The Relationship Between Personal Unsecured Debt and Mental and Physical Health: A Systematic Review and Meta-Analysis," *Clinical Psychology Review* 33, no. 8 (2013), doi.org/10.1016/j.cpr.2013.08.009.

43. Elizabeth Sweet, Christopher W. Kuzawa, and Thomas W. McDade, "Short-Term Lending: Payday Loans as Risk Factors for Anxiety, Inflammation and Poor Health," *SSM—Population Health* 5 (2018): 115, doi.org/10.1016/j.ssmph.2018.05.009.

44. Ibid.

45. G. D. Batty et al., "Association of Systemic Inflammation with Risk of Completed Suicide in the General Population," *JAMA Psychiatry* 73, no. 9 (2016), doi.org/10.1001/jamapsychiatry.2016.1805; G. David Batty et al., "Systemic Inflammation and Suicide Risk: Cohort Study of 419 527 Korean Men and Women," *Journal of Epidemiology and Community Health* 72, no. 7 (2018), doi.org/10.1136/jech-2017-210086.

46. Elizabeth Sweet et al., "The High Price of Debt: Household Financial Debt and Its Impact on Mental and Physical Health," *Social Science and Medicine* 91 (2013), doi.org/10.1016/j.socscimed.2013.05.009.

47. David Harvey, "Roepke Lecture in Economic Geography—Crises, Geographic Disruptions and the Uneven Development of Political Responses," *Economic Geography* 87, no. 1 (2011): 5, doi.org/10.1111/j.1944-8287.2010.01105.x.

48. Sweet et al., "High Price of Debt."

49. Christophe Andre, "Household Debt in OECD Countries: Stylised Facts and Policy Issues," *The Narodowy Bank Polski Workshop: Recent Trends in the*

Real Estate Market and Its Analysis—2015 Edition (2016), ssrn.com/abstract =2841634. Note that debt levels for the rich aren't so much of a concern. If you have assets, then debt is what you use to buy your boat or second home. Debt-to-asset ratio is more of an indicator of distress, if looking at debt alone. More generally, poverty, and the lack of circulation of resources to those who need them most, seems to be what we should be most concerned with. Suicide rates among Chilean pensioners, for instance, are over 10 percent for over-eighties, because of a privatized pension system that discards them once they've circulated through the economy. Suelen Carlos de Oliveira, Cristiani Vieira Machado, and Aléx Alarcón Hein, "Social Security Reforms in Chile: Lessons for Brazil," *Cadernos de saude publica* 35 (2019).

50. Patricia Drentea and Paul J. Lavrakas, "Over the Limit: The Association Among Health, Race and Debt," *Social Science and Medicine* 50, no. 4 (2000), doi.org/10.1016/s0277-9536(99)00298-1.

51. Allan Garland, "Effects of Cardiovascular and Cerebrovascular Health Events on Work and Earnings: A Population-Based Retrospective Cohort Study," *CMAJ* (2019), doi.org/10.1503/cmaj.181238.

52. Javier Valero-Elizondo et al., "Financial Hardship from Medical Bills Among Nonelderly U.S. Adults with Atherosclerotic Cardiovascular Disease," *Journal of the American College of Cardiology* 73, no. 6 (2019), doi.org/10.1016/j.jacc .2018.12.004.

53. Stephen Y. Wang et al., "Longitudinal Associations Between Income Changes and Incident Cardiovascular Disease," *JAMA Cardiology* 4, no. 12 (2019), doi .org/10.1001/jamacardio.2019.3788.

54. Tali Elfassy et al., "Associations of Income Volatility with Incident Cardiovascular Disease and All-Cause Mortality in a US Cohort," *Circulation* 139, no. 7 (2019), doi.org/10.1161/circulationaha.118.035521.

55. Melvin L. Oliver and Thomas M. Shapiro, eds., *Black Wealth, White Wealth: A New Perspective on Racial Inequality* (London: Taylor & Francis, 2006), 7.

56. Edward P. Havranek, "The Influence of Social and Economic Factors on Heart Disease," *JAMA Cardiology* 4, no. 12 (2019), doi.org/10.1001/jamacardio.2019 .3802.

57. Sally C. Curtin, "Trends in Cancer and Heart Disease Death Rates Among Adults Aged 45–64: United States, 1999–2017," *National Vital Statistics Reports* 68, no. 5 (2019), stacks.cdc.gov/view/cdc/78673.

58. G. P. Chrousos, "Stress and Disorders of the Stress System," *Nature Reviews Endocrinology* 5, no. 7 (2009), doi.org/10.1038/nrendo.2009.106.

59. Ilia J. Elenkov and George P. Chrousos, "Stress Hormones, Proinflammatory and Antiinflammatory Cytokines, and Autoimmunity," *Annals of the New York Academy of Sciences* 966, no. 1 (2002), doi.org/10.1111/j.1749-6632.2002 .tb04229.x.

60. S. M. Smith and W. W. Vale, "The Role of the Hypothalamic-Pituitary-Adrenal Axis in Neuroendocrine Responses to Stress," *Dialogues in Clinical Neuroscience* 8, no. 4 (2006), doi.org/10.31887/DCNS.2006.8.4/ssmith.

61. Toral R. Patel, "Anatomy of the Sympathetic Nervous System," in *Nerves and Nerve Injuries* (2015), doi.org/10.1016/B978-0-12-410390-0.00038-X.

62. Bruce S. McEwen, "Stress and the Individual," *Archives of Internal Medicine* 153, no. 18 (1993), doi.org/10.1001/archinte.1993.00410180039004.

63. Andrew Steptoe, Mark Hamer, and Yoichi Chida, "The Effects of Acute

Psychological Stress on Circulating Inflammatory Factors in Humans: A Review and Meta-Analysis," *Brain, Behavior, and Immunity* 21, no. 7 (2007), doi .org/10.1016/j.bbi.2007.03.011; A. L. Marsland et al., "The Effects of Acute Psychological Stress on Circulating and Stimulated Inflammatory Markers: A Systematic Review and Meta-Analysis," *Brain Behavior Immunology* 64 (2017), doi.org/10.1016/j.bbi.2017.01.011.f; Michael Maes et al., "The Effects of Psychological Stress on Humans: Increased Production of Pro-Inflammatory Cytokines and Th1-Like Response in Stress-Induced Anxiety," *Cytokine* 10, no. 4 (1998), doi.org/10.1006/cyto.1997.0290.

64. Steptoe, Hamer, and Chida, "Effects of Acute Psychological Stress"; Simon A. Jones et al., "C-Reactive Protein: A Physiological Activator of Interleukin 6 Receptor Shedding," *Journal of Experimental Medicine* 189, no. 3 (1999), doi.org /10.1084/jem.189.3.599. CRP increases IL-6 receptor shedding, contributing to the pro-inflammatory systemic trans-signaling phenomenon of IL-6.

65. J. Scheller et al., "The Pro- and Anti-Inflammatory Properties of the Cytokine Interleukin-6," *Biochimica et Biophysica Acta* 1813, no. 5 (2011), doi.org /10.1016/j.bbamcr.2011.01.034.

66. C. Gabay, "Interleukin-6 and Chronic Inflammation," *Arthritis Research and Therapy* 8, suppl. 2 (2006), doi.org/10.1186/ar1917; T. Tanaka, M. Narazaki, and T. Kishimoto, "IL-6 in Inflammation, Immunity, and Disease," *Cold Spring Harbor Perspectives in Biology* 6, no. 10 (2014), doi.org/10.1101/cshperspect.a016295.

67. Scheller et al., "Pro-and Anti-Inflammatory Properties."

68. Gabay, "Interleukin-6 and Chronic Inflammation."

69. Scheller et al., "Pro-and Anti-Inflammatory Properties."

70. S. Cohen et al., "Chronic Stress, Glucocorticoid Receptor Resistance, Inflammation, and Disease Risk," *Proceedings of the National Academy of Sciences of the United States of America* 109, no. 16 (2012), doi.org/10.1073/pnas .1118355109.

71. McEwen, "Stress and the Individual."

72. Cohen et al., "Chronic Stress, Glucocorticoid Receptor Resistance."

73. Maes et al., "Effects of Psychological Stress on Humans."

74. Sweet, Kuzawa, and McDade, "Short-Term Lending."

75. Agorastos Agorastos et al., "Early Life Stress and Trauma: Developmental Neuroendocrine Aspects of Prolonged Stress System Dysregulation," *Hormones* 17 (2018), doi.org/10.1007/s42000-018-0065-x; David Bürgin et al., "Compounding Stress: Childhood Adversity as a Risk Factor for Adulthood Trauma Exposure in the Health and Retirement Study," *Journal of Traumatic Stress* (2020), doi.org/10.1002/jts.22617.

76. T. W. Pace et al., "Increased Stress-Induced Inflammatory Responses in Male Patients with Major Depression and Increased Early Life Stress," *American Journal of Psychiatry* 163, no. 9 (2006), doi.org/10.1176/ajp.2006.163.9.1630.

77. Paul H. Black and Lisa D. Garbutt, "Stress, Inflammation and Cardiovascular Disease," *Journal of Psychosomatic Research* 52, no. 1 (2002), doi.org/10.1016 /s0022-3999(01)00302-6.

78. Michael K. Skinner, "Environmental Stress and Epigenetic Transgenerational Inheritance," *BMC Medicine* 12, no. 1 (2014), doi.org/10.1186/s12916-014-0153-y; R. A. Waterland and R. L. Jirtle, "Early Nutrition, Epigenetic Changes at Transposons and Imprinted Genes, and Enhanced Susceptibility to Adult Chronic Diseases," *Nutrition* 20, no. 1 (2004), doi.org/10.1016/j.nut.2003.09

.011; Ian C. G. Weaver et al., "Epigenetic Programming by Maternal Behavior," *Nature Neuroscience* 7, no. 8 (2004), doi.org/10.1038/nn1276.

79. Stephen G. Matthews and David I. Phillips, "Transgenerational Inheritance of Stress Pathology," *Experimental Neurology* 233, no. 1 (2012), doi.org/10.1016/j.expneurol.2011.01.009; Youli Yao et al., "Ancestral Exposure to Stress Epigenetically Programs Preterm Birth Risk and Adverse Maternal and Newborn Outcomes," *BMC Medicine* 12, no. 1 (2014), doi.org/10.1186/s12916-014-0121-6.

80. Masahiro Irie et al., "Relationships Between Perceived Workload, Stress and Oxidative DNA Damage," *International Archives of Occupational and Environmental Health* 74, no. 2 (2001), doi.org/10.1007/s004200000209.

81. Ibid.

82. Naoko Ohtani, "Deciphering the Mechanism for Induction of Senescence-Associated Secretory Phenotype (SASP) and Its Role in Ageing and Cancer Development," *Journal of Biochemistry* 166, no. 4 (2019), doi.org/10.1093/jb/mvz055; Francis Rodier et al., "Persistent DNA Damage Signalling Triggers Senescence-Associated Inflammatory Cytokine Secretion," *Nature Cell Biology* 11, no. 8 (2009), doi.org/10.1038/ncb1909.

83. Ohtani, "Deciphering the Mechanism"; Rodier et al., "Persistent DNA Damage."

84. Frej Fyhrquist, Outi Saijonmaa, and Timo Strandberg, "The Roles of Senescence and Telomere Shortening in Cardiovascular Disease," *Nature Reviews Cardiology* 10, no. 5 (2013), doi.org/10.1038/nrcardio.2013.30.

85. I. Kushner, D. Rzewnicki, and D. Samols, "What Does Minor Elevation of C-Reactive Protein Signify?," *American Journal of Medicine* 119, no. 2 (2006), doi.org/10.1016/j.amjmed.2005.06.057.

86. T. W. Pace et al., "Effect of Compassion Meditation on Neuroendocrine, Innate Immune and Behavioral Responses to Psychosocial Stress," *Psychoneuroendocrinology* 34, no. 1 (2009), doi.org/10.1016/j.psyneuen.2008.08.011.

87. Marc Corbeels et al., "Limits of Conservation Agriculture to Overcome Low Crop Yields in Sub-Saharan Africa," *Nature Food* 1, no. 7 (2020), doi.org/10.1038/s43016-020-0114-x.

88. V. Lorant, "Socioeconomic Inequalities in Depression: A Meta-Analysis," *American Journal of Epidemiology* 157, no. 2 (2003), doi.org/10.1093/aje/kwf182.

89. Though the United States is now just behind Iceland in per capita antidepressant consumption. The OECD publishes data at OECD.Stat on pharmaceutical consumption for its member countries. Although the United States is not listed in the pharmaceutical consumption tables in the 2020 OECD Health Statistics, the CDC provides comparable data. In 2018, Iceland had daily dosage rates of 143.7 per 1000, a little above the average declared over the 2015–18 period in the United States of 13.2 percent of adults having used antidepressant medication in the past thirty days. Debra J. Brody and Qiuping Gu, *National Center for Health Statistics: Antidepressant Use Among Adults: United States, 2015–2018* (Atlanta: Centers for Disease Control and Prevention, 2020), www.cdc.gov/nchs/data/databriefs/db377-H.pdf; Hans-Christoph Steinhausen, "Recent International Trends in Psychotropic Medication Prescriptions for Children and Adolescents," *European Child and Adolescent Psychiatry* 24, no. 6 (2015), doi.org/10.1007/s00787-014-0631-y.

90. Laura A. Brody, Debra J. Pratt, and Qiuping Gu, *National Center for Health Statistics: Antidepressant Use Among Adults: United States, 2005–2008* (Hyattsville,

MD: National Center for Health Statistics, 2011), www.cdc.gov/nchs/data /databriefs/db377-H.pdf.

91. Steven Woloshin et al., "Direct-to-Consumer Advertisements for Prescription Drugs: What Are Americans Being Sold?," *The Lancet* 358, no. 9288 (2001), doi.org/10.1016/S0140-6736(01)06254-7; Michael Ahn, Michael Batty, and Ralf Meisenzahl (2018). "Household Debt-to-Income Ratios in the Enhanced Financial Accounts," *FEDS Notes*. (Washington, DC: Board of Governors of the Federal Reserve System, 2018), doi.org/10.17016/2380 -7172.2138.

92. Shmuel Tiosano et al., "The Impact of Tocilizumab on Anxiety and Depression in Patients with Rheumatoid Arthritis," *European Journal of Clinical Investigation* 50, no. 9 (2020), doi.org/10.1111/eci.13268.

93. Canadian Agency for Drugs and Technologies in Health, *Tocilizumab (Actemra): Adult Patients with Moderately to Severely Active Rheumatoid Arthritis: Common Drug Review* (Ottawa: Canadian Agency for Drugs and Technologies in Health, 2015), table 1.

94. J. Semega et al., *Income and Poverty in the United States: 2019*, Current Population Reports (P60-270), US Census (2020).

95. David U. Himmelstein et al., "Medical Bankruptcy: Still Common Despite the Affordable Care Act," *American Journal of Public Health* 109, no. 3 (2019), doi.org/10.2105/ajph.2018.304901.

96. Andrew Steptoe and Mika Kivimäki, "Stress and Cardiovascular Disease," *Nature Reviews Cardiology* 9, no. 6 (2012), doi.org/10.1038/nrcardio.2012.45.

97. Black and Garbutt, "Stress, Inflammation and Cardiovascular Disease."

98. Paul M. Ridker et al., "C-Reactive Protein and Other Markers of Inflammation in the Prediction of Cardiovascular Disease in Women," *New England Journal of Medicine* 342, no. 12 (2000), doi.org/10.1056/nejm200003233421202.

99. James E. Dalen et al., "The Epidemic of the 20th Century: Coronary Heart Disease," *American Journal of Medicine* 127, no. 9 (2014), doi.org/10.1016/j .amjmed.2014.04.015.

100. Yoriko Heianza et al., "Duration and Life-Stage of Antibiotic Use and Risk of Cardiovascular Events in Women," *European Heart Journal* 40, no. 47 (2019), doi.org/10.1093/eurheartj/ehz231.

101. David G. Harrison et al., "Inflammation, Immunity, and Hypertension," *Hypertension* 57, no. 2 (2011), doi.org/10.1161/hypertensionaha.110.163576.

102. Göran K. Hansson, "Inflammation, Atherosclerosis, and Coronary Artery Disease," *New England Journal of Medicine* 352, no. 16 (2005), doi.org/10.1056 /nejmra043430.

103. M. Ali et al., "Inflammation and Coronary Artery Disease: From Pathophysiology to Canakinumab Anti-Inflammatory Thrombosis Outcomes Study (CANTOS)," *Coronary Artery Disease* 29, no. 5 (2018), doi.org/10.1097/MCA .0000000000000625.

104. Paul M. Ridker et al., "Rosuvastatin to Prevent Vascular Events in Men and Women with Elevated C-Reactive Protein," *New England Journal of Medicine* 359, no. 21 (2008), doi.org/10.1056/nejmoa0807646.

105. Paul M. Ridker et al., "Antiinflammatory Therapy with Canakinumab for Atherosclerotic Disease," *New England Journal of Medicine* 377, no. 12 (2017), doi .org/10.1056/nejmoa1707914.

106. Alexandros Tsoupras, Ronan Lordan, and Ioannis Zabetakis, "Inflammation,

Not Cholesterol, Is a Cause of Chronic Disease," *Nutrients* 10, no. 5 (2018), doi.org/10.3390/nu10050604.

107. Penny M. Kris-Etherton, William S. Harris, and Lawrence J. Appel, "Omega-3 Fatty Acids and Cardiovascular Disease," *Arteriosclerosis, Thrombosis, and Vascular Biology* 23, no. 2 (2003), doi.org/10.1161/01.atv.0000057393.97337.ae.

108. C. Bates et al., "Plasma Essential Fatty Acids in Pure and Mixed Race American Indians On and Off a Diet Exceptionally Rich in Salmon," *Prostaglandins, Leukotrienes and Medicine* 17, no. 1 (1985), doi.org/10.1016/0262-1746(85)90036-8.

109. S. L. Seierstad et al., "Dietary Intake of Differently Fed Salmon; The Influence on Markers of Human Atherosclerosis," *European Journal of Clinical Investigation* 35, no. 1 (2005), doi.org/10.1111/j.1365-2362.2005.01443.x.

110. James M. Helfield and Robert J. Naiman, "Effects of Salmon-Derived Nitrogen on Riparian Forest Growth and Implications for Stream Productivity," *Ecology* 82, no. 9 (2001), doi.org/10.1890/0012-9658(2001)082[2403:EOSDNO]2.0.CO;2.

111. Piers Mitchell, *Sanitation, Latrines and Intestinal Parasites in Past Populations* (London: Routledge, 2015).

112. Patrick McCully, *Silenced Rivers: The Ecology and Politics of Large Dams*, enlarged & updated ed. (London: Zed Books, 2001).

113. The International Commission on Large Dams defines large dams as those at least four stories high. Marcus Nüsser, "Political Ecology of Large Dams: A Critical Review," *Petermanns Geographische Mitteilungen* 147, no. 1 (2003).

114. Andreas Maeck et al., "Sediment Trapping by Dams Creates Methane Emission Hot Spots," *Environmental Science and Technology* 47, no. 15 (2013), doi.org/10.1021/es4003907.

115. McCully, *Silenced Rivers*.

116. Peter Molnár and Jorge A. Ramírez, "Energy Dissipation Theories and Optimal Channel Characteristics of River Networks," *Water Resources Research* 34, no. 7 (1998), doi.org/10.1029/98wr00983.

117. G. M. Kondolf, "Profile: Hungry Water: Effects of Dams and Gravel Mining on River Channels," *Environmental Management* 21, no. 4 (1997), doi.org/10.1007/s002679900048.

118. Bidisha Banerjee, *Superhuman River: Stories of the Ganga* (New Delhi: Aleph Book Company, 2020).

119. Cheryl Darlene Sanderson, "Nipiy Wasekimew / Clear Water: The Meaning of Water, from the Words of the Elders: The Interconnections of Health, Education, Law and the Environment," Ph.D. diss, Simon Fraser University, 2008, 93.

120. Jane Griffith, "Do Some Work for Me: Settler Colonialism, Professional Communication, and Representations of Indigenous Water," *Decolonization: Indigeneity, Education and Society* 7, no. 1 (2018).

121. T. E. Reimchen, "Isotopic Evidence for Enrichment of Salmon-Derived Nutrients in Vegetation, Soil, and Insects in Riparian Zones in Coastal British Columbia," *American Fisheries Society* 34 (2003), sfu.ca/~ianh/geog315/readings/Reimchen.pdf.

122. William Jobin, *Sustainable Management for Dams and Waters* (Boca Raton, FL: CRC Press, 1998), 191.

123. Maureen Nandini Mitra, "The Long Run Home," *Earth Island Journal*, Spring 2018.

124. Reimchen, "Isotopic Evidence for Enrichment."

125. P. C. Calder, "Omega-3 Fatty Acids and Inflammatory Processes," *Nutrients* 2, no. 3 (2010), doi.org/10.3390/nu2030355.

126. Ramin Farzaneh-Far, "Association of Marine Omega-3 Fatty Acid Levels with Telomeric Aging in Patients with Coronary Heart Disease," *JAMA* 303, no. 3 (2010), doi.org/10.1001/jama.2009.2008.

127. L. Eve Armentrout-Ma, "Chinese in California's Fishing Industry, 1850–1941," *California History* 60, no. 2 (1981), online.ucpress.edu/ch/article-abstract/60/2 /142/32089/Chinese-in-California-s-Fishing-Industry-1850-1941.

128. Barton DeLoach, "Important Factors Affecting the Marketing of Canned Salmon," *American Marketing Journal* (1935), doi.org/10.2307/4291477.

129. Alan Lufkin, *California's Salmon and Steelhead: The Struggle to Restore an Imperiled Resource* (Berkeley: University of California Press, 1990).

130. Earl Leitritz, *A History of California's Fish Hatcheries 1870–1960* (Sacramento: California Department of Fish and Game, 1970), tinyurl.com/14wgzw79.

131. Lufkin, *California's Salmon and Steelhead.*

132. Earl Leitritz, *Trout and Salmon Culture (Hatchery Methods)* (Sacramento: California Department of Fish and Game, 1969), tinyurl.com/19tcbkw4; Livingston Stone, *Domesticated Trout: How to Breed and Grow Them* (Boston: James R. Osgood & Co., 1873), 78.

133. Gary Meffe, "Techno-Arrogance and Halfway Technologies: Salmon Hatcheries on the Pacific Coast of North America," *Conservation Biology* 6, no. 3 (1992), conbio.onlinelibrary.wiley.com/doi/abs/10.1046/j.1523-1739.1992.06030350.x.

134. Andrew Simms, *Ecological Debt: Global Warming and the Wealth of Nations,* 2nd ed. (London: Pluto Press, 2009).

135. Lufkin, *California's Salmon and Steelhead,* 82.

136. Emiliano Di Cicco et al., "Heart and Skeletal Muscle Inflammation (Hsmi) Disease Diagnosed on a British Columbia Salmon Farm Through a Longitudinal Farm Study," *PLOS One* 12, no. 2 (2017), doi.org/10.1371/journal.pone .0171471.

137. R. A. Hites, "Global Assessment of Organic Contaminants in Farmed Salmon," *Science* 303, no. 5655 (2004), doi.org/10.1126/science.1091447.

138. Anne-Katrine Lundebye et al., "Lower Levels of Persistent Organic Pollutants, Metals and the Marine Omega 3-Fatty Acid Dha in Farmed Compared to Wild Atlantic Salmon (Salmo Salar)," *Environmental Research* 155 (2017), doi.org/10 .1016/j.envres.2017.01.026.

139. Lisa Kolden Midtbø et al., "Intake of Farmed Atlantic Salmon-Fed Soybean Oil Increases Hepatic Levels of Arachidonic Acid-Derived Oxylipins and Ceramides in Mice," *Journal of Nutritional Biochemistry* 26, no. 6 (2015), doi .org/10.1016/j.jnutbio.2014.12.005.

140. Armentrout-Ma, "Chinese in California's Fishing Industry."

141. Chris Friday, *Organizing Asian American Labor: The Pacific Coast Canned-Salmon Industry, 1870–1942* (Philadelphia: Temple University Press, 1994).

142. Bruce Nelson, "Class, Race and Democracy in the CIO: The 'New' Labor History Meets the 'Wages of Whiteness,'" *International Review of Social History* 41, no. 3 (1996), doi.org/10.1017/S0020859000114051.

143. Yushi Yamazaki, "Radical Crossings: From Peasant Rebellions to Internationalist Multiracial Labor Organizing Among Japanese Immigrant Communities in Hawaii and California, 1885–1935," Ph.D. diss., University of Southern California, 2015.

144. W. F. Elkins, "Black Power in the British West Indies: The Trinidad Long-shoremen's Strike of 1919," *Science and Society* 33, no. 1 (1969), www.jstor.org/stable/40401392.

145. Johnna Montgomerie, "Giving Credit Where It's Due: Public Policy and Household Debt in the United States, the United Kingdom and Canada," *Policy and Society* 25, no. 3 (2006), doi.org/10.1016/S1449-4035(06)70085-6.

146. Courtney Boen and Y. Claire Yang, "The Physiological Impacts of Wealth Shocks in Late Life: Evidence from the Great Recession," *Social Science and Medicine* 150 (2016), doi.org/10.1016/j.socscimed.2015.12.029.

147. Aliza D. Richman, "Concurrent Social Disadvantages and Chronic Inflammation: The Intersection of Race and Ethnicity, Gender, and Socioeconomic Status," *Journal of Racial and Ethnic Health Disparities* 5, no. 4 (2018), doi.org/10.1007/s40615-017-0424-3.

148. Jesse Bricker et al., "Changes in U.S. Family Finances from 2013 to 2016: Evidence from the Survey of Consumer Finances," *Federal Reserve Bulletin* 103, no. 3 (2017): 13, www.federalreserve.gov/publications/files/scf17.pdf.

149. Jason Hickel, *The Divide: A Brief Guide to Global Inequality and Its Solutions* (London: William Heinemann, 2017); Patrisse Cullors, "Abolition and Reparations: Histories of Resistance, Transformative Justice, and Accountability," *Harvard Law Review* 132, no. 6 (2018): 1729.

150. UN Special Rapporteur on Extreme Poverty and Human Rights, "Report on the Parlous State of Poverty Eradication," *A/HRC/44/40* (2020), ohchr.org/EN/Issues/Poverty/Pages/parlous.aspx.

151. David H. Rehkopf et al., "The Impact of a Private Sector Living Wage Intervention on Consumption and Cardiovascular Disease Risk Factors in a Middle Income Country," *BMC Public Health* 18, no. 1 (2018/01/25 2018), doi.org/10.1186/s12889-018-5052-2. There is also evidence that higher blood pressure is associated with cash transfers, and that obesity rates are driven by "resource scarcity" among the poor. I. Forde et al., "The Impact of Cash Transfers to Poor Women in Colombia on BMI and Obesity: Prospective Cohort Study," *International Journal of Obesity* 36, no. 9 (2012), doi.org/10.1038/ijo.2011.234; L. C. Fernald, P. J. Gertler, and X. Hou, "Cash Component of Conditional Cash Transfer Program Is Associated with Higher Body Mass Index and Blood Pressure in Adults," *Journal of Nutrition* 138, no. 11 (Nov 2008), doi.org/10.3945/jn.108.090506; Emily J. Dhurandhar, "The Food-Insecurity Obesity Paradox: A Resource Scarcity Hypothesis," *Physiology and Behavior* 162 (2016), doi.org/10.1016/j.physbeh.2016.04.025.

152. Emmanuel Jimenez et al., "School Effects and Costs for Private and Public Schools in the Dominican Republic," *International Journal of Educational Research* 15, no. 5 (1991), doi.org/10.1016/0883-0355(91)90021-J.

153. Sarah Babb, "The Social Consequences of Structural Adjustment: Recent Evidence and Current Debates," *Annual Review of Sociology* 31, no. 1 (2005), doi.org/10.1146/annurev.soc.31.041304.122258.

154. James Banks et al., "The SES Health Gradient on Both Sides of the Atlantic," in *Developments in the Economics of Aging*, ed. David A. Wise (Chicago: University of Chicago Press, 2009); Raj Patel, *Stuffed and Starved: Markets, Power and the Hidden Battle for the World Food System* (London: Portobello Books, 2007).

155. Elizabeth A. Donnelly, "Making the Case for Jubilee: The Catholic Church

and the Poor-Country Debt Movement," *Ethics and International Affairs* 21, no. S1 (2007), doi.org/10.1111/j.1747-7093.2007.00090.x; Stan Cox, *The Green New Deal and Beyond: Ending the Climate Emergency While We Still Can* (San Francisco: City Lights, 2020); Jason Hickel, *Less Is More: How Degrowth Will Save the World* (London: William Heinemann, 2020).

156. Cullors, "Abolition and Reparations."

157. Joel Millward-Hopkins et al., "Providing Decent Living with Minimum Energy: A Global Scenario," *Global Environmental Change* 65 (2020), doi.org/10.1016/j.gloenvcha.2020.102168.

158. Sweet, Kuzawa, and McDade, "Short-Term Lending."

159. Thanh Lu and Mark Stabile, "The Effect of Payday Lending Restrictions on Suicide and Fatal Poisonings," paper presented at the ninth annual conference of the American Society of Health Economists, 2020, 3.

160. Deborah M. Figart and Mariam Majd, "The Public Bank Movement: A Response to Local Economic Development and Infrastructure Needs in Three U.S. States," *Challenge* 59, no. 6 (2016), doi.org/10.1080/05775132.2016.1239962.

161. Data on debt relief providing respite are from Bernhard G. Gunter, "What's Wrong with the HIPC Initiative and What's Next?," *Development Policy Review* 20, no. 1 (2002), doi.org/10.1111/1467-7679.00154.

162. Angela T. Bednarek, "Undamming Rivers: A Review of the Ecological Impacts of Dam Removal," *Environmental Management* 27, no. 6 (2001), doi.org/10.1007/s002670010189.

163. Thomas P. Quinn et al., "Re-Awakening Dormant Life History Variation: Stable Isotopes Indicate Anadromy in Bull Trout Following Dam Removal on the Elwha River, Washington," *Environmental Biology of Fishes* 100, no. 12 (2017), doi.org/10.1007/s10641-017-0676-0.

164. Liuyong Ding et al., "Global Trends in Dam Removal and Related Research: A Systematic Review Based on Associated Datasets and Bibliometric Analysis," *Chinese Geographical Science* 29, no. 1 (2019), doi.org/10.1007/s11769-018-1009-8.

165. Anna V. Smith, "The Klamath River Now Has the Legal Rights of a Person," *High Country News*, 2019, tinyurl.com/ybgu89jr.

166. Hannah Gosnell and Erin Clover Kelly, "Peace on the River? Social-Ecological Restoration and Large Dam Removal in the Klamath Basin, USA," *Water Alternatives* 3, no. 2 (2010).

3. DIGESTIVE SYSTEM

1. Jean-Jacques Rousseau, *A Discourse Upon the Origins and Foundation of the Inequality Among Mankind* (London, 1761), 97.

2. Stephen Best and Saidiya Hartman, "Fugitive Justice," *Representations* 92, no. 1 (2005): 11, doi.org/10.1525/rep.2005.92.1.1.

3. Ron Sender, Shai Fuchs, and Ron Milo, "Are We Really Vastly Outnumbered? Revisiting the Ratio of Bacterial to Host Cells in Humans," *Cell* 164, no. 3 (2016), doi.org/10.1016/j.cell.2016.01.013.

4. Sudabeh Alatab et al., "The Global, Regional, and National Burden of Inflammatory Bowel Disease in 195 Countries and Territories, 1990–2017: A Systematic Analysis for the Global Burden of Disease Study 2017," *Lancet Gastroenterology and Hepatology* 5, no. 1 (2020), doi.org/10.1016/s2468-1253(19)30333-4.

5. D. G. Thompson, "Structure and Function of the Gut," in *Oxford Textbook of*

Medicine, ed. Timothy M. Cox and David A. Warrell (Oxford: Oxford University Press, 2012).

6. Ricardo Cavicchioli et al., "Scientists' Warning to Humanity: Microorganisms and Climate Change," *Nature Reviews Microbiology* 17, no. 9 (2019), doi.org/10.1038/s41579-019-0222-5.

7. A. Almeida et al., "A New Genomic Blueprint of the Human Gut Microbiota," *Nature* 568, no. 7753 (2019), doi.org/10.1038/s41586-019-0965-1.

8. Lynn Margulis and René Fester, *Symbiosis as a Source of Evolutionary Innovation: Speciation and Morphogenesis* (Cambridge, MA: MIT Press, 1991).

9. Gabriele Berg et al., "Microbiome Definition Re-Visited: Old Concepts and New Challenges," *Microbiome* 8, no. 1 (2020), doi.org/10.1186/s40168-020-00875-0.

10. J. M. Whipps, Karen Lewis, and R. C. Cooke, "Mycoparasitism and Plant Disease Control," in *Fungi in Biological Control Systems*, ed. N. M. Burge (Manchester: Manchester University Press, 1988), 176.

11. Cassandra Willyard, "Expanded Human Gene Tally Reignites Debate," *Nature* 558, no. 7710 (2018), doi.org/10.1038/d41586-018-05462-w.

12. B. T. Tierney et al., "The Landscape of Genetic Content in the Gut and Oral Human Microbiome," *Cell Host and Microbe* 26, no. 2 (2019), doi.org/10.1016/j.chom.2019.07.008.

13. Jason Lloyd-Price et al., "Strains, Functions and Dynamics in the Expanded Human Microbiome Project," *Nature* 550, no. 7674 (2017), doi.org/10.1038/nature23889.

14. Tierney et al., "Landscape of Genetic Content."

15. Maria Rooseboom, "Leeuwenhoek, the Man: A Son of His Nation and His Time," *Bulletin of the British Society for the History of Science* 1, no. 4 (1950), www.jstor.org/stable/4024784.

16. P. Smit and J. Heniger, "Antoni Van Leeuwenhoek (1632–1723) and the Discovery of Bacteria," *Antonie van Leeuwenhoek* 41, no. 1 (1975), doi.org/10.1007/bf02565057.

17. E. J. T. Collins, "Food Adulteration and Food Safety in Britain in the 19th and Early 20th Centuries," *Food Policy* 18, no. 2 (1993), doi.org/10.1016/0306-9192(93)90018-7; Friedrich Christian Accum, *A Treatise on Adulterations of Food, and Culinary Poisons . . .* (London, 1820).

18. John Strachan, "The Pasteurization of Algeria?," *French History* 20, no. 3 (2006), doi.org/10.1093/fh/crl011; Bruno Latour, *The Pasteurization of France* (Cambridge, MA: Harvard University Press, 1988).

19. Helen Tilley, "Medicine, Empires, and Ethics in Colonial Africa," *AMA Journal of Ethics* 18, no. 7 (2016), doi.org/10.1001/journalofethics.2016.18.7.mhst1-1607.

20. Lucile H. Brockway, "Science and Colonial Expansion: The Role of the British Royal Botanic Gardens," *American Ethnologist* 6, no. 3 (1979): 456, doi.org/10.1525/ae.1979.6.3.02a00030.

21. Ibid., 452; Anonymous, "Kew Gardens," *Journal of Horticulture* (1878): 265, books.google.com/books?id=QRLKcLC97sgC.

22. R. S. Phillips, "Current Status of Malaria and Potential for Control," *Clinical Microbiology Reviews* 14, no. 1 (2001), doi.org/10.1128/cmr.14.1.208-226.2001.

23. Paul Farmer, *Fevers, Feuds, and Diamonds: Ebola and the Ravages of History* (New York: Farrar, Straus & Giroux, 2020), 345.

24. Stephane Leduc, "Les conditions sanitaires en France," *Revue scientifique* 20, no. 2 (1892), 234, cited in Latour, *Pasteurization of France*, 35.

25. Michel Foucault et al., *Society Must Be Defended: Lectures at the Collège de France, 1975–76* (New York: Picador, 2003); Laurent Mucchielli, "Criminology, Hygienism, and Eugenics in France, 1870–1914," in *Criminals and Their Scientists: The History of Criminology in International Perspective*, ed. Peter Becker and Richard F. Wetzell (Cambridge: Cambridge University Press, 2006).

26. J. Six et al., "Bacterial and Fungal Contributions to Carbon Sequestration in Agroecosystems," *Soil Science Society of America Journal* 70, no. 2 (2006), doi .org/10.2136/sssaj2004.0347.

27. Danny K. Asami et al., "Comparison of the Total Phenolic and Ascorbic Acid Content of Freeze-Dried and Air-Dried Marionberry, Strawberry, and Corn Grown Using Conventional, Organic, and Sustainable Agricultural Practices," *Journal of Agricultural and Food Chemistry* 51, no. 5 (2003), doi.org/10 .1021/jf020635c.

28. Joan Wennstrom Bennett, *Microbiomes of the Built Environment: A Research Agenda for Indoor Microbiology, Human Health and Buildings* (Washington, DC: National Academies Press, 2017).

29. Lucette Flandroy et al., "The Impact of Human Activities and Lifestyles on the Interlinked Microbiota and Health of Humans and of Ecosystems," *Science of the Total Environment* 627 (2018), doi.org/10.1016/j.scitotenv.2018.01.288.

30. David P. Strachan, "Hay Fever, Hygiene, and Household Size," *BMJ* 299, no. 6710 (1989), doi.org/10.1136/bmj.299.6710.1259.

31. H. Okada et al., "The 'Hygiene Hypothesis' for Autoimmune and Allergic Diseases: An Update," *Clinical and Experimental Immunology* 160, no. 1 (2010), doi.org/10.1111/j.1365-2249.2010.04139.x.

32. P. J. Turnbaugh et al., "The Effect of Diet on the Human Gut Microbiome: A Metagenomic Analysis in Humanized Gnotobiotic Mice," *Science Translational Medicine* 1, no. 6 (2009), doi.org/10.1126/scitranslmed.3000322.

33. N. T. Baxter et al., "Dynamics of Human Gut Microbiota and Short-Chain Fatty Acids in Response to Dietary Interventions with Three Fermentable Fibers," *mBio* 10, no. 1 (2019), doi.org/10.1128/mBio.02566-18; Gijs Den Besten et al., "The Role of Short-Chain Fatty Acids in the Interplay Between Diet, Gut Microbiota, and Host Energy Metabolism," *Journal of Lipid Research* 54, no. 9 (2013), doi.org/10.1194/jlr.r036012; P. J. Parekh, L. A. Balart, and D. A. Johnson, "The Influence of the Gut Microbiome on Obesity, Metabolic Syndrome and Gastrointestinal Disease," *Clinical and Translational Gastroenterology* 6 (2015), doi.org/10.1038/ctg.2015.16; M. Sochocka et al., "The Gut Microbiome Alterations and Inflammation-Driven Pathogenesis of Alzheimer's Disease—A Critical Review," *Molecular Neurobiology* 56, no. 3 (2019), doi.org/10.1007/s12035-018-1188-4.

34. R Bentley, "Biosynthesis of Vitamin K (Menaquinone) in Bacteria," *Microbiology Reviews* 46, no. 3 (1982); J. M. Conly and K. Stein, "Quantitative and Qualitative Measurements of K Vitamins in Human Intestinal Contents," *American Journal of Gastroenterology* 87, no. 3 (1992), www.ncbi.nlm.nih.gov /pubmed/1539565; M. J. Shearer, "Vitamin K," 345, no. 8944 (1995), doi.org /10.1016/s0140-6736(95)90227-9.

35. Hiroshi Maeda and Natalia Dudareva, "The Shikimate Pathway and Aromatic Amino Acid Biosynthesis in Plants," *Annual Review of Plant Biology* 63 (2012), doi.org/10.1146/annurev-arplant-042811-105439.

36. Klaus M. Herrmann and Lisa M. Weaver, "The Shikimate Pathway," *Annual*

Review of Plant Physiology and Plant Molecular Biology 50, no. 1 (1999), doi.org /10.1146/annurev.arplant.50.1.473.

37. J. Conly and K. Stein, "Reduction of Vitamin K2 Concentrations in Human Liver Associated with the Use of Broad Spectrum Antimicrobials," *Clinical and Investigative Medicine* 17, no. 6 (1994), www.ncbi.nlm.nih.gov/pubmed/7895417; S. J. Ford et al., "Iatrogenic Vitamin K Deficiency and Life Threatening Coagulopathy," *BMJ Case Rep* 2008 (2008), doi.org/10.1136/bcr.06.2008.0008.

38. C. A. Lozupone et al., "Diversity, Stability and Resilience of the Human Gut Microbiota," *Nature* 489, no. 7415 (2012), doi.org/10.1038/nature11550.

39. Diwakar Davar et al., "Fecal Microbiota Transplant Overcomes Resistance to Anti-PD-1 Therapy in Melanoma Patients," *Science* 371, no. 6529 (2021), doi .org/10.1126/science.abf3363.

40. I. Rowland et al., "Gut Microbiota Functions: Metabolism of Nutrients and Other Food Components," *European Journal of Nutrition* 57, no. 1 (2018), doi .org/10.1007/s00394-017-1445-8; N. Kamada et al., "Role of the Gut Microbiota in Immunity and Inflammatory Disease," *Nature Reviews Immunology* 13, no. 5 (2013), doi.org/10.1038/nri3430.

41. Yasmine Belkaid and Timothy W. Hand, "Role of the Microbiota in Immunity and Inflammation," *Cell* 157, no. 1 (2014), doi.org/10.1016/j.cell.2014.03.011.

42. Lozupone et al., "Diversity, Stability and Resilience"; J. Lloyd-Price, G. Abu-Ali, and C. Huttenhower, "The Healthy Human Microbiome," *Genome Medicine* 8, no. 1 (2016), doi.org/10.1186/s13073-016-0307-y.

43. E. Le Chatelier et al., "Richness of Human Gut Microbiome Correlates with Metabolic Markers," *Nature* 500, no. 7464 (2013), doi.org/10.1038 /nature12506; Sochocka et al., "Gut Microbiome Alterations."

44. C. Manichanh, "Reduced Diversity of Faecal Microbiota in Crohn's Disease Revealed by a Metagenomic Approach," *Gut* 55, no. 2 (2006), doi.org/10.1136 /gut.2005.073817; Tanya T. Nguyen et al., "Overview and Systematic Review of Studies of Microbiome in Schizophrenia and Bipolar Disorder," *Journal of Psychiatric Research* 99 (2018), doi.org/10.1016/j.jpsychires.2018.01.013; Jane A. Foster and Karen-Anne McVey Neufeld, "Gut-Brain Axis: How the Microbiome Influences Anxiety and Depression," *Trends in Neurosciences* 36, no. 5 (2013), doi .org/10.1016/j.tins.2013.01.005; Xinpu Chen and Sridevi Devaraj, "Gut Microbiome in Obesity, Metabolic Syndrome, and Diabetes," *Current Diabetes Reports* 18, no. 12 (2018), doi.org/10.1007/s11892-018-1104-3; Christina E. West et al., "The Gut Microbiota and Inflammatory Noncommunicable Diseases: Associations and Potentials for Gut Microbiota Therapies," *Journal of Allergy and Clinical Immunology* 135, no. 1 (2015), doi.org/10.1016/j.jaci.2014.11.012.

45. Belkaid and Hand, "Role of Microbiota in Immunity."

46. Erica D. Sonnenburg and Justin L. Sonnenburg, "The Ancestral and Industrialized Gut Microbiota and Implications for Human Health," *Nature Reviews Microbiology* 17, no. 6 (2019), doi.org/10.1038/s41579-019-0191-8.

47. J. L. Sonnenburg and F. Backhed, "Diet-Microbiota Interactions as Moderators of Human Metabolism," *Nature* 535, no. 7610 (2016), doi.org/10.1038 /nature18846.

48. S. L. Schnorr et al., "Gut Microbiome of the Hadza Hunter-Gatherers," *Nature Commununications* 5 (2014), doi.org/10.1038/ncomms4654.

49. Alexandra J. Obregon-Tito et al., "Subsistence Strategies in Traditional Societies Distinguish Gut Microbiomes," *Nature Communications* 6, no. 1 (2015), doi

.org/10.1038/ncomms7505; Raul Y. Tito et al., "Insights from Characterizing Extinct Human Gut Microbiomes," *PLOS One* 7, no. 12 (2012), doi.org/10.1371/journal.pone.0051146.

50. Belkaid and Hand, "Role of Microbiota in Immunity."
51. Erica D. Sonnenburg et al., "Diet-Induced Extinctions in the Gut Microbiota Compound over Generations," *Nature* 529, no. 7585 (2016), doi.org/10.1038/nature16504.
52. J. S. Paula, N. H. Medina, and A. A. V. Cruz, "Trachoma Among the Yanomami Indians," *Brazilian Journal of Medical and Biological Research* 35 (2002), tinyurl.com/qdjml94l.
53. L. S. Weyrich et al., "Neanderthal Behaviour, Diet, and Disease Inferred from Ancient DNA in Dental Calculus," *Nature* 544, no. 7650 (2017), doi.org/10.1038/nature21674; E. R. Davenport et al., "The Human Microbiome in Evolution," *BMC Biology* 15, no. 1 (2017), doi.org/10.1186/s12915-017-0454-7.
54. Marsha C. Wibowo et al., *Large-Scale Reconstruction of Ancient Microbial Genomes from the Human Gut* (London: SMBE, 2019).
55. Sonnenburg and Sonnenburg, "Ancestral and Industrialized Gut Microbiota."
56. Kari E. North, Lisa J. Martin, and Michael H. Crawford, "The Origins of the Irish Travellers and the Genetic Structure of Ireland," *Annals of Human Biology* 27, no. 5 (2000), doi.org/10.1080/030144600419297; E. Gilbert et al., "Genomic Insights into the Population Structure and History of the Irish Travellers," *Scientific Reports* 7 (2017): 9, doi.org/10.1038/srep42187; David M. Keohane et al., "Microbiome and Health Implications for Ethnic Minorities after Enforced Lifestyle Changes," *Nature Medicine* 26 (2020), doi.org/10.1038/s41591-020-0963-8.
57. Keohane et al., "Microbiome and Health Implications."
58. Suzanne Devkota, "The Gut Microbiome During Acute Lifestyle Transition," *Nature Medicine* 26 (2020), doi.org/10.1038/s41591-020-0980-7.
59. Keohane et al., "Microbiome and Health Implications."
60. S. Carding et al., "Dysbiosis of the Gut Microbiota in Disease," *Microbial Ecology in Health and Disease* 26 (2015), doi.org/10.3402/mehd.v26.26191.
61. R. E. Ley et al., "Microbial Ecology: Human Gut Microbes Associated with Obesity," *Nature* 444, no. 7122 (2006), doi.org/10.1038/4441022a; Peter J. Turnbaugh et al., "An Obesity-Associated Gut Microbiome with Increased Capacity for Energy Harvest," *Nature* 444, no. 7122 (2006), doi.org/10.1038/nature05414.
62. Turnbaugh et al., "Obesity-Associated Gut Microbiome."
63. Ley et al., "Microbial Ecology."
64. Carding et al., "Dysbiosis of the Gut Microbiota."
65. A. Hviid, H. Svanstron, and M. Frisch, "Antibiotic Use and Inflammatory Bowel Disease in Childhood," *Gut* 60, no. 1 (2011), doi.org/10.1136/gut.2010.219683.
66. Xiao Zhang et al., "Changes of Soil Prokaryotic Communities after Clear Cutting in a Karst Forest: Evidences for Cutting-Based Disturbance Promoting Deterministic Processes," *FEMS Microbiology Ecology* 92, no. 3 (2016), doi.org/10.1093/femsec/fiw026.
67. S. L. Gorbach, "Antibiotics and *Clostridium difficile*," *New England Journal of Medicine* 341, no. 22 (1999), doi.org/10.1056/NEJM199911253412211.
68. Braden T. Tierney et al., *The Predictive Power of the Microbiome Exceeds That*

of Genome-Wide Association Studies in the Discrimination of Complex Human Disease (New York: Cold Spring Harbor Laboratory, 2020).

69. E. Rackaityte et al., "Viable Bacterial Colonization Is Highly Limited in the Human Intestine in Utero," *Nature Medicine* (2020), doi.org/10.1038/s41591 -020-0761-3.

70. M. Francino, "Early Development of the Gut Microbiota and Immune Health," *Pathogens* 3, no. 3 (2014), doi.org/10.3390/pathogens3030769.

71. Rackaityte et al., "Viable Bacterial Colonization Is Highly Limited."

72. Fredrik Bäckhed et al., "Dynamics and Stabilization of the Human Gut Microbiome During the First Year of Life," *Cell Host and Microbe* 17, no. 5 (2015), doi.org/10.1016/j.chom.2015.04.004.

73. A. Sevelsted et al., "Cesarean Section and Chronic Immune Disorders," *Pediatrics* 135, no. 1 (2015), doi.org/10.1542/peds.2014-0596.

74. K. E. Fujimura et al., "Neonatal Gut Microbiota Associates with Childhood Multisensitized Atopy and T Cell Differentiation," *Nature Medicine* 22, no. 10 (2016), doi.org/10.1038/nm.4176; Bäckhed et al., "Dynamics and Stabilization."

75. Fujimura et al., "Neonatal Gut Microbiota."

76. Hans Hildebrand et al., "Early-Life Exposures Associated with Antibiotic Use and Risk of Subsequent Crohn's Disease," *Scandinavian Journal of Gastroenterology* 43, no. 8 (2008), doi.org/10.1080/00365520801971736.

77. Maciej Chichlowski et al., "*Bifidobacterium longum* Subspecies *infantis* (*B. infantis*) in Pediatric Nutrition: Current State of Knowledge," *Nutrients* 12, no. 6 (2020), doi.org/10.3390/nu12061581.

78. Mark A. Underwood et al., "*Bifidobacterium longum* Subspecies *infantis*: Champion Colonizer of the Infant Gut," *Pediatric Research* 77, no. 1–2 (2015), doi.org/10.1038/pr.2014.156.

79. Francino, "Early Development of Gut Microbiota"; Bethany M. Henrick et al., "Colonization by *B. infantis* EVC001 Modulates Enteric Inflammation in Exclusively Breastfed Infants," *Pediatric Research* 86 (2019), doi.org/10.1038 /s41390-019-0533-2.

80. Henrick et al., "Colonization by *B. infantis*"; Chichlowski et al., "*Bifidobacterium longum*."

81. David Groeger et al., "*Bifidobacterium infantis* 35624 Modulates Host Inflammatory Processes Beyond the Gut," *Gut Microbes* 4, no. 4 (2013), doi.org/10 .4161/gmic.25487.

82. F. Zhang et al., "Should We Standardize the 1,700-Year-Old Fecal Microbiota Transplantation?," *American Journal of Gastroenterology* 107, no. 11 (2012), doi .org/10.1038/ajg.2012.251.

83. Ruben J. Colman and David T. Rubin, "Fecal Microbiota Transplantation as Therapy for Inflammatory Bowel Disease: A Systematic Review and Meta-Analysis," *Journal of Crohn's and Colitis* 8, no. 12 (2014), doi.org/10.1016/j .crohns.2014.08.006; L. J. Brandt et al., "Long-Term Follow-up of Colonoscopic Fecal Microbiota Transplant for Recurrent *Clostridium difficile* Infection," *American Journal of Gastroenterology* 107, no. 7 (2012), doi.org/10.1038 /ajg.2012.60; Johan S. Bakken et al., "Treating *Clostridium difficile* Infection with Fecal Microbiota Transplantation," *Clinical Gastroenterology and Hepatology* 9, no. 12 (2011), doi.org/10.1016/j.cgh.2011.08.014.

84. Aurora Pop-Vicas and Marguerite A. Neill, "*Clostridium difficile*: The Increasingly Difficult Pathogen," *BMC Critical Care* 12, no. 1 (2008), doi.org/10.1186/cc6773.

85. J. Jalanka et al., "The Long-Term Effects of Faecal Microbiota Transplantation for Gastrointestinal Symptoms and General Health in Patients with Recurrent Clostridium Difficile Infection," *Alimentary Pharmacology and Therapeutics* 47, no. 3 (2018), doi.org/10.1111/apt.14443.

86. Davar et al., "Fecal Microbiota Transplant."

87. Jalanka et al., "Long-Term Effects of Faecal Microbiota Transplantation."

88. P. F. De Groot et al., "Fecal Microbiota Transplantation in Metabolic Syndrome: History, Present and Future," *Gut Microbes* 8, no. 3 (2017), doi.org/10.1080/19490976.2017.1293224.

89. Luke K. Ursell et al., "Defining the Human Microbiome," *Nutrition Reviews* 70 (2012), doi.org/10.1111/j.1753-4887.2012.00493.x.

90. F. De Filippis et al., "High-Level Adherence to a Mediterranean Diet Beneficially Impacts the Gut Microbiota and Associated Metabolome," *Gut* 65, no. 11 (2016), doi.org/10.1136/gutjnl-2015-309957.

91. Aleksandra Tomova, "The Effects of Vegetarian and Vegan Diets on Gut Microbiota," *Frontiers in Nutrition* 6, no. 47 (2019), doi.org/10.3389/fnut.2019.00047/full.

92. Yangbo Sun, "Inverse Association Between Organic Food Purchase and Diabetes Mellitus in US Adults," *Nutrients* 10 (2018), doi.org/10.3390/nu10121877; Evangelos Evangelou et al., "Exposure to Pesticides and Diabetes: A Systematic Review and Meta-Analysis," *Environment International* 91 (2016), doi.org/10.1016/j.envint.2016.02.013.

93. C. Sara and Robert A. Britton, "Adaptation of the Gut Microbiota to Modern Dietary Sugars and Sweeteners," *Advances in Nutrition* 11, no. 3 (2019), doi.org/10.1093/advances/nmz118.

94. RoundUp is also comprised of inactive ingredients which may interact with one another or glyphosate, though it's hard to tell—the precise mix of these inactive ingredients is a trade secret which Monsanto guards fiercely. Charles M. Benbrook, "Trends in Glyphosate Herbicide Use in the United States and Globally," *Environmental Sciences Europe* 28, no. 1 (2016), doi.org/10.1186/s12302-016-0070-0.

95. T. N. Lapkovskaya, S. V. Soroka, and O. K. Lobach, "Application of a Herbicide Tornado 500 in Cereal Crop Plantings and for a Preceding Crop," *Agriculture and Plant Protection: Scientific-Practical Journal* (2010), agris.fao.org/agris-search/search.do?recordID=BY2010000952.

96. A. A. Shehata et al., "The Effect of Glyphosate on Potential Pathogens and Beneficial Members of Poultry Microbiota in Vitro," *Current Microbiology* 66, no. 4 (2013), doi.org/10.1007/s00284-012-0277-2.

97. Robin Mesnage et al., "Use of Shotgun Metagenomics and Metabolomics to Evaluate the Impact of Glyphosate or Roundup MON 52276 on the Gut Microbiota and Serum Metabolome of Sprague-Dawley Rats," *Environmental Health Perspectives* 129, no. 1 (2021), doi.org/10.1289/ehp6990.

98. Erick V. S. Motta, Kasie Raymann, and Nancy A. Moran, "Glyphosate Perturbs the Gut Microbiota of Honey Bees," *Proceedings of the National Academy of Sciences of the United States of America* 115, no. 41 (2018), doi.org/10.1073/pnas.1803880115.

99. Shehata et al., "Effect of Glyphosate on Potential Pathogens."

100. Ibid.

101. E. Ofori et al., "Community-Acquired *Clostridium difficile*: Epidemiology, Ri-

botype, Risk Factors, Hospital and Intensive Care Unit Outcomes, and Current and Emerging Therapies," *Journal of Hospital Infection* 99, no. 4 (2018), doi.org/10.1016/j.jhin.2018.01.015.

102. Fernando Rubio, "Survey of Glyphosate Residues in Honey, Corn and Soy Products," *Journal of Environmental and Analytical Toxicology* 5, no. 1 (2014), doi.org/10.4172/2161-0525.1000249.

103. Jaime Rendon-Von Osten and Ricardo Dzul-Caamal, "Glyphosate Residues in Groundwater, Drinking Water and Urine of Subsistence Farmers from Intensive Agriculture Localities: A Survey in Hopelchén, Campeche, Mexico," *International Journal of Environmental Research and Public Health* 14, no. 6 (2017), doi.org/10.3390/ijerph14060595.

104. John R. Kelly et al., "Breaking Down the Barriers: The Gut Microbiome, Intestinal Permeability and Stress-Related Psychiatric Disorders," *Frontiers in Cellular Neuroscience* 9 (2015), doi.org/10.3389/fncel.2015.00392; J. P. Karl et al., "Effects of Psychological, Environmental and Physical Stressors on the Gut Microbiota," *Front Microbiology* 9 (2018), doi.org/10.3389/fmicb.2018.02013; Jane A. Foster, Linda Rinaman, and John F. Cryan, "Stress and the Gut-Brain Axis: Regulation by the Microbiome," *Neurobiology of Stress* 7 (2017), doi.org/10.1016/j.ynstr.2017.03.001.

105. A. Farhadi et al., "Intestinal Barrier: An Interface Between Health and Disease," *Journal of Gastroenterology and Hepatology* 18, no. 5 (2003), doi.org/10.1046/j.1440-1746.2003.03032.x.

106. Nobuyuki Sudo et al., "Postnatal Microbial Colonization Programs the Hypothalamic-Pituitary-Adrenal System for Stress Response in Mice," *Journal of Physiology* 558, no. 1 (2004), doi.org/10.1113/jphysiol.2004.063388.

107. Ibid.

108. G. A. Rook, "Regulation of the Immune System by Biodiversity from the Natural Environment: An Ecosystem Service Essential to Health," *Proceedings of the National Academy of Sciences of the United States of America* 110, no. 46 (2013), doi.org/10.1073/pnas.1313731110; Stephanie G. Cheung et al., "Systematic Review of Gut Microbiota and Major Depression," *Frontiers in Psychiatry* 10 (2019), doi.org/10.3389/fpsyt.2019.00034.

109. Ross M. Maltz et al., "Social Stress Affects Colonic Inflammation, the Gut Microbiome, and Short-Chain Fatty Acid Levels and Receptors," *Journal of Pediatric Gastroenterology and Nutrition* 68, no. 4 (2019), doi.org/10.1097/mpg.0000000000002226; Kelly et al., "Breaking Down Barriers."

110. Maltz et al., "Social Stress Affects Colonic Inflammation."

111. Kelly et al., "Breaking Down Barriers."

112. S. Da Silva et al., "Stress Disrupts Intestinal Mucus Barrier in Rats Via Mucin O-Glycosylation Shift: Prevention by a Probiotic Treatment," *American Journal of Physiology—Gastrointestinal and Liver Physiology* 307, no. 4 (2014), doi.org/10.1152/ajpgi.00290.2013.

113. Kelly et al., "Breaking Down Barriers."

114. J. D. Soderholm et al., "Neonatal Maternal Separation Predisposes Adult Rats to Colonic Barrier Dysfunction in Response to Mild Stress," *American Journal of Physiology—Gastrointestinal and Liver Physiology* 283, no. 6 (2002), doi.org/10.1152/ajpgi.00314.2002.

115. Vincent J. Felitti et al., "Relationship of Childhood Abuse and Household Dysfunction to Many of the Leading Causes of Death in Adults," *American*

Journal of Preventive Medicine 14, no. 4 (1998), doi.org/10.1016/s0749 -3797(98)00017-8.

116. Liisa Hantsoo et al., "Childhood Adversity Impact on Gut Microbiota and Inflammatory Response to Stress During Pregnancy," *Brain, Behavior, and Immunity* 75 (2019), doi.org/10.1016/j.bbi.2018.11.005; Andrea Danese and Jessie R. Baldwin, "Hidden Wounds? Inflammatory Links Between Childhood Trauma and Psychopathology," *Annual Review of Psychology* 68, no. 1 (2017), doi.org/10 .1146/annurev-psych-010416-044208.

117. Hantsoo et al., "Childhood Adversity Impact."

118. Bridget L. Callaghan et al., "Mind and Gut: Associations Between Mood and Gastrointestinal Distress in Children Exposed to Adversity," *Development and Psychopathology* 32, no. 1 (2020), doi.org/10.1017/s0954579419000087.

119. Saad Y. Salim, Gilaad G. Kaplan, and Karen L. Madsen, "Air Pollution Effects on the Gut Microbiota," *Gut Microbes* 5, no. 2 (2014), doi.org/10.4161/gmic.27251.

120. Limin Zhang et al., "Perfluorooctane Sulfonate Alters Gut Microbiota-Host Metabolic Homeostasis in Mice," *Toxicology* 431 (2020), doi.org/10.1016/j.tox.2020 .152365.

121. David Trudel et al., "Estimating Consumer Exposure to PFOS and PFOA," *Risk Analysis* 28, no. 2 (2008), doi.org/10.1111/j.1539-6924.2008.01017.x.

122. M. M. Stein et al., "Innate Immunity and Asthma Risk in Amish and Hutterite Farm Children," *New England Journal of Medicine* 375, no. 5 (2016), doi.org /10.1056/NEJMoa1508749.

123. Jeffrey M. Craig, Alan C. Logan, and Susan L. Prescott, "Natural Environments, Nature Relatedness and the Ecological Theater: Connecting Satellites and Sequencing to Shinrin-Yoku," *Journal of Physiological Anthropology* 35, no. 1 (2016), doi.org/10.1186/s40101-016-0083-9; Margaret M. Hansen, Reo Jones, and Kirsten Tocchini, "Shinrin-Yoku (Forest Bathing) and Nature Therapy: A State-of-the-Art Review," *International Journal of Environmental Research and Public Health* 14, no. 8 (2017), doi.org/10.3390/ijerph14080851.

124. Mike MacEacheran, "The Birthplace of Alpine Hay Bathing," *BBC*, December 8, 2020, www.bbc.com/travel/story/20201208-is-this-europes-new-wellness-trend.

125. David G. Smith et al., "Identification and Characterization of a Novel Anti-Inflammatory Lipid Isolated from *Mycobacterium vaccae*, a Soil-Derived Bacterium with Immunoregulatory and Stress Resilience Properties," *Psychopharmacology* 236 (2019), doi.org/10.1007/s00213-019-05253-9.

126. Dorothy M. Matthews and Susan M. Jenks, "Ingestion of *Mycobacterium vaccae* Decreases Anxiety-Related Behavior and Improves Learning in Mice," *Behavioural Processes* 96 (2013), doi.org/10.1016/j.beproc.2013.02.007.

127. Joan Wennstrom Bennett, *Microbiomes of the Built Environment: A Research Agenda for Indoor Microbiology, Human Health and Buildings* (Washington, DC: National Academies Press, 2017); N. Segata, "Gut Microbiome: Westernization and the Disappearance of Intestinal Diversity," *Current Biology* 25, no. 14 (2015), doi.org/10.1016/j.cub.2015.05.040.

128. And also how we move. Elite marathon runners possess an overabundance of *Veillonella atypica*, which is absent in other runners. Mice that were fed this organism ran 13 percent longer than control mice. Signs of inflammation were lowered in the *Veillonella*-treated mice as well. *Veillonella atypica* transforms lactic acid into the short-chain fatty acid propionate, turning the molecule that gives us sore muscles into one with an anti-inflammatory advantage. Jonathan

Scheiman et al., "Meta-omics Analysis of Elite Athletes Identifies a Performance-Enhancing Microbe That Functions via Lactate Metabolism," *Nature Medicine* 25, no. 7 (2019), doi.org/10.1038/s41591-019-0485-4.

129. J. H. Hehemann et al., "Transfer of Carbohydrate-Active Enzymes from Marine Bacteria to Japanese Gut Microbiota," *Nature* 464, no. 7290 (2010), doi .org/10.1038/nature08937.

130. J. C. D. Hotopp et al., "Widespread Lateral Gene Transfer from Intracellular Bacteria to Multicellular Eukaryotes," *Science* 317, no. 5845 (2007), doi.org/10 .1126/science.1142490.

131. World Economic Forum, *The New Plastics Economy: Rethinking the Future of Plastics* (Davos: World Economic Forum, 2015).

132. Shosuke Yoshida et al., "A Bacterium That Degrades and Assimilates Poly(ethylene Terephthalate)," *Science* 351, no. 6278 (2016), doi.org/10.1126/science .aad6359; M. G. Luciani-Torres, D. H. Moore, W. H. Goodson, 3rd, and S. H. Dairkee, "Exposure to the Polyester PET Precursor—Terephthalic Acid Induces and Perpetuates DNA Damage-Harboring Non-Malignant Human Breast Cells," *Carcinogenesis* 36, no. 1 (2015): 168–76, https://doi.org/10.1093/carcin/bgu234.

133. Kieran D. Cox et al., "Human Consumption of Microplastics," *Environmental Science and Technology* 53, no. 12 (2019), doi.org/10.1021/acs.est.9b01517.

134. John D. Meeker, Sheela Sathyanarayana, and Shanna H. Swan, "Phthalates and Other Additives in Plastics: Human Exposure and Associated Health Outcomes," *Philosophical Transactions of the Royal Society B: Biological Sciences* 364, no. 1526 (2009), doi.org/10.1098/rstb.2008.0268.

135. Sandrine P. Claus, Hervé Guillou, and Sandrine Ellero-Simatos, "The Gut Microbiota: A Major Player in the Toxicity of Environmental Pollutants?," *NPJ Biofilms and Microbiomes* 2, no. 1 (2016), doi.org/10.1038/npjbiofilms.2016.3.

136. Erica D. Sonnenburg and Justin L. Sonnenburg, "The Ancestral and Industrialized Gut Microbiota and Implications for Human Health," *Nature Reviews Microbiology* 17, no. 6 (2019), doi.org/10.1038/s41579-019-0191-8.

137. Gwyneira Isaac et al., "Native American Perspectives on Health and Traditional Ecological Knowledge," *Environmental Health Perspectives* 126, no. 12 (2018), doi.org/10.1289/ehp1944.

138. Segata, "Gut Microbiome."

139. Peter J. Ucko and G. W. Dimbleby, *The Domestication and Exploitation of Plants and Animals* (New Brunswick, N.J.: AldineTransaction, 2008).

140. Erik Axelsson et al., "The Genomic Signature of Dog Domestication Reveals Adaptation to a Starch-Rich Diet," *Nature* 495, no. 7441 (2013), doi.org/10 .1038/nature11837.

141. Bernardo Chessa et al., "Revealing the History of Sheep Domestication Using Retrovirus Integrations," *Science* 324, no. 5926 (2009), doi.org/10.1126/science .1170587.

142. T. J. Wilkinson et al., "Contextualizing Early Urbanization: Settlement Cores, Early States and Agro-Pastoral Strategies in the Fertile Crescent During the Fourth and Third Millennia BC," *Journal of World Prehistory* 27, no. 1 (2014), doi.org/10.1007/s10963-014-9072-2.

143. Bruce D. Smith, "Documenting Plant Domestication: The Consilience of Biological and Archaeological Approaches," *Proceedings of the National Academy of Sciences of the United States of America* 98, no. 4 (2001), doi.org/10.1073/pnas .98.4.1324t; Umberto Lombardo et al., "Early Holocene Crop Cultivation and

Landscape Modification in Amazonia," *Nature* 581 (2020), doi.org/10.1038 /s41586-020-2162-7; James L. A. Webb, *The Guts of the Matter: A Global History of Human Waste and Infectious Intestinal Disease* (Cambridge: Cambridge University Press, 2019); Greger Larson and Dorian Q. Fuller, "The Evolution of Animal Domestication," *Annual Review of Ecology, Evolution, and Systematics* 45, no. 1 (2014), doi.org/10.1146/annurev-ecolsys-110512-135813.

144. Stan Cox, "Crop Domestication and the First Plant Breeders," in *Plant Breeding and Farmer Participation,* ed. S. Ceccarelli, E. P. Guimarães, and E. Weltzien (Rome: UN Food and Agricultural Organization, 2009), 3; J. G. Hawkes, *The Ecological Background of Plant Domestication* (London: Gerald Duckworth & Co., 1969). These were early examples of humans' botany of desire. Michael Pollan, *The Botany of Desire: A Plant's-Eye View of the World* (New York: Random House, 2001).

145. John Smalley, Michael Blake, and Warren R DeBoer, "Sweet Beginnings: Stalk Sugar and the Domestication of Maize," *Current Anthropology* 44, no. 5 (2003), doi.org/10.1086/377664.

146. Madhav Gadgil, Fikret Berkes, and Carl Folke, "Indigenous Knowledge for Biodiversity Conservation," *Ambio* 22, no. 2–3 (1993), www.jstor.org/stable /4314060.

147. Nancy J. Turner, *Ancient Pathways, Ancestral Knowledge: Ethnobotany and Ecological Wisdom of Indigenous Peoples of Northwestern North America* (Montreal: McGill-Queen's University Press, 2014), 117.

148. Ibid., 121.

149. Ibid., 151.

150. Pekka Hämäläinen, *The Comanche Empire* (New Haven, CT: Yale University Press, 2008).

151. Cole Harris, *Making Native Space: Colonialism, Resistance, and Reserves in British Columbia* (Vancouver: University of British Columbia Press, 2002).

152. Colonists held—and continue to hold—dim views about local capacities for land management, whose Western form is a discipline founded on the idea that well-informed experts can counsel locals on how to arrest the declining health of the ground beneath their feet. One classic study gave the lie to this notion by using aerial photographs taken by the French as they mapped out their claims to Guinée. By comparing forest cover in the 1950s and the early '90s, researchers showed how forest area had *increased* through farmers' active land management. Niek Koning and Eric Smaling, "Environmental Crisis or 'Lie of the Land'? The Debate on Soil Degradation in Africa," *Land Use Policy* 22, no. 1 (2005), doi.org/10.1016/j.landusepol.2003.08.003; James Fairhead and Melissa Leach, *Misreading the African Landscape: Society and Ecology in a Forest-Savanna Mosaic* (Cambridge: Cambridge University Press, 1996).

153. "God's Own Country" (editorial), *Clarence and Richmond Examiner,* January 21, 1902, trove.nla.gov.au/newspaper/article/61385036.

154. Bruce Pascoe, *Dark Emu: Black Seeds: Agriculture or Accident?* (Broome, Western Australia: Magabala Books, 2014).

155. John N. Warner, "Sugar Cane: An Indigenous Papuan Cultigen," *Ethnology* 1, no. 4 (1962), doi.org/10.2307/3772848.

156. S. Mahdihassan, "A Comparative Study of the Word *Sugar* and of Its Equivalents in Hindustani as Traceable to Chinese," *American Journal of Chinese Medicine* 9, no. 3 (1981), doi.org/10.1142/S0192415X8100024X.

157. Rebecca Catz, *Christopher Columbus and the Portuguese, 1476–1498* (Westport, CT: Greenwood, 1993); Sidney M. Greenfield, "Madeira and the Beginnings of New World Sugar Cane Cultivation and Plantation Slavery: A Study in Institution Building," *Annals of the New York Academy of Sciences* 292, no. 1 (1977), doi.org/10.1111/j.1749-6632.1977.tb47771.x; Jason W. Moore, "Madeira, Sugar, and the Conquest of Nature in the 'First' Sixteenth Century: Part I: From 'Island of Timber' to Sugar Revolution, 1420–1506," *Review (Fernand Braudel Center)* 32, no. 4 (2009), www.jstor.org/stable/41427474; Stuart B. Schwartz, "Indian Labor and New World Plantations: European Demands and Indian Responses in Northeastern Brazil," *American Historical Review* 83, no. 1 (1978), doi.org/10.2307/1865902; Stuart B. Schwartz, "A Commonwealth Within Itself: The Early Brazilian Sugar Industry, 1550–1670," in *Tropical Babylons: Sugar and the Making of the Atlantic World, 1450–1680,* ed. Stuart B. Schwartz (Chapel Hill: University of North Carolina Press, 2004); Charles Verlinden, *The Beginnings of Modern Colonization* (Ithaca, NY: Cornell University Press, 1970); Alberto Vieira, "Sugar Islands. The Sugar Economy of Madeira and the Canaries, 1450–1650," in Schwartz, *Tropical Babylons.*

158. Sidney Wilfred Mintz, *Sweetness and Power: The Place of Sugar in Modern History* (New York: Penguin, 1985), 82.

159. Raj Patel and Jason W. Moore, *A History of the World in Seven Cheap Things: A Guide to Capitalism, Nature, and the Future of the Planet* (Berkeley: University of California Press, 2017).

160. K. J. Newens and J. Walton, "A Review of Sugar Consumption from Nationally Representative Dietary Surveys across the World," *Journal of Human Nutrition and Dietetics* 29, no. 2 (2016), doi.org/10.1111/jhn.12338.

161. Laura A. Schmidt, "New Unsweetened Truths About Sugar," *JAMA Internal Medicine* 174, no. 4 (2014), doi.org/10.1001/jamainternmed.2013.12991; Robert Lustig, *Metabolical* (New York: HarperWave, 2021); M. L. Slattery et al., "Dietary Sugar and Colon Cancer," *Cancer Epidemiology, Biomarkers and Prevention* 6, no. 9 (1997), www.ncbi.nlm.nih.gov/pubmed/9298574.

162. R. K. Singh et al., "Influence of Diet on the Gut Microbiome and Implications for Human Health," *Journal of Translational Medicine* 15, no. 1 (2017), doi.org/10.1186/s12967-017-1175-y.

163. Mike Davis, *Late Victorian Holocausts: El Nino Famines and the Making of the Third World* (New York: Verso, 2001).

164. C. K. Khoury et al., "Increasing Homogeneity in Global Food Supplies and the Implications for Food Security," *Proceedings of the National Academy of Sciences of the United States of America* 111, no. 11 (2014), doi.org/10.1073/pnas.1313490111.

165. Jennifer Cole, "Agriculture: Land Use, Food Systems and Biodiversity," in *Planetary Health: Human Health in an Era of Global Environmental Change,* ed. Jennifer Cole et al. (Oxford: CAB International, 2019).

166. Y. M. Bar-On, R. Phillips, and R. Milo, "The Biomass Distribution on Earth," *Proceedings of the National Academy of Sciences of the United States of America* 115, no. 25 (2018), doi.org/10.1073/pnas.1711842115.

167. Gerardo Ceballos et al., "Accelerated Modern Human-Induced Species Losses: Entering the Sixth Mass Extinction," *Science Advances* 1, no. 5 (2015), doi.org/10.1126/sciadv.1400253; Jonathan L. Payne et al., "Ecological Selectivity of

the Emerging Mass Extinction in the Oceans," *Science* 353, no. 6305 (2016), doi.org/10.1126/science.aaf2416.

168. Rachel Carson, *Silent Spring* (Boston: Houghton Mifflin, 1962); Jorge Fernandez-Cornejo et al., "Pesticide Use in U.S. Agriculture: 21 Selected Crops, 1960–2008," *USDA-ERS Economic Information Bulletin* no. 124 (2014), doi.org/10.2139/ssrn.2502986; Donald Atwood and Claire Paisley-Jones, *Pesticides Industry Sales and Usage: 2008–2012 Market Estimates* (Washington, DC: US Environmental Protection Agency, 2017), tinyurl.com/2rl8gjh8.

169. United Nations FAO, "Pesticides Use," FAOSTAT (Rome: UN Food and Agriculture Organization, 2021), www.fao.org/faostat/en/#data/RP.

170. Nancy J. Turner et al., "Edible and Tended Wild Plants, Traditional Ecological Knowledge and Agroecology," *Critical Reviews in Plant Sciences* 30, no. 1–2 (2011), doi.org/10.1080/07352689.2011.554492; Nancy J. Turner and Katherine L. Turner, "Where Our Women Used to Get the Food: Cumulative Effects and Loss of Ethnobotanical Knowledge and Practice; Case Study from Coastal British Columbia," *Botany* 86, no. 2 (2008): 86, doi.org/10.1139/b07-020; Miguel A. Altieri, *Agroecology: The Scientific Basis of Alternative Agriculture* (Boulder, CO: Westview Press, 1987); Jennifer C. Sowerwine, "Effects of Economic Liberalization on Dao Women's Traditional Knowledge, Ecology, and Trade of Medicinal Plants in Northern Vietnam," *Advances in Economic Botany* 15 (2004), www.jstor.org/stable/43927646; Nancy Turner, "'Passing on the News': Women's Work, Traditional Knowledge and Plant Resource Management in Indigenous Societies of North-Western North America," in *Women and Plants: Gender Relations in Biodiversity Management and Conservation*, ed. Patricia L. Howard (London: Zed Books, 2003).

171. A. D. Luis, A. J. Kuenzi, and J. N. Mills, "Species Diversity Concurrently Dilutes and Amplifies Transmission in a Zoonotic Host-Pathogen System Through Competing Mechanisms," *Proceedings of the National Academy of Sciences of the United States of America* 115, no. 31 (2018), doi.org/10.1073/pnas.1807106115; Fernandez-Cornejo et al., "Pesticide Use in U.S. Agriculture."

172. E. Ofori et al., "Community-Acquired *Clostridium difficile*: Epidemiology, Ribotype, Risk Factors, Hospital and Intensive Care Unit Outcomes, and Current and Emerging Therapies," *Journal of Hospital Infection* 99, no. 4 (2018), doi.org/10.1016/j.jhin.2018.01.015.

173. Deverick J. Anderson et al., "Identification of Novel Risk Factors for Community-Acquired *Clostridium difficile* Infection Using Spatial Statistics and Geographic Information System Analyses," *PLOS One* 12, no. 5 (2017), doi.org/10.1371/journal.pone.0176285.

174. Johan S. Bakken et al., "Treating *Clostridium difficile* Infection with Fecal Microbiota Transplantation," *Clinical Gastroenterology and Hepatology* 9, no. 12 (2011), doi.org/10.1016/j.cgh.2011.08.014.

175. John Fagan et al., "Organic Diet Intervention Significantly Reduces Urinary Glyphosate Levels in U.S. Children and Adults," *Environmental Research* 189 (2020), doi.org/10.1016/j.envres.2020.109898.

176. John Bellamy Foster, "Marx's Theory of Metabolic Rift: Classical Foundations for Environmental Sociology," *American Journal of Sociology* 105, no. 2 (1999), www.jstor.org/stable/10.1086/210315?seq = 1; Jason W. Moore, "Transcending the Metabolic Rift: A Theory of Crises in the Capitalist World-Ecology," *Journal of Peasant Studies* 38, no. 1 (January 2011), doi.org/10.1080/03066150.2010

.538579; Mindi Schneider and Philip McMichael, "Deepening, and Repairing, the Metabolic Rift," *Journal of Peasant Studies* 37, no. 3 (2010), doi.org/10.1080 /03066150.2010.494371; Michael Friedman, "Metabolic Rift and the Human Microbiome," *Monthly Review* 70, no. 3 (2018), monthlyreview.org/2018/07 /01/metabolic-rift-and-the-human-microbiome. In farming at least, there are movements that are looking to move beyond that rift. Hannah Wittman, "Reworking the Metabolic Rift: La Vía Campesina, Agrarian Citizenship, and Food Sovereignty," *Journal of Peasant Studies* 36, no. 4 (2009), doi.org/10.1080 /03066150903353991.

177. Philip Mackowiak, "Recycling Metchnikoff: Probiotics, the Intestinal Microbiome and the Quest for Long Life," *Frontiers in Public Health* 1, no. 52 (2013), doi.org/10.3389/fpubh.2013.00052.

178. Les Dethlefsen, Margaret McFall-Ngai, and David A. Relman, "An Ecological and Evolutionary Perspective on Human-Microbe Mutualism and Disease," *Nature* 449, no. 7164 (2007), doi.org/10.1038/nature06245; Ali K. Yetisen, "Biohacking," *Trends in Biotechnology* 36, no. 8 (2018), doi.org/10.1016/j.tibtech.2018.02.011.

179. Dan Buettner and Sam Skemp, "Blue Zones," *American Journal of Lifestyle Medicine* 10, no. 5 (2016), doi.org/10.1177/1559827616637066.

180. Bradley J. Willcox, Donald Craig Willcox, and Makoto Suzuki, "Demographic, Phenotypic, and Genetic Characteristics of Centenarians in Okinawa and Japan: Part 1—Centenarians in Okinawa," *Mechanisms of Ageing and Development* 165 (2017), doi.org/10.1016/j.mad.2016.11.001.

181. Miriam Capri et al., "Human Longevity within an Evolutionary Perspective: The Peculiar Paradigm of a Post-Reproductive Genetics," *Experimental Gerontology* 43, no. 2 (2008), doi.org/10.1016/j.exger.2007.06.004.

182. Adriana Lleras-Muney, "The Relationship Between Education and Adult Mortality in the United States," *Review of Economic Studies* 72, no. 1 (2005), doi.org /10.1111/0034-6527.00329; Howard S. Friedman and Leslie R. Martin, *The Longevity Project: Surprising Discoveries for Health and Long Life from the Landmark Eight-Decade Study* (New York: Hudson Street Press, 2011).

183. This is an explanation popular since the eighteenth century. Georges Louis Leclerc de Buffon, *De la vieillesse et de la mort*, vol. 12 of *Œuvres complètes de Buffon* (Paris: F. D. Pillot, 1831).

184. B. J. Willcox et al., "Caloric Restriction, the Traditional Okinawan Diet, and Healthy Aging," *Annals of the New York Academy of Sciences* 1114, no. 1 (2007), doi.org/10.1196/annals.1396.037; D. Craig Willcox et al., "The Okinawan Diet: Health Implications of a Low-Calorie, Nutrient-Dense, Antioxidant-Rich Dietary Pattern Low in Glycemic Load," *Journal of the American College of Nutrition* 28, no. 4 (2009), doi.org/10.1080/07315724.2009.10718117.

185. S. Miyagi et al., "Longevity and Diet in Okinawa, Japan: The Past, Present and Future," *Asia Pacific Journal of Public Health* 15, no. 1 (2003), doi.org/10 .1177/101053950301500s03.

186. Aike P. Rots, "Strangers in the Sacred Grove: The Changing Meanings of Okinawan Utaki," *Religions* 10, no. 5 (2019), www.mdpi.com/2077-1444/10/5/298.

187. George Feifer, "The Rape of Okinawa," *World Policy Journal* 17, no. 3 (2000), www.jstor.org/stable/40209702.

188. Michel Poulain, "Exceptional Longevity in Okinawa: A Plea for in-Depth Validation," *Demographic Research* 25, no. 7 (2011), www.demographic-research .org/volumes/vol25/7/.

189. Norimitsu Onishi, "On U.S. Fast Food, More Okinawans Grow Super-Sized," *The New York Times*, March 30, 2004, tinyurl.com/psofeg6f; Y. Matsushita et al., "Overweight and Obesity Trends Among Japanese Adults: A 10-Year Follow-up of the JPHC Study," *International Journal of Obesity* 32, no. 12 (2008), doi.org/10.1038/ijo.2008.188.

190. Willcox et al., "Caloric Restriction, Traditional Okinawan Diet"; D. Craig Willcox et al., "The Okinawan Diet: Health Implications of a Low-Calorie, Nutrient-Dense, Antioxidant-Rich Dietary Pattern Low in Glycemic Load," *Journal of the American College of Nutrition* 28 (2009), tinyurl.com/4n2xqxh9; Bradley J. Willcox, D. Craig Willcox, and Makoto Suzuki, *The Okinawa Way: How to Improve Your Health and Longevity Dramatically* (London: Michael Joseph, 2001).

191. Pasupuleti Visweswara Rao et al., "Biological and Therapeutic Effects of Honey Produced by Honey Bees and Stingless Bees: A Comparative Review," *Revista brasileira de farmacognosia* 26, no. 5 (2016), doi.org/10.1016/j.bjp.2016.01.012.

192. M. Barone et al., "Gut Microbiome Response to a Modern Paleolithic Diet in a Western Lifestyle Context," *PLOS One* 14, no. 8 (2019), doi.org/10.1371/journal.pone.0220619.

193. Michelle A. Morris et al., "What Is the Cost of a Healthy Diet? Using Diet Data from the UK Women's Cohort Study," *Journal of Epidemiology and Community Health* 68, no. 11 (2014), doi.org/10.1136/jech-2014-204039.

194. Marialaura Bonaccio et al., "High Adherence to the Mediterranean Diet Is Associated with Cardiovascular Protection in Higher but Not in Lower Socioeconomic Groups: Prospective Findings from the Moli-sani Study," *International Journal of Epidemiology* 46, no. 5 (2017), doi.org/10.1093/ije/dyx145.

195. Walter Willett et al., "Food in the Anthropocene: The EAT-*Lancet* Commission on Healthy Diets from Sustainable Food Systems," *The Lancet* 393, no. 10170 (2019), doi.org/10.1016/S0140-6736(18)31788-4.

196. S. Nishijima et al., "The Gut Microbiome of Healthy Japanese and Its Microbial and Functional Uniqueness," *DNA Research* 23, no. 2 (2016), doi.org/10.1093/dnares/dsw002.

197. See, for instance, David T. Suzuki and Keibō Ōiwa, *The Other Japan: Voices Beyond the Mainstream* (Golden, CO: Fulcrum, 1999).

198. Takuya Yamanouchi, Atsumu Ohnishi, and Shoichi Tashiro, "Tolerated Cultivation and the Postwar Period Processing Problem:A Case Study on Yomitan Village in Okinawa Prefecture," *Bulletin of the Faculty of Agriculture*, no. 54 (2004).

199. He may have been older, but Ahagon's father recorded his birth date with the Japanese authorities as 1903—possibly so he could avoid the draft. Ahagon Shoko and C. Douglas Lummis, "I Lost My Only Son in the War: Prelude to the Okinawan Anti-Base Movement," *Asia-Pacific Journal* 8, no. 23 (2010), apjjf.org/-C.-Douglas-Lummis/3369/article.html.

200. Suzuki and Ōiwa, *Other Japan*.

201. Stéphane M. McLachlan, *"Water Is a Living Thing": Environmental and Human Health Implications of the Athabasca Oil Sands for the Mikisew Cree First Nation and Athabasca Chipewyan First Nation in Northern Alberta* (Winnipeg: University of Manitoba, 2014), https://tinyurl.com/efj7uy9f.

202. L. Eggertson, "High Cancer Rates Among Fort Chipewyan Residents," *Canadian Medical Association Journal* 181, no. 12 (2009), doi.org/10.1503/cmaj.090248.

203. Committee on Oversight and Reform, U.S. House of Representatives, *Baby Foods Are Tainted with Dangerous Levels of Arsenic, Lead, Cadmium, and Mercury* (2021), oversight.house.gov/sites/democrats.oversight.house.gov/files/2021-02-04% 20ECP%20Baby%20Food%20Staff%20Report.pdf.

204. Erik Lacitis, "Last Few Whulshootseed Speakers Spread the Word," *Seattle Times*, February 8, 2005, tinyurl.com/rluksnzv.

205. Heidi G. Bruce, "Muckleshoot Foods and Culture: Pre-20th Century Stka-mish, Skopamish, Smulkamish, and Allied Longhouses," *Fourth World Journal* 16, no. 1 (2017).

206. P. A. Moore, J. C. Zgibor, and A. P. Dasanayake, "Diabetes: A Growing Epidemic of All Ages," *Journal of the American Dental Association* 134, suppl. 1 (2003), doi.org/10.14219/jada.archive.2003.0369.

4. RESPIRATORY SYSTEM

1. Melinda Mitchell Jones, Kathleen M. Kearney, and Carrie Edwards, "Seeking PPE Protection: Is the Law on Your Side?," *Nursing Made Incredibly Easy* 18, no. 6 (2020), journals.lww.com/nursingmadeincrediblyeasy/Fulltext/2020 /11000/Seeking_PPE_protection__Is_the_law_on_your_side_.4.aspx.

2. Leslie Marmon Silko, *Ceremony* (New York: Viking Press, 1977).

3. Ben Okri, *Birds of Heaven* (London: Phoenix, 1996), 18.

4. Ralph Kahn, "A Global Perspective on Wildfires," *Eos*, January 27, 2020, doi .org/10.1029/2020EO138260.

5. Brigitte Rooney et al., "Air Quality Impact of the Northern California Camp Fire of November 2018," *Atmospheric Chemistry and Physics* 20, no. 23 (2020), acp.copernicus.org/articles/20/14597/2020/acp-20-14597-2020.pdf.

6. Rizzlyn Terri M. Melo, "We Didn't Start the Fire . . . Did We? Analyzing Why California Cannot Seem to Extinguish Its Worsening Wildfire Problem," *Villanova Environmental Law Journal* 31, no. 1 (2020), digitalcommons.law .villanova.edu/elj/vol31/iss1/5/.

7. High blood pressure, smoking, and poor diet are the greater risk factors, though as we'll see, they're all linked. Health Effects Institute, *State of Global Air 2020* (Boston: Health Effects Institute, 2020).

8. A. Park Williams et al., "Observed Impacts of Anthropogenic Climate Change on Wildfire in California," *Earth's Future* 7, no. 8 (2019), doi.org/10.1029/2019ef0 01210.

9. H. Orru, K. L. Ebi, and B. Forsberg, "The Interplay of Climate Change and Air Pollution on Health," *Current Environmental Health Reports* 4, no. 4 (2017), doi .org/10.1007/s40572-017-0168-6; Y. Fang et al., "Air Pollution and Associated Human Mortality: The Role of Air Pollutant Emissions, Climate Change and Methane Concentration Increases from the Preindustrial Period to Present," *Atmospheric Chemistry and Physics* 13, no. 3 (2013), doi.org/10.5194/acp-13-1377-2013.

10. Hina is a composite of several people and cases from across the waste-picking world. When we began this book, we had planned to visit several groups in Delhi to conduct research. Lockdown thwarted those plans, and multiplied the suffering of waste pickers. For more on the impact of Covid on waste pickers, see Bharati Chaturvedi, *The Covid-19 Impact on Waste Pickers in Delhi* (Delhi: Oxfam India, 2020), tinyurl.com/cnhhcnlt.

11. Anamika Pandey et al., "Health and Economic Impact of Air Pollution in the

States of India: The Global Burden of Disease Study 2019," *Lancet Planetary Health* 5, no. 1 (2021), doi.org/10.1016/s2542-5196(20)30298-9.

12. Navarro Ferronato and Vincenzo Torretta, "Waste Mismanagement in Developing Countries: A Review of Global Issues," *International Journal of Environmental Research and Public Health* 16, no. 6 (2019), doi.org/10.3390/ijerph16061060; Federico Demaria and Seth Schindler, "Contesting Urban Metabolism: Struggles over Waste-to-Energy in Delhi, India," *Antipode* 48, no. 2 (2016), doi.org/10.1111/anti.12191.

13. Re-Centering Delhi Team, "Mapping Delhi Landfills," *Yamuna River Project*, Fall 2016, www.yamunariverproject.org/mapping-delhi-landfills.html.

14. J. S. Grewal, "Historical Geography of the Punjab," *Journal of Punjab Studies* 11, no. 1 (2004), tinyurl.com/yn3qh3me.

15. David E. Ludden, *An Agrarian History of South Asia* (New York: Cambridge University Press, 1999); Dorian Q. Fuller, "Agricultural Origins and Frontiers in South Asia: A Working Synthesis," *Journal of World Prehistory* 20, no. 1 (2006), doi.org/10.1007/s10963-006-9006-8; Prathama Banerjee, "Writing the Adivasi: Some Historiographical Notes," *Indian Economic and Social History Review* 53, no. 1 (2016); Chetan Singh, "Conformity and Conflict: Tribes and the 'Agrarian System' of Mughal India," *Indian Economic and Social History Review* 25, no. 3 (1988), doi.org/10.1177/001946468802500302.

16. Krishna-Dwaipayana Vyasa, *The Mahabharata*, trans. Kisari Mohan Ganguli (1883), sec. 230, www.sacred-texts.com/hin/m01/m01231.htm.

17. Madhav Gadgil, "India's Deforestation: Patterns and Processes," *Society and Natural Resources* 3, no. 2 (1990), doi.org/10.1080/08941929009380713.

18. Jean Birrell, "Common Rights in the Medieval Forest: Disputes and Conflicts in the Thirteenth Century," *Past and Present*, no. 117 (1987), www.jstor.org/stable/650787. The tragedy of the commons lies in the fact that the commons were destroyed, not that they were unowned. For more, see e.g., Raj Patel, *The Value of Nothing* (New York: Picador, 2010).

19. Peter Blickle, *The Revolution of 1525: The German Peasants' War from a New Perspective* (Baltimore: Johns Hopkins University Press, 1981).

20. Peter Linebaugh, *The Magna Carta Manifesto: Liberties and Commons for All* (Berkeley: University of California Press, 2008).

21. Alexander Mather, "The Transition from Deforestation to Reforestation in Europe," in *Agricultural Technologies and Tropical Deforestation*, ed. Arild Angelsen and David Kaimowitz (Wallingford, UK: CABI Publishing, 2001).

22. Shashank Kela, "Adivasi and Peasant: Reflections on Indian Social History," *Journal of Peasant Studies* 33, no. 3 (2006), doi.org/10.1080/03066150601063074. And in Great Britain, they remain. In a recent report on the state of nature in the UK, 97 percent of wildflower meadows were reported lost in the past century, among other findings. D. B. Hayhow et al., *The State of Nature 2019* (Nottingham, UK: National Biodiversity Network for the State of Nature Partnership, 2019).

23. Romila Thapar, "Perceiving the Forest: Early India," *Studies in History* 17, no. 1 (2001), doi.org/10.1177/025764300101700101.

24. Michael R. Dove, "The Dialectical History of 'Jungle' in Pakistan: An Examination of the Relationship Between Nature and Culture," *Journal of Anthropological Research* 48, no. 3 (1992), doi.org/10.1086/jar.48.3.3630636.

25. Ramachandra Guha, "Forestry in British and Post-British India: A Histori-

cal Analysis," *Economic and Political Weekly* 18, no. 44 (1983): www.jstor.org /stable/4372653.

26. Ibid.

27. Ibid.

28. Amiya Kumar Bagchi, "Land Tax, Property Rights and Peasant Insecurity in Colonial India," *Journal of Peasant Studies* 20, no. 1 (1992), doi.org/10.1080 /03066159208438500; Mike Davis, *Late Victorian Holocausts: El Nino Famines and the Making of the Third World* (New York: Verso, 2001).

29. Cormac Ó Gráda and Andrés Eiríksson, *Ireland's Great Famine: Interdisciplinary Perspectives* (Dublin: University College Dublin Press, 2006).

30. "Notes from India: The Effect of Famine on the Population of India," *The Lancet* 157, no. 4059 (1901), doi.org/10.1016/S0140-6736(01)89212-6.

31. Raj Patel, "The Long Green Revolution," *Journal of Peasant Studies* 40, no. 1 (2013).

32. Ibid., 5.

33. Vandana Shiva, *The Violence of the Green Revolution: Ecological Degradation and Political Conflict in Punjab* (Dehra Dun: Research Foundation for Science and Ecology, 1989); Utsa Patnaik, "Neoliberalism and Rural Poverty in India," *Economic and Political Weekly* 42, no. 30 (2007), www.jstor.org/stable /4419844.

34. Ludden, *Agrarian History of South Asia.*

35. For the planetary nature of this phenomenon, see Matti Kummu et al., "Is Physical Water Scarcity a New Phenomenon? Global Assessment of Water Shortage over the Last Two Millennia," *Environmental Research Letters* 5, no. 3 (2010), doi.org/10.1088/1748-9326/5/3/034006.

36. Seema Singh, "Pumping Punjab Dry," *IEEE Spectrum* 47, no. 6 (2010), doi.org /10.1109/mspec.2010.5466794.

37. The naturally occurring mineral salts in the groundwater and the residues from industrial chemicals combine to make a toxic mix. Khalid Mahmood et al., "Groundwater Uptake and Sustainability of Farm Plantations on Saline Sites in Punjab Province, Pakistan," *Agricultural Water Management* 48, no. 1 (2001), doi.org/10.1016/S0378-3774(00)00114-1; Amarnath Tripathi, Ashok K. Mishra, and Geetanjali Verma, "Impact of Preservation of Subsoil Water Act on Groundwater Depletion: The Case of Punjab, India," *Environmental Management* 58, no. 1 (2016), doi.org/10.1007/s00267-016-0693-3.

38. Sucha S. Gill, "Economic Distress and Farmer Suicides in Rural Punjab," *Journal of Punjab Studies* 12, no. 2 (2006), tinyurl.com/y68vjtev.

39. Kiran Chand Thumaty et al., "Spatio-Temporal Characterization of Agriculture Residue Burning in Punjab and Haryana, India, Using MODIS and Suomi NPP VIIRS Data," *Current Science* 109, no. 10 (2015), doi.org/10.18520 /v109/i10/1850-1868.

40. Navroz K. Dubash and Sarath Guttikunda, "Delhi Has a Complex Air Pollution Problem," *Hindustan Times*, December 22, 2018, tinyurl.com/10qd0yal.

41. Michael D. Hays et al., "Open Burning of Agricultural Biomass: Physical and Chemical Properties of Particle-Phase Emissions," *Atmospheric Environment* 39, no. 36 (2005), doi.org/10.1016/j.atmosenv.2005.07.072. See also Andrew C. Scott, *Burning Planet: The Story of Fire Through Time* (Oxford: Oxford University Press, 2018).

42. P. Kulshreshtha, M. Khare, and P. Seetharaman, "Indoor Air Quality Assessment

in and Around Urban Slums of Delhi City, India," *Indoor Air* 18, no. 6 (2008), doi .org/10.1111/j.1600-0668.2008.00550.x.

43. U. C. Kulshrestha et al., "Emissions and Accumulation of Metals in the Atmosphere Due to Crackers and Sparkles During Diwali Festival in India," *Atmospheric Environment* 38, no. 27 (2004), doi.org/10.1016/j.atmosenv.2004.05.044.

44. Sourangsu Chowdhury et al., "'Traffic Intervention' Policy Fails to Mitigate Air Pollution in Megacity Delhi," *Environmental Science and Policy* 74 (2017), doi.org/10.1016/j.envsci.2017.04.018.

45. Srinivas Bikkina et al., "Air Quality in Megacity Delhi Affected by Countryside Biomass Burning," *Nature Sustainability* 2, no. 3 (2019), doi.org/10.1038 /s41893-019-0219-0.

46. Chowdhury et al., "'Traffic Intervention' Policy Fails."

47. Kalpana Balakrishnan et al., "The Impact of Air Pollution on Deaths, Disease Burden, and Life Expectancy across the States of India: The Global Burden of Disease Study 2017," *Lancet Planetary Health* 3, no. 1 (2019), doi.org/10.1016 /s2542-5196(18)30261-4.

48. Ibid.

49. Jincy Mathew et al., "Air Pollution and Respiratory Health of School Children in Industrial, Commercial and Residential Areas of Delhi," *Air Quality, Atmosphere and Health* 8, no. 4 (2015), doi.org/10.1007/s11869-014-0299-y; Shabana Siddique, Manas R. Ray, and Twisha Lahiri, "Effects of Air Pollution on the Respiratory Health of Children: A Study in the Capital City of India," *Air Quality, Atmosphere and Health* 4, no. 2 (2011), doi.org/10.1007/s11869 -010-0079-2.

50. Y. F. Xing et al., "The Impact of $PM_{2.5}$ on the Human Respiratory System," *Journal of Thoracic Disease* 8, no. 1 (2016), doi.org/10.3978/j.issn.2072-1439 .2016.01.19.

51. Douglas W. Dockery et al., "An Association Between Air Pollution and Mortality in Six U.S. Cities," *New England Journal of Medicine* 329 (1993), doi.org /10.1056/nejm199312093292401.

52. M. A. Zoran et al., "Assessing the Relationship Between Ground Levels of Ozone (O3) and Nitrogen Dioxide (NO2) with Coronavirus (Covid-19) in Milan, Italy," *Science of the Total Environment* 740 (2020), doi.org/10.1016/j .scitotenv.2020.140005; Leonardo Setti, "SARS-Cov-2 RNA Found on Particulate Matter of Bergamo in Northern Italy: First Evidence," *Environmental Research* 188 (2020), doi.org/10.1016/j.envres.2020.109754.

53. G. W. Hammond, R. L. Raddatz, and D. E. Gelskey, "Impact of Atmospheric Dispersion and Transport of Viral Aerosols on the Epidemiology of Influenza," *Clinical Infectious Diseases* 11, no. 3 (1989), doi.org/10.1093/clinids/11 .3.494.

54. Dockery et al., "Association Between Air Pollution."

55. C. Arden Pope III et al., "Lung Cancer, Cardiopulmonary Mortality, and Long-Term Exposure to Fine Particulate Air Pollution," *JAMA* 287, no. 9 (2002), doi .org/10.1001/jama.287.9.1132.

56. C. Arden Pope III, M. Ezzati, and D. W. Dockery, "Fine-Particulate Air Pollution and Life Expectancy in the United States," *New England Journal of Medicine* 360, no. 4 (2009), doi.org/10.1056/NEJMsa0805646.

57. Dean E. Schraufnagel et al., "Air Pollution and Noncommunicable Diseases," *Chest* 155, no. 2 (2019), doi.org/10.1016/j.chest.2018.10.042.

58. J. Schwartz, "Lung Function and Chronic Exposure to Air Pollution: A Cross-Sectional Analysis of NHANES II," *Environmental Research* 50, no. 2 (1989), doi.org/10.1016/s0013-9351(89)80012-x; B. Brunekreef and S. T. Holgate, "Air Pollution and Health," *The Lancet* 360, no. 9341 (2002), doi.org/10.1016/S0140-6736(02)11274-8; P. T. King, "Inflammation in Chronic Obstructive Pulmonary Disease and Its Role in Cardiovascular Disease and Lung Cancer," *Clinical and Translational Medicine* 4, no. 1 (2015), doi.org/10.1186/s40169-015-0068-z.

59. M. S. Link et al., "Acute Exposure to Air Pollution Triggers Atrial Fibrillation," *Journal of the American College of Cardiology* 62, no. 9 (2013), doi.org/10.1016/j.jacc.2013.05.043; C. Arden Pope III et al., "Short-Term Exposure to Fine Particulate Matter Air Pollution Is Preferentially Associated with the Risk of St-Segment Elevation Acute Coronary Events," *Journal of the American Heart Association* 4, no. 12 (2015), doi.org/10.1161/JAHA.115.002506.

60. Hammond, Raddatz, and Gelskey, "Impact of Atmospheric Dispersion."

61. X. Wu et al., "Air Pollution and Covid-19 Mortality in the United States: Strengths and Limitations of an Ecological Regression Analysis," *Science Advances* 6, no. 45 (2020), doi.org/10.1126/sciadv.abd4049.

62. Chaomin Wu et al., "Risk Factors Associated with Acute Respiratory Distress Syndrome and Death in Patients with Coronavirus Disease 2019 Pneumonia in Wuhan, China," *JAMA Internal Medicine* 180, no. 7 (2020), doi.org/10.1001/jamainternmed.2020.0994; Chuan Qin et al., "Dysregulation of Immune Response in Patients with Coronavirus 2019 (Covid-19) in Wuhan, China," *Clinical Infectious Diseases* 71, no. 15 (2020), doi.org/10.1093/cid/ciaa248.

63. Pratik Sinha, Michael A. Matthay, and Carolyn S. Calfee, "Is a 'Cytokine Storm' Relevant to Covid-19?," *JAMA Internal Medicine* 180, no. 9 (2020), doi.org/10.1001/jamainternmed.2020.3313.

64. Lijuan Qian, Jie Yu, and Heshui Shi, "Severe Acute Respiratory Disease in a Huanan Seafood Market Worker: Images of an Early Casualty," *Radiology: Cardiothoracic Imaging* 2, no. 1 (2020), doi.org/10.1148/ryct.2020200033.

65. Xiao Wu et al., "Exposure to Air Pollution and COVID-19 Mortality in the United States," *Science Advances* 6, no. 45 (2020), doi.org/10.1126/sciadv.abd4049.

66. Kota Katanoda, "An Association Between Long-Term Exposure to Ambient Air Pollution and Mortality from Lung Cancer and Respiratory Diseases in Japan," *Journal of Epidemiology* 21, no. 2 (2011), doi.org/10.2188/jea.je20100098; Karen Clay, "Pollution, Infectious Disease, and Mortality: Evidence from the 1918 Spanish Influenza Pandemic," *Journal of Economic History* 78, no. 4 (2018), doi.org/10.1017/s002205071800058x.

67. Clay, "Pollution, Infectious Disease, and Mortality."

68. Y. Cui et al., "Air Pollution and Case Fatality of SARS in the People's Republic of China: An Ecologic Study," *Environmental Health* 2, no. 1 (2003), doi.org/10.1186/1476-069X-2-15.

69. Anamika Pandey et al., "Health and Economic Impact of Air Pollution in the States of India: The Global Burden of Disease Study 2019," *Lancet Planetary Health* 5, no. 1 (2021), doi.org/10.1016/s2542-5196(20)30298-9.

70. Neil Genzlinger, "Kious Kelly, 48," *The New York Times*, March 31, 2020, tinyurl.com/425crfcu.

71. Melinda Mitchell Jones, Kathleen M. Kearney, and Carrie Edwards, "Seeking PPE Protection: Is the Law on Your Side?," *Nursing Made Incredibly Easy* 18, no. 6 (2020), tinyurl.com/4clueoux.

72. Daniele Fattorini and Francesco Regoli, "Role of the Chronic Air Pollution Levels in the Covid-19 Outbreak Risk in Italy," *Environmental Pollution* 264 (2020), doi.org/10.1016/j.envpol.2020.114732.

73. Kaveri Gill, "The Informal Waste Sector: 'Surplus' Labour, Detritus, and the Right to the Post-Colonial City" in *Research Handbook on Law, Environment and the Global South* (Cheltenham, UK: Edward Elgar, 2019).

74. For an excellent analysis, see Kaveri Gill, *Of Poverty and Plastic: Scavenging and Scrap Trading Entrepreneurs in India's Urban Informal Economy* (New Delhi: Oxford University Press, 2010).

75. Praveen Chokhandre, Shrikant Singh, and Gyan Chandra Kashyap, "Prevalence, Predictors and Economic Burden of Morbidities Among Waste-Pickers of Mumbai, India: A Cross-Sectional Study," *Journal of Occupational Medicine and Toxicology* 12, no. 1 (2017), doi.org/10.1186/s12995-017-0176-3; Thayyil Jayakrishnan, Mathummal Jeeja, and Rao Bhaskar, "Occupational Health Problems of Municipal Solid Waste Management Workers in India," *International Journal of Environmental Health Engineering* 2, no. 1 (2013), doi.org/10.4103/2277-9183.122430.

76. Federico Demaria and Seth Schindler, "Contesting Urban Metabolism: Struggles over Waste-to-Energy in Delhi, India," *Antipode* 48, no. 2 (2016), doi.org/10.1111/anti.12191.

77. F. M. Walters, *The Principles of Health Control* (Lexington, KY: D.C. Heath & Company, 1920), 102.

78. Matthias Ochs et al., "The Number of Alveoli in the Human Lung," *American Journal of Respiratory and Critical Care Medicine* 169, no. 1 (2004), doi.org/10.1164/rccm.200308-1107OC.

79. Ibid.; Rebecca Dezube, "Overview of the Respiratory System," 2019, tinyurl.com/1v0nkkee.

80. C. C. Hsia, D. M. Hyde, and E. R. Weibel, "Lung Structure and the Intrinsic Challenges of Gas Exchange," *Comprehensive Physiology* 6, no. 2 (2016), doi.org/10.1002/cphy.c150028.

81. Dezube, "Overview of Respiratory System."

82. Lien Ai Pham-Huy, Hua He, and Chuong Pham-Huy, "Free Radicals, Antioxidants in Disease and Health," *International Journal of Biomedical Science* 4, no. 2 (2008), pubmed.ncbi.nlm.nih.gov/23675073.

83. N. Azad, Y. Rojanasakul, and V. Vallyathan, "Inflammation and Lung Cancer: Roles of Reactive Oxygen/Nitrogen Species," *Journal of Toxicology and Environmental Health Part B: Critical Reviews* 11, no. 1 (2008), doi.org/10.1080/10937400701436460.

84. I. Rahman and I. M. Adcock, "Oxidative Stress and Redox Regulation of Lung Inflammation in COPD," *European Respiratory Journal* 28 (2006), doi.org/10.1183/09031936.06.00053805.

85. Xing et al., "Impact of $PM_{2.5}$ on Human Respiratory System"; Azad, Rojanasakul, and Vallyathan, "Inflammation and Lung Cancer."

86. R. K. Wolff, "Effects of Airborne Pollutants on Mucociliary Clearance," *Environmental Health Perspectives* 66 (1986), doi.org/10.1289/ehp.8666223.

87. Yu Cao et al., "Environmental Pollutants Damage Airway Epithelial Cell Cilia: Implications for the Prevention of Obstructive Lung Diseases," *Thoracic Cancer* 11, no. 3 (2020), doi.org/10.1111/1759-7714.13323.

88. C. Arden Pope III et al., "Exposure to Fine Particulate Air Pollution Is Asso-

ciated with Endothelial Injury and Systemic Inflammation," *Circulation Research* 119, no. 11 (2016), doi.org/10.1161/CIRCRESAHA.116.309279.

89. B. A. Franklin, R. Brook, and C. Arden Pope III, "Air Pollution and Cardiovascular Disease," *Current Problems in Cardiology* 40, no. 5 (2015), doi.org/10.1016/j.cpcardiol.2015.01.003; Robert D. Brook et al., "Particulate Matter Air Pollution and Cardiovascular Disease," *Circulation* 121, no. 21 (2010), doi.org/10.1161/cir.0b013e3181dbece1; Stephen S. Lim et al., "A Comparative Risk Assessment of Burden of Disease and Injury Attributable to 67 Risk Factors and Risk Factor Clusters in 21 Regions, 1990–2010: A Systematic Analysis for the Global Burden of Disease Study 2010," *The Lancet* 380, no. 9859 (2012), doi.org/10.1016/s0140-6736(12)61766-8.

90. H. Qiu et al., "Long-Term Exposure to Fine Particulate Matter Air Pollution and Type 2 Diabetes Mellitus in Elderly: A Cohort Study in Hong Kong," *Environment International* 113 (2018), doi.org/10.1016/j.envint.2018.01.008.

91. John F. Pearson et al., "Association Between Fine Particulate Matter and Diabetes Prevalence in the U.S.," *Diabetes Care* 33, no. 10 (2010), doi.org/10.2337/dc10-0698.

92. Carol Potera, "Toxicity Beyond the Lung: Connecting PM2.5, Inflammation, and Diabetes," *Environmental Health Perspectives* 122, no. 1 (2014), doi.org/10.1289/ehp.122-a29.

93. L. Calderón-Garcidueñas et al., "Air Pollution and Brain Damage," *Toxicologic Pathology* 30, no. 3 (2002), doi.org/10.1080/01926230252929954.

94. Lilian Calderón-Garcidueñas et al., "Brain Inflammation and Alzheimer's-Like Pathology in Individuals Exposed to Severe Air Pollution," *Toxicologic Pathology* 32, no. 6 (2004), doi.org/10.1080/01926230490520232.

95. Ibid.

96. P. V. Moulton and W. Yang, "Air Pollution, Oxidative Stress, and Alzheimer's Disease," *Journal of Environmental Public Health* 2012 (2012), doi.org/10.1155/2012/472751.

97. Lilian Calderón-Garcidueñas et al., "Hallmarks of Alzheimer Disease Are Evolving Relentlessly in Metropolitan Mexico City Infants, Children and Young Adults. Apoe4 Carriers Have Higher Suicide Risk and Higher Odds of Reaching NFT Stage V at ≤ 40 Years of Age," *Environmental Research* 164 (2018), doi.org/10.1016/j.envres.2018.03.023.

98. Lilian Calderón-Garcidueñas et al., "Exposure to Severe Urban Air Pollution Influences Cognitive Outcomes, Brain Volume and Systemic Inflammation in Clinically Healthy Children," *Brain and Cognition* 77, no. 3 (2011), doi.org/10.1016/j.bandc.2011.09.006.

99. Michael Gilraine, "Air Filters, Pollution and Student Achievement," *EdWorkingPapers.com* (2020), www.edworkingpapers.com/ai20-188.

100. Heather E. Volk et al., "Traffic-Related Air Pollution, Particulate Matter, and Autism," *JAMA Psychiatry* 70, no. 1 (2013), doi.org/10.1001/jamapsychiatry.2013.266.

101. Barbara A. Maher et al., "Magnetite Pollution Nanoparticles in the Human Brain," *Proceedings of the National Academy of Sciences of the United States of America* 113, no. 39 (2016), doi.org/10.1073/pnas.1605941113.

102. Ibid.

103. L. A. Calderón-Garcidueñas et al. "Quadruple Abnormal Protein Aggregates in Brainstem Pathology and Exogenous Metal-Rich Magnetic Nanoparticles.

The Substantia Nigrae Is a Very Early Target in Young Urbanites and the Gastrointestinal Tract Likely a Key Brainstem Portal," *Environmental Research* (2020): 110139, doi.org/10.1016/j.envres.2020.110139; Scott Weichenthal et al. "Within-City Spatial Variations in Ambient Ultrafine Particle Concentrations and Incident Brain Tumors in Adults," *Epidemiology* 31, no. 2 (2020): 177–83, doi.org/10.1097/ede.0000000000001137.

104. Azad, Rojanasakul, and Vallyathan, "Inflammation and Lung Cancer."

105. Meng Wang et al., "Association Between Long-Term Exposure to Ambient Air Pollution and Change in Quantitatively Assessed Emphysema and Lung Function," *JAMA* 322, no. 6 (2019), doi.org/10.1001/jama.2019.10255.

106. Robert A. Rohde and Richard A. Muller, "Air Pollution in China: Mapping of Concentrations and Sources," *PLOS One* 10, no. 8 (2015), doi.org/10.1371/journal .pone.0135749; Richard A. Muller and Elizabeth A. Muller, "Air Pollution and Cigarette Equivalence," *Berkeley Earth*, December 17, 2015, berkeleyearth.org /air-pollution-and-cigarette-equivalence/.

107. Ahmad Rafay Alam, "The Lahore Smog Isn't Indian Farmers' Fault Alone. Pakistan Should Look Within," *The Print*, November 19, 2019, theprint.in /opinion/the-lahore-smog-isnt-indian-farmers-fault-alone-pakistan-should -look-within/323094/.

108. Vanessa Resende Nogueira Cruvinel et al., "Health Conditions and Occupational Risks in a Novel Group: Waste Pickers in the Largest Open Garbage Dump in Latin America," *BMC Public Health* 19, no. 1 (2019), doi.org/10.1186 /s12889-019-6879-x; Doyle Rice, "New Delhi's Toxic, Polluted Air Chokes City's 20 Million People, and the Haze Can Be Seen from Space," *USA Today*, November 5, 2019, tinyurl.com/1wdhpku1. If you want to know how bad you have it where you live, there's an app to translate your city's particulate matter readings into cigarettes, called "Sh**t! I Smoke," at shootismoke.app.

109. Sunil K. Chhabra et al., "Ambient Air Pollution and Chronic Respiratory Morbidity in Delhi," *Archives of Environmental Health* 56, no. 1 (2001), doi.org/10 .1080/00039890109604055.

110. Francesco Forastiere et al., "Socioeconomic Status, Particulate Air Pollution, and Daily Mortality: Differential Exposure or Differential Susceptibility," *American Journal of Industrial Medicine* 50, no. 3 (2007), doi.org/10.1002/ajim .20368; Isabelle Romieu et al., "Multicity Study of Air Pollution and Mortality in Latin America (the Escala Study)," *Research Report | (Health Effects Institute)*, no. 171 (2012), pubmed.ncbi.nlm.nih.gov/23311234; Sabit Cakmak et al., "The Modifying Effect of Socioeconomic Status on the Relationship Between Traffic, Air Pollution and Respiratory Health in Elementary Schoolchildren," *Journal of Environmental Management* 177 (2016), doi.org/10.1016/j .jenvman.2016.03.051.

111. Anjum Hajat, Charlene Hsia, and Marie S. O'Neill, "Socioeconomic Disparities and Air Pollution Exposure: A Global Review," *Current Environmental Health Reports* 2, no. 4 (2015), doi.org/10.1007/s40572-015-0069-5.

112. Philip J. Landrigan et al., "The *Lancet* Commission on Pollution and Health," *The Lancet* 391, no. 10119 (2018): 13, doi.org/10.1016/s0140-6736(17)32345-0.

113. Stephen Graham, "Life Support: The Political Ecology of Urban Air," *City* 19, no. 2–3 (2015), doi.org/10.1080/13604813.2015.1014710; Alana Hansen et al., "Residential Air-Conditioning and Climate Change: Voices of the Vulnerable," *Health Promotion Journal of Australia* 22, no. 4 (2011), doi.org/10.1071/he11413.

114. Sunil Kumar, Sanjeev Kumar Gupta, and Manish Rawat, "Resources and Utilization of Geothermal Energy in India: An Eco-Friendly Approach Towards Sustainability," *Materials Today: Proceedings* 26 (2020), doi.org/10.1016/j.matpr.2020.02.347.

115. Jitendra Pandey et al., "Environmental and Socio-Economic Impacts of Fire in Jharia Coalfield, Jharkhand, India: An Appraisal," *Current Science* 110, no. 9 (2016), doi.org/10.18520/cs/v110/i9/1639-1650.

116. Smita Gupta, "Jharia's Century-Old Fire Kept Ablaze by Crime and Politics," in *The Wild East: Criminal Political Economies in South Asia*, ed. Barbara Harriss-White and Lucia Michelutti (London: UCL Press, 2019).

117. Research Collective, *Coallateral: A Report of the Independent People's Tribunal on the MoU Signed Between Rajmahal Pahad Bachao Andolan and PANEM Coal Mines* (New Delhi: Programme for Social Action, 2015), static1.squarespace.com/static/559b6c31e4b02802c8b26ce9/t/55bc97dde4b0c4bdc34f9ae2/1438671153846/Coallateral+-+English.pdf.

118. Nandini Sundar, *The Burning Forest: India's War Against the Maoists* (London: Verso, 2019).

119. Sanjay G. Reddy, "All That Is Wrong with Modi Govt's Obsession with Ease of Doing Business Rankings," *ThePrint*, November 27, 2018, theprint.in/opinion/all-that-is-wrong-with-modi-govts-obsession-with-ease-of-doing-business-rankings/155160; Sangheon Lee, Deirdre McCann, and Nina Torm, "The World Bank's 'Employing Workers' Index: Findings and Critiques—A Review of Recent Evidence," *International Labour Review* 147, no. 4 (2008), doi.org/10.1111/j.1564-913X.2008.00043.x; Rush Doshi, Judith G. Kelley, and Beth A. Simmons, "The Power of Ranking: The Ease of Doing Business Indicator and Global Regulatory Behavior," *International Organization* 73, no. 3 (2019), doi.org/10.1017/s0020818319000158.

120. To understand how structural violence kills 2 million people a year in India through malnutrition and morbidity alone, see Akhil Gupta, *Red Tape: Bureaucracy, Structural Violence, and Poverty in India* (Durham, NC: Duke University Press, 2012).

121. Alpa Shah, *Nightmarch: Among India's Revolutionary Guerrillas* (Chicago: University of Chicago Press, 2019), 38; Jason Miklian, "The Purification Hunt: The Salwa Judum Counterinsurgency in Chhattisgarh, India," *Dialectical Anthropology* 33, no. 3 (2009), doi.org/10.1007/s10624-009-9138-1.

122. Sanjay Nigam, "Disciplining and Policing the 'Criminals by Birth,' Part 1: The Making of a Colonial Stereotype—The Criminal Tribes and Castes of North India," *Indian Economic and Social History Review* 27, no. 2 (1990), doi.org/10.1177/001946469002700201. This is not to argue that India was some undifferentiated paradise before the British arrived. The kinds of social contempt reserved for those groups who, for instance, dispose of the dead weren't manufactured by the British. Arnold describes, for instance, how one criminal tribe—Doms—became a fixture of dissecting rooms, precisely because of their association with tending to corpses. See David Arnold, *Colonizing the Body: State Medicine and Epidemic Disease in Nineteenth-Century India* (Berkeley: University of California Press, 1993), 5. But in creating the administrative categories through which precolonial social divisions might be managed, the bureaucracy of the post-Independence Indian state created new kinds of power to discriminate. The death toll of British divide-and-rule policies, from the Middle East to East

Africa to South Asia, is in the millions. A. J. Christopher, "'Divide and Rule': The Impress of British Separation Policies," *Area* 20, no. 3 (1988), www.jstor .org/stable/20002624.

123. Rahi Gaikwad, "Manmohan: Naxalism the Greatest Internal Threat," *Hindu*, October 11, 2009, tinyurl.com/gwo31086.

124. "Singh Sees 'Vital Interest' in Peace with Pakistan," *Dawn*, June 10, 2009, tinyurl.com/1slsmt8l.

125. Sandeep Bamzai, "Chidambaram's 2007 Flip-Flop Let Anil Agarwal's Vedanta Take over Sesa Goa," *India Today*, January 23, 2012, tinyurl.com/1kawt0q9.

126. Praful Bidwai, "War on Maoists," *Frontline*, March 26, 2010, tinyurl.com /4v9guuj3.

127. Ramachandra Guha, *The Unquiet Woods: Ecological Change and Peasant Resistance in the Himalaya* (Berkeley: University of California Press, 1990).

128. S. K. Sahu, T. Ohara, and G. Beig, "The Role of Coal Technology in Redefining India's Climate Change Agents and Other Pollutants," *Environmental Research Letters* 12, no. 10 (2017), doi.org/10.1088/1748-9326/aa814a.

129. Kuntala Lahiri-Dutt, *The Coal Nation: Histories, Ecologies and Politics of Coal in India* (Surrey, UK: Ashgate, 2014).

130. Rikard Warlenius, "Decolonizing the Atmosphere: The Climate Justice Movement on Climate Debt," *Journal of Environment and Development* 27, no. 2 (2018), doi.org/10.1177/1070496517744593.

131. Suzanne M. Simkovich et al., "The Health and Social Implications of Household Air Pollution and Respiratory Diseases," *NPJ Primary Care Respiratory Medicine* 29, no. 1 (2019), doi.org/10.1038/s41533-019-0126-x.

132. Sumeet Saksena, Raj Kumar Prasad, and V. Ravi Shankar, "Daily Exposure to Air Pollutants in Indoor, Outdoor and In-Vehicle Micro-Environments: A Pilot Study in Delhi," *Indoor and Built Environment* 16, no. 1 (2007), doi.org/10 .1177/1420326X06074715.

133. Jyoti Parikh, Kirk Smith, and Laxmi Vijay, "Indoor Air Pollution: A Reflection on Gender Bias," *Economic and Political Weekly* 34, no. 9 (1999), www.jstor .org/stable/4407707.

134. Sarah Bradshaw and Maureen Fordham, "Double Disaster: Disaster Through a Gender Lens," in *Hazards, Risks and Disasters in Society*, ed. Andrew E. Collins et al. (Amsterdam: Elsevier, 2015).

135. Cecilia Sorensen et al., "Climate Change and Women's Health: Impacts and Opportunities in India," *GeoHealth* 2, no. 10 (2018), doi.org/10.1029/2018GH000163.

136. Max Ajl, "Eco-Fascisms and Eco-Socialisms," *Verso Blog*, August 12, 2019, www.versobooks.com/blogs/4404-eco-fascisms-and-eco-socialisms; Bernhard Forchtner, "Climate Change and the Far Right," *WIREs Climate Change* 10, no. 5 (2019), doi.org/10.1002/wcc.604.

137. Graham Lawton, "The Rise of Real Eco-Fascism," *New Scientist* 243, no. 3243 (2019), doi.org/10.1016/S0262-4079(19)31529-5.

138. Jordan Dyett and Cassidy Thomas, "Overpopulation Discourse: Patriarchy, Racism, and the Specter of Ecofascism," *Perspectives on Global Development and Technology* 18, no. 1–2 (2019), doi.org/10.1163/15691497 -12341514.

139. Bailey Richards, Krishna Rao, and David Bishai, *Disparities in Child Mortality Among Religious Minorities in the Districts of India* (Washington, DC: World Bank, 2016), tinyurl.com/543x5kcv; Sana Contractor and Tejal Barai-Jaitly,

"Social Exclusion and Health of Muslim Communities in Maharashtra," *eSocialSciences and Humanities* 1, no. 2 (2018), tinyurl.com/x13k6mvs.

140. Contractor and Barai-Jaitly, "Social Exclusion and Health."

141. Jason Cons, *Sensitive Space: Fragmented Territory at the India-Bangladesh Border* (Seattle: University of Washington Press, 2016).

142. Mirel Zaman, "The Surprising Ways Climate Change Is Already Affecting Our Health," *Refinery29*, September 25, 2020, tinyurl.com/15v4sz6g.

143. Ye-Seul Lee et al., "Understanding Mind-Body Interaction from the Perspective of East Asian Medicine," *Evidence-Based Complementary and Alternative Medicine* no. 1 (2017), doi.org/10.1155/2017/7618419.

144. Carina J. Gronlund et al., "Vulnerability to Renal, Heat and Respiratory Hospitalizations During Extreme Heat Among U.S. Elderly," *Climatic Change* 136, no. 3–4 (2016), doi.org/10.1007/s10584-016-1638-9; Manish Pareek et al., "Ethnicity and Covid-19: An Urgent Public Health Research Priority," *The Lancet* 395, no. 10234 (2020), doi.org/10.1016/s0140-6736(20)30922-3.

145. Stephane Hallegatte and Julie Rozenberg, "Climate Change Through a Poverty Lens," *Nature Climate Change* 7, no. 4 (2017), doi.org/10.1038/nclimate3253; F. Canouï-Poitrine et al., "Excess Deaths During the August 2003 Heat Wave in Paris, France," *Revue d'épidémiologie et de santé publique* 54, no. 2 (2006), doi.org/10.1016/s0398-7620(06)76706-2; Jan C. Semenza et al., "Heat-Related Deaths During the July 1995 Heat Wave in Chicago," *New England Journal of Medicine* 335, no. 2 (1996), doi.org/10.1056/nejm199607113350203.

146. International Panel on Climate Change, *Climate Change 2007—Impacts, Adaptation and Vulnerability: Contribution of Working Group II to the Fourth Assessment Report of the IPCC* (Cambridge: Cambridge University Press, 2007), tinyurl.com/1glpms58; Steven W. Running, "The 5 Stages of Climate Grief," *Numerical Terradynamic Simulation Group Publications* 173 (2007), scholarworks.umt.edu/ntsg_pubs/173.

147. Elisabeth Kübler-Ross, *On Grief and Grieving: Finding the Meaning of Grief Through the Five Stages of Loss*, ed. David Kessler (New York: Simon & Schuster, 2005).

148. Parita Mukta, "The 'Civilizing Mission': The Regulation and Control of Mourning in Colonial India," *Feminist Review* 63, no. 1 (1999): 37, doi.org/10.1080/014177899339045.

149. Shah, *Nightmarch*, 33–34.

150. Shiri Pasternak and Dayna Nadine Scott, "Introduction: Getting Back the Land," *South Atlantic Quarterly* 119, no. 2 (2020), doi.org/10.1215/00382876-8177723.

151. Paul Trawick, "Against the Privatization of Water: An Indigenous Model for Improving Existing Laws and Successfully Governing the Commons," *World Development* 31, no. 6 (2003), doi.org/10.1016/s0305-750x(03)00049-4; Ashwini Chhatre and Arun Agrawal, "Forest Commons and Local Enforcement," *Proceedings of the National Academy of Sciences of the United States of America* 105, no. 36 (2008), doi.org/10.1073/pnas.0803399105; Arun Agrawal, Ashwini Chhatre, and Rebecca Hardin, "Changing Governance of the World's Forests," *Science* 320, no. 5882 (2008), doi.org/10.1126/science.1155369; Sergio Villamayor-Tomas and Gustavo García-López, "Social Movements as Key Actors in *Governing the Commons*: Evidence from Community-Based Resource Management Cases across the World," *Global Environmental Change* 53 (2018), doi.org/doi.org/10.1016/j.gloenvcha.2018.09.005.

152. Elizabeth Rata, "Encircling the Commons: Neotribal Capitalism in New Zealand Since 2000," *Anthropological Theory* 11, no. 3 (2011), doi.org/10.1177/1463499611416724.

153. Anirban Akhand et al., "High Cadmium Contamination at the Gateway to Sundarban Ecosystem Driven by Kolkata Metropolitan Sewage in India," *Current Science* 110, no. 3 (2016), www.jstor.org/stable/24906783.

154. Amitav Ghosh, *The Great Derangement: Climate Change and the Unthinkable* (Chicago: University of Chicago Press, 2016), 172.

155. Kate C. McLean et al., "The Empirical Structure of Narrative Identity: The Initial Big Three," *Journal of Personality and Social Psychology* 119, no. 4 (2020), doi.org/10.1037/pspp0000247.

156. Jo-Ann Archibald, *Indigenous Storywork: Educating the Heart, Mind, Body and Spirit* (Vancouver: University of British Columbia Press, 2008); Jonathan A. Draper, *Orality, Literacy, and Colonialism in Antiquity* (Atlanta, GA: Society of Biblical Literature, 2004); Asoka Kumar Sen, *Indigeneity, Landscape and History: Adivasi Self-Fashioning in India* (London: Routledge, 2018).

157. Archibald, *Indigenous Storywork*.

158. LeAnne Howe, "Tribalography: The Power of Native Stories," *Journal of Dramatic Theory and Criticism* 14, no. 1 (1999), journals.ku.edu/jdtc/article/view/3325/3254.

159. Robin Wall Kimmerer, *Braiding Sweetgrass* (Minneapolis: Milkweed, 2013).

160. Louise Fowler-Smith, "Adorning and Adoring: The Sacred Trees of India," *Journal for the Study of Religion, Nature and Culture* 12, no. 3 (2018), doi.org/10.1558/jsrnc.33347; K. S. Singh, "The Munda Epic: An Interpretation," *India International Centre Quarterly* 19, no. 1–2 (1992), www.jstor.org/stable/23002221; Vivian M. Jiménez Estrada, "The Tree of Life as a Research Methodology," *Australian Journal of Indigenous Education* 34 (2005), doi.org/10.1017/S1326011100003951; Renee M. Borges, "The Sacred in Forests, Trees, and Seeds: Boon or Bane of Ecosystem Services?," in *Anthropology, Nutrition and Wildlife Conservation*, ed. Edmond Dounias, Igor de Garine, and Valérie de Garine (Guadalajara: University of Guadalajara, forthcoming); George Lechler, "The Tree of Life in Indo-European and Islamic Cultures," *Ars Islamica* 4 (1937), www.jstor.org/stable/25167048; Padmaja Sen, "The Culture of Present: An Understanding of the Adivasi Aesthetics," *Journal of Adivasi and Indigenous Studies* 1, no. 1 (2014).

161. S. B. Chandrasekar et al., "Phytopharmacology of *Ficus religiosa*," *Pharmacognosy Reviews* 4, no. 8 (2010), doi.org/10.4103/0973-7847.70918.

162. H. W. Jung et al., "Methanol Extract of Ficus Leaf Inhibits the Production of Nitric Oxide and Proinflammatory Cytokines in LPS-Stimulated Microglia via the MAPK Pathway," *Phytotherapy Research* 22, no. 8 (2008), doi.org/10.1002/ptr.2442.

163. Hugo Asselin, "Indigenous Forest Knowledge," in *Routledge Handbook of Forest Ecology*, ed. Kelvin S. H. Peh (London: Routledge, 2015).

164. Claudia Sobrevila, *The Role of Indigenous Peoples in Biodiversity Conservation* (Washington, DC: World Bank, 2008); S. T. Garnett, "A Spatial Overview of the Global Importance of Indigenous Lands for Conservation," *Nature Sustainability* 1, no. 7 (2018), doi:10.1038/s41893-018-0100-6.

165. Mark Spence, *Dispossessing the Wilderness: Indian Removal and the Making of the National Parks* (Oxford: Oxford University Press, 1999), 4.

166. Eric Michael Johnson, "How John Muir's Brand of Conservation Led to the Decline of Yosemite," *Scientific American*, August 13, 2014, blogs.scientificamerican .com/primate-diaries/how-john-muir-s-brand-of-conservation-led-to-the -decline-of-yosemite/.

167. John Muir, *The Mountains of California* (New York: Century, 1894), chap. 5.

168. William D. Nikolakis and Emma Roberts, "Indigenous Fire Management: A Conceptual Model from Literature," *Ecology and Society* 25, no. 4 (2020): 11, doi.org/10.5751/ES-11945-250411.

169. Andrew E. Scholl and Alan H. Taylor, "Fire Regimes, Forest Change, and Self-Organization in an Old-Growth Mixed-Conifer Forest, Yosemite National Park, USA," *Ecological Applications* 20, no. 2 (2010), doi.org/10.1890/08-2324.1.

170. Ibid.

171. Archibald, *Indigenous Storywork*.

172. Naykky Singh Ospina et al., "Eliciting the Patient's Agenda—Secondary Analysis of Recorded Clinical Encounters," *Journal of General Internal Medicine* 34, no. 1 (2019), doi.org/10.1007/s11606-018-4540-5.

173. Archibald, *Indigenous Storywork*.

5. REPRODUCTIVE SYSTEM

1. Alameda County Public Health Department, "Healthy Alameda County: Life Expectancy Tables" (Oakland, CA, 2021), tinyurl.com/1bnfd2es.

2. Malcolm Margolin, *The Ohlone Way* (Berkeley, CA: Heyday Books, 1978).

3. Nels Christina Nelson, *Shellmounds of the San Francisco Bay Region* (Berkeley: University of California Press, 1909).

4. Alison Griner, "'On My Ancestors' Remains': The Fight for Sacred Lands," *Al Jazeera*, December 16, 2019, tinyurl.com/1h71k8sq.

5. K. E. French and W. R. Stanley,. "A Game of European Colonization in Africa," *Journal of Geography* 73, no. 7 (1974): 44–48.

6. Silvia Federici, *Caliban and the Witch* (New York: Autonomedia, 2004).

7. Lauren Cross, Lauren Seitz, and Shannon Walter, "The First of Its Kind," *Digital Literature Review* 3 (2016); Catherine Hodeir, ed., *Decentering the Gaze at French Colonial Exhibitions* (Berkeley: University of California Press, 2002); Karen Sotiropoulos, "'Town of God': Ota Benga, the Batetela Boys, and the Promise of Black America," *Journal of World History* 26, no. 1 (2016), doi .org/10.1353/jwh.2016.0002; Pamela Newkirk, "Ota Benga in the Archives: Unmaking Myths, Mapping Resistance in the Margins of History," *Journal of Contemporary African Art* 2016, no. 38–39 (2016): 172.

8. Federici, *Caliban and the Witch*.

9. Wallace Notestein, *A History of Witchcraft in England from 1558 to 1718* (Washington, DC: American Historical Association, 1911), 49.

10. Erika Gasser, "Witchcraft, Possession, and the Unmaking of Women and Men: A Late-Sixteenth-Century English Case Study," *Magic, Ritual, and Witchcraft* 11, no. 2 (2016): 156, doi.org/10.1353/mrw.2016.0013. Historians have wondered what the girl had read in order for her to convincingly perform demonic possession. Frantz Fanon's doctoral work suggests that it's possible for there to have been an underlying neurological condition, and for its manifestation to be culturally tuned. Frantz Fanon and Asselah Slimane, "The Phenomenon of Agitation in the Psychiatric Milieu: General Considerations, Psychopathological Meaning," in *Alienation and Freedom*, ed. Jean

Khalfa and Robert J. C. Young, trans. Steven Corcoran (London: Bloomsbury, 2018).

11. Gasser, "Witchcraft, Possession."
12. Barbara Rosen, ed., *Witchcraft in England, 1558–1618* (Amherst: University of Massachusetts Press, 1991), 241.
13. Lady Cromwell was the second wife of Sir Henry Cromwell, Oliver Cromwell's grandfather, and a friend of the girls' father, Robert Throckmorton. Orna Alyagon Darr, "Experiments in the Courtroom: Social Dynamics and Spectacles of Proof in Early Modern English Witch Trials," *Law and Social Inquiry* 39, no. 1 (2014): 157, doi.org/10.1111/lsi.12054.
14. Gasser, "Witchcraft, Possession," 155.
15. Ibid., 163.
16. Anne Reiber DeWindt, "Witchcraft and Conflicting Visions of the Ideal Village Community," *Journal of British Studies* 34, no. 4 (1995), www.jstor.org/stable/175779.
17. Rosen, *Witchcraft in England,* 296–97.
18. J. A. Dossett, "The Nature of Breast Secretion in Infancy," *Journal of Pathology and Bacteriology* 80, no. 1 (1960); T. R. Forbes, "Witch's Milk and Witches' Marks," *Yale Journal of Biology and Medicine* 22, no. 3 (1950), pubmed.ncbi.nlm.nih.gov/15399986.
19. Keith Thomas, "The Relevance of Social Anthropology to the Historical Study of English Witchcraft," in *Witchcraft Confessions and Accusations*, ed. Mary Douglas (London: Tavistock, 1970).
20. Carolyn Merchant, "The Scientific Revolution and *The Death of Nature*," *Isis* 97, no. 3 (2006), doi.org/doi:10.1086/508090.
21. Darr, "Experiments in the Courtroom."
22. Silvia Federici, *Re-Enchanting the World: Feminism and the Politics of the Commons* (Oakland: PM Press, 2018).
23. American Physical Society, "August 1620: Kepler's Mother Imprisoned for Witchcraft," *APS News* 24, no. 8 (2015), www.aps.org/publications/apsnews/201508/physicshistory.cfm; Jeremy Bernstein, "Heaven's Net: The Meeting of John Donne and Johannes Kepler," *American Scholar* 66, no. 2 (1997), www.jstor.org/stable/41212614; James A. Connor, *Kepler's Witch: An Astronomer's Discovery of Cosmic Order amid Religious War, Political Intrigue, and the Heresy Trial of His Mother* (San Francisco: HarperSanFrancisco, 2004).
24. Bernstein, "Heaven's Net," 180.
25. Silvia Federici, *Witches, Witch-Hunting, and Women* (Oakland: PM Press, 2018), 35.
26. Fred Charles Moten, *The Poetics of the Undercommons* (New York: Sputnik & Fizzle, 2016).
27. Miranda Fricker, *Epistemic Injustice: Power and the Ethics of Knowing* (Oxford: Oxford University Press, 2007), 7.
28. Susan Brownmiller, *In Our Time: Memoir of a Revolution* (New York: Dial Press, 1999), cited in Miranda Fricker, *Epistemic Injustice: Power and the Ethics of Knowing* (New York: Oxford University Press, 2009), 148–49.
29. Jeff Wicks, "Helena, the Desolate Exile, Has Become Known as the 'Place of Witches,'" *Sunday Times*, April 14, 2019, tinyurl.com/3c9l9l2u; Lucia Newman, "Brazilian Social Group Alleges Witch-Hunt Since Bolsonaro's Win," *Aljazeera*, December 30, 2018, tinyurl.com/3mfxgkqp; Andrea Martinelli, "Witch Hunts

Are Back—And This Time They're Targeting Female Activists," *HuffPost Brazil*, October 1, 2019, tinyurl.com/eu6yk403.

30. Samar Bosu Mullick, "Gender Relations and Witches Among the Indigenous Communities of Jharkhand, India," *Gender, Technology and Development* 4, no. 3 (2000), doi.org/10.1080/09718524.2000.11909975.

31. Tanvi Yadav, "Witch Hunting: A Form of Violence Against Dalit Women in India," *CASTE/A Global Journal on Social Exclusion* 1, no. 2 (2020); Silvia Federici, "Women, Witch-Hunting and Enclosures in Africa Today," *Sozial .Geschichte Online* 3 (2010); Friday A. Eboiyehi, "Convicted Without Evidence: Elderly Women and Witchcraft Accusations in Contemporary Nigeria," *Journal of International Women's Studies* 18, no. 4 (2017), vc.bridgew.edu/jiws/vol18/iss4/18; Sharit K. Bhowmik, "Review: Adivasi Women Workers in Tea Plantations," *Economic and Political Weekly* 49, no. 49 (2014), www.jstor.org/stable/24481050.

32. Federici, *Witches, Witch-Hunting, and Women*, 42.

33. "The Bull *Romanus Pontifex*, January 8, 1455," in *European Treaties Bearing on the History of the United States and Its Dependencies to 1648*, ed. Frances Gardiner Davenport (Washington, DC: Carnegie Institution, 1917), 23.

34. Special Rapporteur, *Preliminary Study of the Impact on Indigenous Peoples of the International Legal Construct Known as the Doctrine of Discovery*, E/C.19/2010/13 (New York: UN General Assembly, 2010).

35. Tonya Gonnella Frichner, "The Preliminary Study on the Doctrine of Discovery Symposium on the Prospects for the United Nations Declaration on the Rights of Indigenous Peoples," *Pace Environmental Law Review* 28, no. 1 (2010): 345, heinonline.org/HOL/P?h = hein.journals/penv28&i = 341.

36. Blake A. Watson, "The Impact of the American Doctrine of Discovery on Native Land Rights in Australia, Canada, and New Zealand," *Seattle University Law Review* 34, no. 2 (2010): 552.

37. Robert J. Miller et al., *Discovering Indigenous Lands: The Doctrine of Discovery in the English Colonies* (Oxford: Oxford University Press, 2010); Jacinta Ruru, "Lenses of Comparison Across Continents: Understanding Modern Aboriginal Title in Tsilhqot'in Nation and Ngati Apa," *UBC Law Review* 48, no. 3 (2015): 942.

38. United Nations, *Preliminary Study Shows "Doctrine of Discovery" Legal Construct Historical Root for Ongoing Violations of Indigenous Peoples' Rights, Permanent Forum Told* (New York: United Nations, 2010).

39. Susan M. Hill, *The Clay We Are Made Of: Haudenosaunee Land Tenure on the Grand River* (Winnipeg: University of Manitoba Press, 2017), 11.

40. Barbara A. Mann and Jerry L. Fields, "A Sign in the Sky: Dating the League of the Haudenosaunee," *American Indian Culture and Research Journal* 21, no. 2 (1997), doi.org/10.17953/aicr.21.2.k36m1485r3062510.

41. Robin Wall Kimmerer, *Braiding Sweetgrass* (Minneapolis: Milkweed, 2013), chap. 1.

42. Barbara A. Mann, "The Lynx in Time: Haudenosaunee Women's Traditions and History," *American Indian Quarterly* 21, no. 3 (1997), doi.org/10.2307/1185516.

43. Laiwan, "Return to the Water: First Nations Relations with Salmon," Hydrologic blog, January 29, 2021, www2.laiwanette.net/fountain/return-to-the-water-first-nations-relations-with-salmon/.

44. Irene Silverblatt, *Moon, Sun, and Witches: Gender Ideologies and Class in Inca and Colonial Peru* (Princeton, N.J.: Princeton University Press, 1987), 172–73.

45. Brian Levack, *The Witch-Hunt in Early Modern Europe* (London: Pearson Education, 2006).

46. Heidi I. Hartmann, "The Family as the Locus of Gender, Class, and Political Struggle: The Example of Housework," *Signs* 6, no. 3 (1981), doi.org/10.1086/493813.

47. Daniel Scott Smith, "The Curious History of Theorizing About the History of the Western Nuclear Family," *Social Science History* 17, no. 3 (1993), doi.org/10.1017/S0145553200018629.

48. Richard Phillips, "Settler Colonialism and the Nuclear Family," *Canadian Geographer* 53, no. 2 (2009), doi.org/10.1111/j.1541-0064.2009.00256.x.

49. Richard Allen Chapman, *"Leviathan* Writ Small: Thomas Hobbes on the Family," *American Political Science Review* 69, no. 1 (1975), doi.org/10.2307/1957886.

50. bell hooks and Tanya McKinnon, "Sisterhood: Beyond Public and Private," *Signs* 21, no. 4 (1996), www.jstor.org/stable/3175025; Stephanie Coontz, *The Social Origins of Private Life: A History of American Families, 1600–1900* (London: Verso, 1988). On the "Great Domestication," see C. A. Bayly, *The Birth of the Modern World, 1780–1914: Global Connections and Comparisons* (Malden, MA: Blackwell, 2004); and Raj Patel and Jason W. Moore, *A History of the World in Seven Cheap Things: A Guide to Capitalism, Nature, and the Future of the Planet* (Berkeley: University of California Press, 2017), chap. 4.

51. Friederike Habermann, "Hegemonie, Identität und der *homo oeconomicus* Oder: Warum feministische Ökonomie nicht ausreicht," in *Gender and Economics*, ed. Christine Bauhardt and Gülay Çaglar (Berlin: Springer, 2010), doi.org/10.1007/978-3-531-92347-5; Maria Mies, *Patriarchy and Accumulation on a World Scale: Women in the International Division of Labour* (London: Zed, 1986).

52. Oyèrónké Oyěwùmí, *The Invention of Women: Making an African Sense of Western Gender Discourses* (Minneapolis: University of Minnesota Press, 1997).

53. Sue-Ellen Jacobs and Jason Cromwell, "Visions and Revisions of Reality: Reflections on Sex, Sexuality, Gender, and Gender Variance," *Journal of Homosexuality* 23, no. 4 (1992), doi.org/10.1300/J082v23n04_03.

54. Sandra E. Hollimon, "The Third Gender in Native California: Two-Spirit Undertakers Among the Chumash and Their Neighbors," in *Women in Prehistory: North America and Mesoamerica*, ed. Cheryl Claassen and Rosemary A. Joyce (Philadelphia: University of Pennsylvania Press, 1994); Scott Lauria Morgensen, *Spaces Between Us: Queer Settler Colonialism and Indigenous Decolonization* (Minneapolis: University of Minnesota Press, 2011).

55. Anne Fausto-Sterling, *Sexing the Body: Gender Politics and the Construction of Sexuality*, 2nd ed. (New York: Basic Books, 2020). Those same tools today are being used to liberate some people in gender quandaries, showing how it is not the tools themselves that are problematic, but the mindset behind their application.

56. Gervase Markham and Michael R. Best, *The English Housewife* (Kingston: McGill-Queen's University Press, 1986); Kristin A. Collins, "Federalism's Fallacy: The Early Tradition of Federal Family Law and the Invention of States' Rights," *Cardozo Law Review* 26, no. 5 (2005): 1866.

57. UN Office on Drugs and Crime, *Global Study on Homicide: Gender-Related Killing of Women and Girls* (UN Office on Drugs and Crime, 2019).

58. Claudia Garcia-Moreno et al., "Prevalence of Intimate Partner Violence: Findings from the WHO Multi-Country Study on Women's Health and Domestic Violence," *The Lancet* 368, no. 9543 (2006): 1264, doi.org/10.1016/S0140-6736(06)69523-8.

59. Shannon Speed, "States of Violence: Indigenous Women Migrants in the Era of Neoliberal Multicriminalism," *Critique of Anthropology* 36, no. 3 (2016), doi.org/10.1177/0308275x16646834.

60. George P. Chrousos, "Stress, Chronic Inflammation, and Emotional and Physical Well-Being: Concurrent Effects and Chronic Sequelae," *Journal of Allergy and Clinical Immunology* 106, no. 5 (2000), doi.org/10.1067/mai.2000.110163.

61. Evan Stark, Anne Flitcraft, and William Frazier, "Medicine and Patriarchal Violence: The Social Construction of a 'Private' Event," *International Journal of Health Services* 9, no. 3 (1979): 484, doi.org/10.2190/KTLU-CCU7-BMNQ-V2KY.

62. Debra Houry et al., "Violence-Inflicted Injuries: Reporting Laws in the Fifty States," *Annals of Emergency Medicine* 39, no. 1 (2002), doi.org/10.1067/mem.2002.117759; Eileen F. Baker et al., "Law Enforcement and Emergency Medicine: An Ethical Analysis," *Annals of Emergency Medicine* 68, no. 5 (2016), doi.org/10.1016/j.annemergmed.2016.02.013; Henriette Roscam Abbing, "Medical Confidentiality and Patient Safety: Reporting Procedures," *European Journal of Health Law* 21, no. 3 (2014), doi.org/10.1163/15718093-12341319.

63. Vivian Ho, "SF Man Found Guilty of Killing Girlfriend, Throwing Body in Bay," *SFGate*, June 15, 2017, tinyurl.com/t3c9h289.

64. San Francisco Police Department, *Officer Involved Shootings Historical Data*, 2020, tinyurl.com/1398yjw4.

65. See, e.g., A. Negro, "Christian Missions in West Africa," *Fraser's Magazine* 14, no. 82 (1876).

66. "'Brasil é uma virgem que todo tarado de fora quer,' diz Bolsonaro ao falar sobre Amazônia," *Globo.com*, July 6, 2019, g1.globo.com/politica/noticia/2019/07/06/brasil-e-uma-virgem-que-todo-tarado-de-fora-quer-diz-bolsonaro-ao-falar-sobre-amazonia.ghtml.

67. Rick Ruddell et al., "Drilling Down: An Examination of the Boom-Crime Relationship in Resource-Based Boom Counties," *Western Criminology Review* 15 (2014), www.westerncriminology.org/documents/WCR/v15n1/Ruddell.pdf.

68. R. Bachman, *Violence Against American Indian and Alaska Native Women and the Criminal Justice Response: What Is Known* (Washington, DC: US Department of Justice, 2008), www.ncjrs.gov/pdffiles1/nij/grants/223691.pdf.

69. Sarah Bradshaw, Brian Linneker, and Lisa Overton, "Extractive Industries as Sites of Supernormal Profits and Supernormal Patriarchy?," *Gender and Development* 25, no. 3 (2017), doi.org/10.1080/13552074.2017.1379780; Itzá Castañeda Camey et al., *Gender-Based Violence and Environment Linkages: The Violence of Inequality* (Gland, Switzerland: International Union for the Conservation of Nature, 2020); Adriana Eftimie, Katherine Heller, and John Strongman, *Gender Dimensions of the Extractive Industries: Mining for Equity* (Washington, DC: World Bank, 2009).

70. André Rosay, "Violence Against American Indian and Alaska Native Women and Men," *National Institute of Justice Journal* (2016), tinyurl.com/zjmkhwzm.

71. Ibid.; Bachman, *Violence Against American Indian*.

72. Danielle L. McGuire, "'It Was Like All of Us Had Been Raped': Sexual

Violence, Community Mobilization, and the African American Freedom Struggle," *Journal of American History* 91, no. 3 (2004), doi.org/10.2307 /3662860.

73. Mies, *Patriarchy and Accumulation*; Carolyn Merchant, *The Death of Nature: Women, Ecology, and the Scientific Revolution* (San Francisco: Harper & Row, 1980).

74. Haywood L. Brown et al., "Black Women Health Inequity: The Origin of Perinatal Health Disparity," *Journal of the National Medical Association* (forthcoming), doi.org/10.1016/j.jnma.2020.11.008.

75. P. Dasgupta et al., "Variations in Outcomes for Indigenous Women with Breast Cancer in Australia: A Systematic Review," *European Journal of Cancer Care* 26, no. 6 (2017), doi.org/10.1111/ecc.12662.

76. Claudia R. Valeggia and J. Josh Snodgrass, "Health of Indigenous Peoples," *Annual Review of Anthropology* 44, no. 1 (2015), doi.org/10.1146/annurev-anthro-102214 -013831.

77. Miriam Rich, "The Curse of Civilised Woman: Race, Gender and the Pain of Childbirth in Nineteenth-Century American Medicine," *Gender and History* 28, no. 1 (2016): 60, doi.org/10.1111/1468-0424.12177.

78. Dorothy E. Roberts, *Killing the Black Body: Race, Reproduction, and the Meaning of Liberty* (New York: Pantheon, 1997); Molly R. Altman et al., "Listening to Women: Recommendations from Women of Color to Improve Experiences in Pregnancy and Birth Care," *Journal of Midwifery and Women's Health* 65, no. 4 (2020), doi.org/10.1111/jmwh.13102; Brittany D. Chambers et al., "Black Women's Perspectives on Structural Racism Across the Reproductive Lifespan: A Conceptual Framework for Measurement Development," *Maternal and Child Health Journal* (2021), doi.org/10.1007/s10995-020-03074-3.

79. Jennifer L. Morgan, *Laboring Women: Reproduction and Gender in New World Slavery* (Philadelphia: University of Pennsylvania Press, 2004).

80. Stephanie E. Jones-Rogers, *They Were Her Property: White Women as Slave Owners in the American South* (New Haven, CT: Yale University Press, 2019).

81. Eric Foner, *Gateway to Freedom: The Hidden History of the Underground Railroad* (New York: Norton, 2016).

82. Martia Graham Goodson, "Enslaved Africans and Doctors in South Carolina," *Journal of the National Medical Association* 95, no. 3 (2003), www.ncbi .nlm.nih.gov/pmc/articles/PMC2594411.

83. Martia G. Goodson, "Medical-Botanical Contributions of African Slave Women to American Medicine," *Western Journal of Black Studies* 11, no. 4 (1987).

84. Francis Peyre Porcher, "A Medico-Botanical Catalogue of the Plants and Ferns of St. John's, Berkly, South-Carolina" (Medical College of the State of South-Carolina, 1847), 13, tinyurl.com/25c9j5v5.

85. Mareike Maas, Alexandra M. Deters, and Andreas Hensel, "Anti-Inflammatory Activity of *Eupatorium perfoliatum* L. Extracts, Eupafolin, and Dimeric Guaianolide via iNOS Inhibitory Activity and Modulation of Inflammation-Related Cytokines and Chemokines," *Journal of Ethnopharmacology* 137, no. 1 (2011), doi.org/10.1016/j.jep.2011.05.040.

86. Francis Peyre Porcher, *Resources of the Southern Fields and Forests, Medical, Economical, and Agricultural* (Charleston, SC: Walker, Evans & Cogswell, 1869), 202.

87. Wagner, Ernst. *A Manual of General Pathology: For the Use of Students and Practitioners of Medicine* (New York: William Wood, 1876), 769.

88. Paul F. Mundé, "Dr. J. Marion Sims—The Father of Modern Gynecology: Being an Address Delivered October 20, 1894, in Bryant Park, New York, on the Unveiling of the Statue of Dr. J. Marion Sims," *Medical Record (1866–1922)* 46, no. 17 (1894); Jeffrey S. Sartin, "J. Marion Sims, the Father of Gynecology: Hero or Villain?," *Southern Medical Journal* 97, no. 5 (2004), doi.org/10.1097 /00007611-200405000-00017.

89. James Marion Sims, *The Story of My Life* (New York: D. Appleton, 1884), 234.

90. G. L. Smith and G. Williams, "Vesicovaginal Fistula," *BJU International* 83, no. 5 (2001), doi.org/10.1046/j.1464-410x.1999.00006.x.

91. L. Lewis Wall, "The Controversial Dr. J. Marion Sims (1813–1883)," *International Urogynecology Journal* 31, no. 7 (2020), doi.org/10.1007/s00192-020 -04301-9.

92. Stephen C. Kenny, "'I Can Do the Child No Good': Dr. Sims and the Enslaved Infants of Montgomery, Alabama," *Social History of Medicine* 20, no. 2 (2007), doi.org/10.1093/shm/hkm036; Sims, *Story of My Life*, 230.

93. Terri Kapsalis, *Public Privates: Performing Gynecology from Both Ends of the Speculum* (Durham, NC: Duke University Press, 1997), 43.

94. D. Ojanuga, "The Medical Ethics of the 'Father of Gynaecology,' Dr. J. Marion Sims," *Journal of Medical Ethics* 19, no. 1 (1993), doi.org/10.1136/jme.19.1.28; L. L. Wall, "The Medical Ethics of Dr. J. Marion Sims: A Fresh Look at the Historical Record," *Journal of Medical Ethics* 32, no. 6 (2006), doi.org/10.1136 /jme.2005.012559.

95. Carlye Chaney et al., "Systematic Review of Chronic Discrimination and Changes in Biology During Pregnancy Among African American Women," *Journal of Racial and Ethnic Health Disparities* 6, no. 6 (2019), doi.org/10.1007 /s40615-019-00622-8.

96. James W. Collins, Jr., Shou-Yien Wu, and Richard J. David, "Differing Intergenerational Birth Weights Among the Descendants of US-Born and Foreign-Born Whites and African Americans in Illinois," *American Journal of Epidemiology* 155, no. 3 (2002), doi.org/10.1093/aje/155.3.210.

97. Youli Yao et al., "Ancestral Exposure to Stress Epigenetically Programs Preterm Birth Risk and Adverse Maternal and Newborn Outcomes," *BMC Medicine* 12, no. 1 (2014), doi.org/10.1186/s12916-014-0121-6.

98. D. C. Owens and S. M. Fett, "Black Maternal and Infant Health: Historical Legacies of Slavery," *American Journal of Public Health* 109, no. 10 (2019): 1343, doi.org/10.2105/AJPH.2019.305243.

99. Rabah Kamal, *What Do We Know About Infant Mortality in the US and Comparable Countries?* (San Francisco: Kaiser Family Foundation, 2019), tinyurl.com/1nrwtrcq.

100. Alice Chen, "Why Is Infant Mortality Higher in the United States Than in Europe?," *American Journal of Economic Policy* 8, no. 2 (2016), doi.org/10.1257 /pol.20140224.

101. Brad N. Greenwood et al., "Physician-Patient Racial Concordance and Disparities in Birthing Mortality for Newborns," *Proceedings of the National Academy of Sciences of the United States of America* 117, no. 35 (2020), doi.org/10 .1073/pnas.1913405117.

102. Chambers et al., "Black Women's Perspectives on Structural Racism."

103. Altman et al., "Listening to Women."

104. Radostina K. Purvanova and John P. Muros, "Gender Differences in Burnout:

A Meta-Analysis," *Journal of Vocational Behavior* 77, no. 2 (2010), doi.org/10
.1016/j.jvb.2010.04.006.

105. Maya Dusenbery, *Doing Harm: The Truth About How Bad Medicine and Lazy
Science Leave Women Dismissed, Misdiagnosed, and Sick* (New York: Harper-
One, 2017), 43.

106. See Michael E. Franks, Gordon R. Macpherson, and William D. Figg,
"Thalidomide," *The Lancet* 363, no. 9423 (2004), doi.org/10.1016/s0140
-6736(04)16308-3; Dusenbery, *Doing Harm.*

107. Paul M. Ridker et al., "The Effect of Chronic Platelet Inhibition with Low-
Dose Aspirin on Atherosclerotic Progression and Acute Thrombosis: Clinical
Evidence from the Physicians' Health Study," *American Heart Journal* 122, no.
6 (1991), doi.org/10.1016/0002-8703(91)90275-M.

108. Brian McKinstry, "Are There Too Many Female Medical Graduates? Yes,"
BMJ 336, no. 7647 (2008), doi.org/10.1136/bmj.39505.491065.94; Association
of American Medical Colleges, *2020 Fall Applicant, Matriculant, and Enroll-
ment Data Tables* (Washington, DC: Association of American Medical Colleges, 2020), www.aamc.org/media/49911/download.

109. Meredith Alberta Palmer, "Land, Family, Body: Measurement and the Racial
Politics of US Colonialism in Haudenosaunee Country," Ph.D. diss., University of California, 2020.

110. Saba Hemmati et al., "Synthesis, Characterization, and Evaluation of Cytotoxic-
ity, Antioxidant, Antifungal, Antibacterial, and Cutaneous Wound Healing Effects of Copper Nanoparticles Using the Aqueous Extract of Strawberry Fruit
and L-Ascorbic Acid," *Polyhedron* 180 (2020), doi.org/10.1016/j.poly.2020.114425.

111. Joy Ann Bilharz, *The Allegany Senecas and Kinzua Dam: Forced Relocation
Through Two Generations* (Lincoln: University of Nebraska Press, 1998).

112. Laurence M. Hauptman, "The Meddlesome Friend: Philip Evan Thomas
Among the Onöndawa´ Ga´:1838-1861," in *Quakers and Native Americans*,
ed. Ignacio Gallup-Diaz and Geoffrey Plank (Leiden: Brill, 2019), brill.com
/view/book/edcoll/9789004388178/BP000009.xml; Lori Quigley, "Thomas Indian School: Social Experiment Resulting in Traumatic Effects." *Judicial No-
tice: A Periodical of New York Court History*, no. 14 (2019): 49–63.

113. Chris Cunneen, "Legal and Political Responses to the Stolen Generations:
Lessons from Ireland?," *Indigenous Law Bulletin* 5, no. 27 (2003); Australian
Institute of Health and Welfare, *Aboriginal and Torres Strait Islander Stolen Gen-
erations and Descendants: Numbers, Demographic Characteristics and Selected
Outcomes* (Canberra: AIHW, 2018); Kirsten Kamphuis and Elise van Nederveen
Meerkerk, "Education, Labour, and Discipline: New Perspectives on Imperial
Practices and Indigenous Children in Colonial Asia," *International Review of
Social History* 65, no. 1 (2020), doi.org/10.1017/S0020859019000750; Bob W.
White, "Talk About School: Education and the Colonial Project in French and
British Africa (1860-1960)," *Comparative Education* 32, no. 1 (1996), doi.org/10
.1080/03050069628902.

114. Donna Haraway, "Anthropocene, Capitalocene, Plantationocene, Chthulu-
cene: Making Kin," *Environmental Humanities* 6, no. 1 (2015), doi.org/10.1215
/22011919-3615934.

115. Beth H. Piatote, *Domestic Subjects: Gender, Citizenship, and Law in Native
American Literature* (New Haven, CT: Yale University Press, 2013), 12.

116. I. Mudnic et al., "Cardiovascular Effects in Vitro of Aqueous Extract of Wild

Strawberry (*Fragaria vesca, L.*) Leaves," *Phytomedicine* 16, no. 5 (2009), doi.org /10.1016/j.phymed.2008.11.004.

117. Sarah L. Surface-Evans, "'I Could Feel Your Heart,'" in *Archaeologies of the Heart*, ed. Kisha Supernant et al. (Cham, Switzerland: Springer International, 2020); Sonya Atalay, "An Archaeology Led by Strawberries," ibid.; and Leanne Simpson, 'Bubbling Like a Beating Heart': Reflections on Nishnaabeg Poetic and Narrative Consciousness," in *Indigenous Poetics in Canada*, ed. Neal McLeod (Waterlook. Ontario: Wilfred Laurier University Press, 2014): 108.

118. Harold A. Johnson, "The Contributions of Private Strawberry Breeders," *Hort-Science* 25, no. 8 (1990), doi.org/10.21273/HORTSCI.25.8.897; Sara Moffatt Schenck and Edward Winslow Gifford, *Karok Ethnobotany* (Berkeley: University of California Press, 1952); Chad E. Finn et al., "The Chilean Strawberry (*Fragaria chiloensis*): Over 1000 Years of Domestication," *HortScience* 48, no. 4 (2013), doi.org/10.21273/hortsci.48.4.418.

119. Naomi Roht-Arriaza, "Of Seeds and Shamans: The Appropriation of the Scientific and Technical Knowledge of Indigenous and Local Communities," *Michigan Journal of International Law* 17, no. 4 (1995): 966, heinonline.org /HOL/P?h = hein.journals/mjil17&i = 929.

120. Julie Guthman, *Wilted: Pathogens, Chemicals, and the Fragile Future of the Strawberry Industry* (Oakland: University of California Press, 2019), 7.

121. Danny K. Asami et al., "Comparison of the Total Phenolic and Ascorbic Acid Content of Freeze-Dried and Air-Dried Marionberry, Strawberry, and Corn Grown Using Conventional, Organic, and Sustainable Agricultural Practices," *Journal of Agricultural and Food Chemistry* 51, no. 5 (2003), doi.org/10.1021 /jf020635c; Agnieszka Najda et al., "Comparative Analysis of Secondary Metabolites Contents in Fragaria Vesca L. Fruits," *Annals of Agricultural and Environmental Medicine* 21, no. 2 (2014).

122. Shamsherjit Kaur et al., "Potential Pharmacological Strategies for the Improved Treatment of Organophosphate-Induced Neurotoxicity," *Canadian Journal of Physiology and Pharmacology* 92, no. 11 (2014), doi.org/10.1139/cjpp -2014-0113; Timothy C Marrs, "Organophosphates: History, Chemistry, Pharmacology," in *Organophosphates and Health*, ed. Stanley Feldman et al. (London: Imperial College Press, 2001).

123. Maryse F. Bouchard et al., "Prenatal Exposure to Organophosphate Pesticides and Iq in 7-Year-Old Children," *Environmental Health Perspectives* 119, no. 8 (04/21 11/08/received 04/13/accepted 2011), doi.org/10.1289/ehp.1003185.

124. D. H. Wall, U. N. Nielsen, and J. Six, "Soil Biodiversity and Human Health," *Nature* 528, no. 7580 (2015), doi.org/10.1038/nature15744.

125. Sara A. Quandt and Thomas A. Arcury, "The Status of Latinx Occupational Health," in *New and Emerging Issues in Latinx Health*, edited by A. D. Martínez and S. D. Rhodes (Cham, Switzerland: Springer International Publishing, 2020), 197–216, doi.org/10.1007/978-3-030-24043-1_9.

126. Rachel Soper, "How Wage Structure and Crop Size Negatively Impact Farmworker Livelihoods in Monocrop Organic Production: Interviews with Strawberry Harvesters in California," *Agriculture and Human Values* (2019): 331.

127. Shanna H. Swan, "Semen Quality in Fertile US Men in Relation to Geographical Area and Pesticide Exposure," *Journal of Pineal Research* 29, no. 1 (2006), doi.org/10.1111/j.1365-2605.2005.00620.x; Youn K. Shim, Steven P. Mlynarek, and Edwin Van Wijngaarden, "Parental Exposure to Pesticides and Childhood

Brain Cancer: U.S. Atlantic Coast Childhood Brain Cancer Study," *Environmental Health Perspectives* 117, no. 6 (2009), doi.org/10.1289/ehp.0800209.

128. Omid Mehrpour et al., "Occupational Exposure to Pesticides and Consequences on Male Semen and Fertility: A Review," *Toxicology Letters* 230, no. 2 (2014), doi.org/10.1016/j.toxlet.2014.01.029.

129. T. Colborn, "A Case for Revisiting the Safety of Pesticides: A Closer Look at Neurodevelopment," *Environ Health Perspectives* 114, no. 1 (2006), doi.org/10.1289/ehp.7940.

130. Asami et al., "Comparison of Phenolic and Ascorbic Acid Content."

131. Wasim Aktar, Dwaipayan Sengupta, and Ashim Chowdhury, "Impact of Pesticides Use in Agriculture: Their Benefits and Hazards," *Interdisciplinary Toxicology* 2, no. 1 (2009), doi.org/10.2478/v10102-009-0001-7.

132. In another twist of the knife, the land endowed to US "land grant" universities was stolen from Indigenous people. Robert Lee and Tristan Ahtone, "Land-Grab Universities," *High Country News*, March 30, 2020, tinyurl.com/1qtb7d30.

133. Community Alliance for Global Justice, *Messengers of Gates' Agenda: A Case Study of the Cornell Alliance for Science Global Leadership Fellows Program* (Seattle, WA: AGRA Watch, 2020); Tim Schwab, "Journalism's Gates Keepers," *Columbia Journalism Review*, August 21, 2020, www.cjr.org/criticism/gates-foundation-journalism-funding.php.

134. Anne-Emanuelle Birn and Elizabeth Fee, "The Rockefeller Foundation and the International Health Agenda," *The Lancet* 381, no. 9878 (2013): 1619.

135. Anne-Emanuelle Birn, "Philanthrocapitalism, Past and Present: The Rockefeller Foundation, the Gates Foundation, and the Setting (S) of the International/Global Health Agenda," *Hypothesis* 12, no. 1 (2014), pdfs.semanticscholar.org/68af/1700ca6cd1a9fc05a611b9dd6fef52e9c06c.pdf.

136. Raj Patel, Eric Holt Giménez, and Annie Shattuck, "Ending Africa's Hunger," *The Nation*, September 21, 2009, www.thenation.com/article/ending-africas-hunger.

137. Jules Pretty et al., "Assessment of the Growth in Social Groups for Sustainable Agriculture and Land Management," *Global Sustainability* 3 (2020), e23, doi.org/10.1017/sus.2020.19.

138. Raj Patel, "Food Sovereignty: Power, Gender, and the Right to Food," *PLOS Medicine* 9, no. 6 (2012), doi.org/doi:10.1371/journal.pmed.1001223; Miranda Imperial, "New Materialist Feminist Ecological Practices: La Via Campesina and Activist Environmental Work," *Social Sciences* 8, no. 8 (2019), doi.org/10.3390/socsci8080235.

139. Eric Okeefe, "Bill Gates: America's Top Farmland Owner," *The Land Report: Magazine of the American Landowner*, January 8, 2021, web.archive.org/web/20210115023510/landreport.com/2021/01/bill-gates-americas-top-farmland-owner/; Madeleine Fairbairn, *Fields of Gold: Financing the Global Land Rush* (Ithaca, NY: Cornell University Press, 2020); Ann Gibbons, "There's No Such Thing as a 'Pure' European—or Anyone Else," *Science Magazine*, May 15, 2017, tinyurl.com/yp9ox4rs.

140. Aoife O'Donovan and Thomas C. Neylan, "Associations of Trauma and Post-traumatic Stress Disorder with Inflammation and Endothelial Function: On Timing, Specificity, and Mechanisms," *Biological Psychiatry* 82, no. 12 (2017), doi.org/10.1016/j.biopsych.2017.10.002; Aoife O'Donovan et al., "Lifetime

Exposure to Traumatic Psychological Stress Is Associated with Elevated In-flammation in the Heart and Soul Study," *Brain, Behavior, and Immunity* 26, no. 4 (2012), doi.org/10.1016/j.bbi.2012.02.003; George P. Chrousos, "Stress, Chronic Inflammation, and Emotional and Physical Well-Being: Concurrent Effects and Chronic Sequelae," *Journal of Allergy and Clinical Immunology* 106, no. 5 (2000), doi.org/10.1067/mai.2000.110163.

141. Natalia S. Harasymowicz et al., "Intergenerational Transmission of Diet-Induced Obesity, Metabolic Imbalance, and Osteoarthritis in Mice," *Arthritis and Rheumatology* 72, no. 4 (2020), doi.org/10.1002/art.41147.

142. M. J. Meaney and M. Szyf, "Environmental Programming of Stress Responses Through DNA Methylation: Life at the Interface Between a Dynamic Environment and a Fixed Genome," *Dialogues in Clinical Neuroscience* 7, no. 2 (2005), www.ncbi.nlm.nih.gov/pubmed/16262207.

143. Rachel Yehuda et al., "Holocaust Exposure Induced Intergenerational Effects on *FKBP5* Methylation," *Biological Psychiatry* 80, no. 5 (2016), doi.org/10.1016/j.biopsych.2015.08.005; confirmed by Linda M. Bierer et al., "Intergenerational Effects of Maternal Holocaust Exposure on *FKBP5* Methylation," *American Journal of Psychiatry* (2020), doi.org/10.1176/appi.ajp.2019.19060618.

144. Maria Mies, *Patriarchy and Accumulation on a World Scale: Women in the International Division of Labour* (London: Zed, 1986).

145. Adam Z. Reynolds et al. "Matriliny Reverses Gender Disparities in Inflammation and Hypertension among the Mosuo of China," *Proceedings of the National Academy of Sciences of the United States of America* 117, no. 48 (2020): 30324–27. doi.org/10.1073/pnas.2014403117.

146. Judith K. Brown, "Economic Organization and the Position of Women Among the Iroquois," *Ethnohistory* 17, no. 3–4 (1970).

147. Carl Van Doren and Julian P. Boyd, eds., *Indian Treaties Printed by Benjamin Franklin, 1735–1762* (Philadelphia: Historical Society of Pennsylvania, 1938); Bruce E. Johansen, "Native American Societies and the Evolution of Democracy in America, 1600–1800," *Ethnohistory* 37, no. 3 (1990), doi.org/10.2307/482447; Elisabeth Tooker, "The United States Constitution and the Iroquois League," *Ethnohistory* 35, no. 4 (1988), doi.org/10.2307/482139; Bruce E. Johansen, *Forgotten Founders: Benjamin Franklin, the Iroquois, and the Rationale for the American Revolution* (Ipswich, MA: Gambit, 1982).

148. Barbara A. Mann, "The Lynx in Time: Haudenosaunee Women's Traditions and History," *American Indian Quarterly* 21, no. 3 (Summer 1997): 440, doi.org/10.2307/1185516.

149. Michael M. Pomedli, "Eighteenth-Century Treaties: Amended Iroquois Condolence Rituals," *American Indian Quarterly* 19, no. 3 (1995), doi.org/10.2307/1185594.

150. Jenni Monet, "Mohawk Women Integrate the Condolence Ceremony into Modern Systems," *Indian Country Today*, March 22 2012, tinyurl.com/27azadbk.

151. Pomedli, "Eighteenth-Century Treaties"; Susan M. Hill, *The Clay We Are Made Of: Haudenosaunee Land Tenure on the Grand River* (Winnipeg: University of Manitoba Press, 2017).

152. Saidiya V. Hartman, "The Time of Slavery," *South Atlantic Quarterly* 101, no. 4 (2002): 758; emphasis in original.

153. María Elena Martínez-Torres and Peter M. Rosset, "La Vía Campesina: The Birth and Evolution of a Transnational Social Movement," *Journal of Peasant*

Studies 37, no. 1 (2010), doi.org/10.1080/03066150903498804; Priscilla Claeys and Marc Edelman, "The United Nations Declaration on the Rights of Peasants and Other People Working in Rural Areas," *Journal of Peasant Studies* 47, no. 1 (2020), doi.org/10.1080/03066150.2019.1672665.

154. UN General Assembly, *United Nations Declaration on the Rights of Indigenous Peoples*, vol. 12 (New York: United Nations, 2007), tinyurl.com/g51vd5wf; Claeys and Edelman, "United Nations Declaration"; *ILO Declaration on Fundamental Principles and Rights at Work* (Geneva: International Labour Organization, 1998), www.ilo.org/declaration/thedeclaration/textdeclaration/lang—en /index.htm; United Nations, *International Convention on the Elimination of All Forms of Racial Discrimination* (1965); World Health Organization, *Preventing Disease Through Healthy Environments: Exposure to Highly Hazardous Pesticides: A Major Public Health Concern* (Geneva: World Health Organization, 2019), apps.who.int/iris/bitstream/handle/10665/329501/WHO-CED-PHE-EPE-19.4 .6-eng.pdf.

155. Craig M. Kauffman and Pamela L. Martin, "Constructing Rights of Nature Norms in the US, Ecuador, and New Zealand," *Global Environmental Politics* 18, no. 4 (2018), doi.org/10.1162/glep_a_00481.

6. CONNECTIVE TISSUE

1. James Baldwin and Nikki Giovanni, *A Dialogue* (Philadelphia: Lippincott, 1973), 26, 30–31.

2. Maya Angelou, *Wouldn't Take Nothing for My Journey Now* (New York: Random House, 1993), 121.

3. Mike Baker et al., "Three Words. 70 Cases. The Tragic History of 'I Can't Breathe,'" *The New York Times*, June 28, 2020, tinyurl.com/rian3399.

4. M. Leider, "On the Weight of the Skin," *Journal of Investigative Dermatology* 12, no. 3 (1949), 187–91.

5. J. Dennis Fortenberry, "The Uses of Race and Ethnicity in Human Microbiome Research," *Trends in Microbiology* 21, no. 4 (2013), doi.org/10.1016/j.tim.2013 .01.001; Clarence C. Gravlee, "How Race Becomes Biology: Embodiment of Social Inequality," *American Journal of Physical Anthropology* 139, no. 1 (2009), doi .org/10.1002/ajpa.20983. Waves of human migrations over sixty thousand years have rendered everyone an impure mix. Gibbons, "There's No Such Thing."

6. Friedrich Engels, *The Condition of the Working Class in England in 1844*, trans. Florence Kelley Wischnewetzky (New York: John W. Lovell Co., 1887), 84.

7. Arline T. Geronimus et al., "'Weathering' and Age Patterns of Allostatic Load Scores Among Blacks and Whites in the United States," *American Journal of Public Health* 96, no. 5 (2006), doi.org/10.2105/ajph.2004.060749.

8. S. Cohen et al., "Chronic Stress, Glucocorticoid Receptor Resistance, Inflammation, and Disease Risk," *Proceedings of the National Academy of Sciences of the United States of America* 109, no. 16 (2012), doi.org/10.1073/pnas.1118355109; M. Gough and K. Godde, "A Multifaceted Analysis of Social Stressors and Chronic Inflammation," *SSM Population Health* 6 (2018), doi.org/10.1016/j .ssmph.2018.09.005; April D. Thames et al., "Corrigendum to 'Experienced Discrimination and Racial Differences in Leukocyte Gene Expression [*Psychoneuroendocrinology* 106 (2019), 277–283],'" *Psychoneuroendocrinology* 109 (2019), doi.org/10.1016/j.psyneuen.2019.104422; B. S. McEwen and T. Seeman, "Protective and Damaging Effects of Mediators of Stress. Elaborating and Testing

the Concepts of Allostasis and Allostatic Load," *Annals of the New York Academy of Sciences* 896 (1999), doi.org/10.1111/j.1749-6632.1999.tb08103.x.

9. Thames et al., "Corrigendum."

10. Kristi Pullen Fedinick, Steve Taylor, and Michele Roberts, *Watered Down Justice* (Washington, DC: Natural Resources Defense Council, 2019).

11. Holly Silverman, "Navajo Nation Surpasses New York State for the Highest Covid-19 Infection Rate in the US," *CNN*, May 18, 2020, tinyurl.com/1hdh87be.

12. Million Women Study Collaborators, "Breast Cancer and Hormone-Replacement Therapy in the Million Women Study," *The Lancet* 362, no. 9382 (2003), doi.org/10.1016/s0140-6736(03)14065-2.

13. Scott M. Stringer, *New York City's Frontline Workers* (New York, 2020), comptroller.nyc.gov/reports/new-york-citys-frontline-workers.

14. Ibid.

15. Department of Health, *Age Adjusted Rate of Fatal Lab Confirmed Covid-19 Cases Per 100,000 by Race/Ethnicity Group as of April 6, 2020* (New York, 2020).

16. N. D. Powell et al., "Social Stress Up-Regulates Inflammatory Gene Expression in the Leukocyte Transcriptome via Beta-Adrenergic Induction of Myelopoiesis," *Proceedings of the National Academy of Sciences of the United States of America* 110, no. 41 (2013), doi.org/10.1073/pnas.1310655110; S. W. Cole, "Social Regulation of Human Gene Expression," *Current Directions in Psychological Science* 18, no. 3 (2009), doi.org/10.1111/j.1467-8721.2009.01623.x.

17. Paul Bastard et al., "Auto-Antibodies against Type I IFNs in Patients with Life-Threatening Covid-19," *Science* 370, no. 6515 (2020), doi.org/10.1126/science.abd4585.

18. Jarvis T. Chen and Nancy Krieger, "Revealing the Unequal Burden of COVID-19 by Income, Race/Ethnicity, and Household Crowding: US County Versus Zip Code Analysis," *Journal of Public Health Management and Practice* 27 (2021), doi.org/10.1097/PHH.0000000000001263; Neeraj Bhala et al., "Sharpening the Global Focus on Ethnicity and Race in the Time of Covid-19," *The Lancet* 395, no. 10238 (2020), doi.org/10.1016/S0140-6736(20)31102-8; Clare Bambra et al., "The Covid-19 Pandemic and Health Inequalities," *Journal of Epidemiology and Community Health* 74, no. 11 (2020), doi.org/10.1136/jech-2020-214401.

19. Ziad Obermeyer et al., "Dissecting Racial Bias in an Algorithm Used to Manage the Health of Populations," *Science* 366, no. 6464 (2019), doi.org/10.1126/science.aax2342.

20. Harsha Walia, *Border and Rule: Global Migration, Capitalism, and the Rise of Racist Nationalism* (Chicago: Haymarket Books, 2021), 2.

21. Cedric J. Robinson, *Black Marxism: The Making of the Black Radical Tradition* (Chapel Hill: University of North Carolina Press, 2000), 62.

22. Stuart Hall et al., eds., *Policing the Crisis: Mugging, the State and Law and Order* (London: Macmillan, 1978), 394. See also Benjamin Balthaser, "When Anti-Zionism Was Jewish: Jewish Racial Subjectivity and the Anti-Imperialist Literary Left from the Great Depression to the Cold War," *American Quarterly* 72, no. 2 (2020), doi.org/10.1353/aq.2020.0019.

23. Aydin Nazmi and Cesar G. Victora, "Socioeconomic and Racial/Ethnic Differentials of C-Reactive Protein Levels: A Systematic Review of Population-Based Studies," *BMC Public Health* 7, no. 1 (2007), doi.org/10.1186/1471-2458-7-212.

24. Geronimus et al., "'Weathering' and Age Patterns"; Thames et al., "Corrigendum."

25. Ronald L. Simons et al., "Discrimination, Segregation, and Chronic Inflammation: Testing the Weathering Explanation for the Poor Health of Black Americans," *Developmental Psychology* 54, no. 10 (2018), doi.org/10.1037/dev0000511; T. T. Lewis et al., "Self-Reported Experiences of Everyday Discrimination Are Associated with Elevated C-Reactive Protein Levels in Older African-American Adults," *Brain Behavior, and Immunity* 24, no. 3 (2010), doi.org/10.1016/j.bbi.2009.11.011.

26. J. C. Chambers et al., "C-Reactive Protein, Insulin Resistance, Central Obesity, and Coronary Heart Disease Risk in Indian Asians from the United Kingdom Compared with European Whites," *Circulation* 104, no. 2 (2001), doi.org/10.1161/01.cir.104.2.145.

27. D. R. Williams, "Miles to Go before We Sleep: Racial Inequities in Health," *Journal of Health and Social Behavior* 53, no. 3 (2012), doi.org/10.1177/0022146512455804.

28. Michael Paalani et al., "Determinants of Inflammatory Markers in a Bi-Ethnic Population," *Ethnicity and Disease* 21, no. 2 (2011), www.ncbi.nlm.nih.gov/pubmed/21749016.

29. Simons et al., "Discrimination, Segregation."

30. Johanna Wald and Daniel J. Losen, "Defining and Redirecting a School-to-Prison Pipeline," *New Directions for Youth Development*, November 5, 2003, doi.org/10.1002/yd.51.

31. "Mapping Police Violence," January 30, 2021, mappingpoliceviolence.org/nationaltrends.

32. Rory Kramer and Brianna Remster, "Stop, Frisk, and Assault? Racial Disparities in Police Use of Force During Investigatory Stops," *Law and Society Review*, November 5, 2018, doi.org/10.1111/lasr.12366.

33. Gabriel L. Schwartz and Jaquelyn L. Jahn, "Mapping Fatal Police Violence across U.S. Metropolitan Areas: Overall Rates and Racial/Ethnic Inequities, 2013–2017," *PLOS One* 15, no. 6 (2020), doi.org/10.1371/journal.pone.0229686.

34. "Mapping Police Violence," 2020, mappingpoliceviolence.org/cities.

35. Justin M. Feldman et al., "Police-Related Deaths and Neighborhood Economic and Racial/Ethnic Polarization, United States, 2015–2016," *American Journal of Public Health* 109, no. 3 (2019), doi.org/10.2105/ajph.2018.304851.

36. F. Edwards, H. Lee, and M. Esposito, "Risk of Being Killed by Police Use of Force in the United States by Age, Race-Ethnicity, and Sex," *Proceedings of the National Academy of Sciences of the United States of America* 116, no. 34 (2019), doi.org/10.1073/pnas.1821204116.

37. Ibid.

38. Julian Mark, "Jamaica Hampton, Shot by SFPD, Has Leg Amputated," *Mission Local* (San Francisco), January 10, 2020, missionlocal.org/2020/01/jamaica-hampton-shot-by-sfpd-has-leg-amputated; Abraham Rodriguez, "Woman Who Says Her Son Was Shot by San Francisco Police Questions Use of Lethal Force," *Mission Local*, December 10, 2019, missionlocal.org/2019/12/woman-who-says-her-son-was-shot-by-san-francisco-police-questions-use-of-lethal-force.

39. Nika Knight, "'People Are Going to Die': Father of Wounded DAPL Activist Sophia Wilansky Speaks Out," *Common Dreams*, November 23, 2016, tinyurl

.com/aypv6lhr; "Father of Activist Injured at Standing Rock Calls on Obama to Stop Dakota Access Pipeline Drilling," *Democracy Now!*, November 23, 2016, tinyurl.com/244yfsn3; Will Parrish, "The Federal Government Is Trying to Imprison These Six Water Protectors," *Dissenter*, 2019, tinyurl.com /1vhweaux.

40. Charles E. Menifield, Geiguen Shin, and Logan Strother, "Do White Law Enforcement Officers Target Minority Suspects?," *Public Administration Review* 79, no. 1 (2019), doi.org/10.1111/puar.12956. Recent research suggests that in Chicago, Black officers may use less force than white, and women less than men, but this result represents an unusual finding. For more, see Bocar A. Ba, Dean Knox, Jonathan Mummolo, and Roman Rivera. "The Role of Officer Race and Gender in Police-Civilian Interactions in Chicago," *Science* 371, no. 6530 (2021), 696. doi.org/10.1126/science.abd8694.

41. Michael German, *Hidden in Plain Sight: Racism, White Supremacy, and Far-Right Militancy in Law Enforcement* (New York: Brennan Center, 2020), tinyurl .com/3cjz7fgz.

42. Katrin Bennhold, "Body Bags and Enemy Lists: How Far-Right Police Officers and Ex-Soldiers Planned for 'Day X,'" *The New York Times*, August 1, 2020, tinyurl.com/29gpoz97.

43. Larry H. Spruill, "Slave Patrols,'Packs of Negro Dogs' and Policing Black Communities," *Phylon* 53, no. 1 (2016), www.jstor.org/stable/phylon1960.53.1.42.

44. Michel Hogue, *Metis and the Medicine Line: Creating a Border and Dividing a People* (Chapel Hill: University of North Carolina Press, 2015), 11.

45. Martin Case, *The Relentless Business of Treaties: How Indigenous Land Became US Property* (St. Paul: Minnesota Historical Society Press, 2018).

46. Čhaŋtémaza (Neil McKay) and Monica Siems McKay, "Where We Stand: The University of Minnesota and Dakhóta Treaty Lands," *Open Rivers* 17 (2020), editions.lib.umn.edu/openrivers/article/where-we-stand.

47. US Government, *An Act to Provide for the Allotment of Lands in Severalty to Indians on the Various Reservations* (General Allotment Act or Dawes Act), Statutes at Large 24, 388–91, NADP Document A1887 (1887).

48. Patrik Lantto, "Borders, Citizenship and Change: The Case of the Sami People, 1751–2008," *Citizenship Studies* 14, no. 5 (2010), doi.org/10.1080/13621025 .2010.506709.

49. Cori Bush, "This Is the America That Black People Know," *The Washington Post*, January 9, 2021, tinyurl.com/1o7wiu0b.

50. Cheryl I. Harris, "Whiteness as Property," *Harvard Law Review* 106, no. 8 (1993): 1174, doi.org/10.2307/1341787.

51. Ibid.

52. J. Edward Chamberlin, *The Harrowing of Eden: White Attitudes Toward Native Americans* (New York: Seabury Press, 1975).

53. See in particular his discussion of the national bourgeoisie in Frantz Fanon, *The Wretched of the Earth*, trans. Constance Farrington (London: Penguin, 1965).

54. Junia Howell and Elizabeth Korver-Glenn, "Neighborhoods, Race, and the Twenty-First-Century Housing Appraisal Industry," *Sociology of Race and Ethnicity* 4, no. 4 (2018): 482, doi.org/10.1177/2332649218755178.

55. Debra Kamin, "Black Homeowners Face Discrimination in Appraisals," *The New York Times*, August 15, 2020, tinyurl.com/gxeo31mc.

56. Keeanga-Yamahtta Taylor, *Race for Profit: How Banks and the Real Estate Industry Undermined Black Homeownership* (Chapel Hill: University of North Carolina Press, 2019); Andre M. Perry, *Know Your Price: Valuing Black Lives and Property in America's Black Cities* (Washington, DC: Brookings Institution Press, 2020).

57. Anthony A. Braga, Andrew V. Papachristos, and David M. Hureau, "The Effects of Hot Spots Policing on Crime: An Updated Systematic Review and Meta-Analysis," *Justice Quarterly* 31, no. 4 (2014), doi.org/10.1080/07418825 .2012.673632; Kathryn Henne and Rita Shah, "Unveiling White Logic in Criminological Research: An Intertextual Analysis," *Contemporary Justice Review* 18, no. 2 (2015), doi.org/10.1080/10282580.2015.1025620. Note too that segregation also means fewer health care facilities in Black neighborhoods. D. Jones Brittni, M. Harris Kelly, and F. Tate William, "Ferguson and Beyond: A Descriptive Epidemiological Study Using Geospatial Analysis," *Journal of Negro Education* 84, no. 3 (2015), doi.org/10.7709/jnegroeducation.84.3.0231.

58. Jeremy S. Hoffman, Vivek Shandas, and Nicholas Pendleton, "The Effects of Historical Housing Policies on Resident Exposure to Intra-Urban Heat: A Study of 108 US Urban Areas," *Climate* 8, no. 1 (2020), doi.org/10.3390 /cli8010012.

59. Quite what the proper body temperature should be is itself a moving target. See Myroslava Protsiv et al., "Decreasing Human Body Temperature in the United States Since the Industrial Revolution," *eLife* 9 (2020), doi.org/10.7554 /elife.49555.

60. Nidhi Singh, Saumya Singh, and R. K. Mall, "Urban Ecology and Human Health: Implications of Urban Heat Island, Air Pollution and Climate Change Nexus," *Urban Ecology* (2020), doi.org/10.1016/B978-0-12-820730-7.00017-3.

61. Jane E. Dematte, "Near-Fatal Heat Stroke During the 1995 Heat Wave in Chicago," *Annals of Internal Medicine* 129, no. 3 (1998): 173, doi.org/10.7326/0003 -4819-129-3-199808010-00001.

62. Jeremy J. Hess et al., "Climate Change and Emergency Medicine: Impacts and Opportunities," *Academic Emergency Medicine* 16, no. 8 (2009), doi.org/10 .1111/j.1553-2712.2009.00469.x.

63. Naomi Klein, *The Shock Doctrine: The Rise of Disaster Capitalism* (New York: Metropolitan Books, 2007).

64. Michelle Alexander, *The New Jim Crow: Mass Incarceration in the Age of Colorblindness* (New York: New Press, 2010); Ruth Wilson Gilmore, *Golden Gulag: Prisons, Surplus, Crisis, and Opposition in Globalizing California* (Berkeley: University of California Press, 2007).

65. Gilmore, *Golden Gulag*, 7.

66. For more on biopolitical Keynesianism, see Gabriel Winant, "'Hard Times Make for Hard Arteries and Hard Livers': Deindustrialization, Biopolitics, and the Making of a New Working Class," *Journal of Social History* 53, no. 1 (2019), doi.org/10.1093/jsh/shy11.

67. Allen M. Hornblum, *Acres of Skin: Human Experiments at Holmesburg Prison: A Story of Abuse and Exploitation in the Name of Medical Science* (New York: Routledge, 1998), xx, l.

68. Howard Goodman, "Studying Prison Experiments Research: For 20 Years, a Dermatologist Used the Inmates of a Philadelphia Prison as the Willing Subjects of Tests on Shampoo, Foot Powder, Deodorant, and Later, Mind-

Altering Drugs and Dioxin," *Baltimore Sun*, July 21, 1998, www.baltimoresun
.com/news/bs-xpm-1998-07-21-1998202099-story.html.

69. Peter Linebaugh, *The London Hanged: Crime and Civil Society in the Eighteenth Century*, 2nd ed. (London: Verso, 2006).

70. Rebecca Smith, Ana Avendaño, and Julie Martínez Ortega, *Iced Out: How Immigration Enforcement Has Interfered with Workers' Rights* (Washington, DC: AFL-CIO, 2009), 19–20.

71. Tianna Spears, "I Was a U.S. Diplomat. Customs and Border Protection Only Cared That I Was Black," *Politico*, August 30, 2020, tinyurl.com/2vd7kfck.

72. Lanre Bakare, "Angela Davis: 'We Knew That the Role of the Police Was to Protect White Supremacy,'" *The Guardian*, June 15, 2020, tinyurl.com /4q7m9nl9.

73. Derek Lutterbeck, "Between Police and Military: The New Security Agenda and the Rise of Gendarmeries," *Cooperation and Conflict* 39, no. 1 (2004), doi .org/10.1177/0010836704040832.

74. Kelly M. Hoffman et al., "Racial Bias in Pain Assessment and Treatment Recommendations, and False Beliefs About Biological Differences Between Blacks and Whites," *Proceedings of the National Academy of Sciences of the United States of America* 113, no. 16 (2016), doi.org/10.1073/pnas.1516047113.

75. Similarly, working-class patients, regardless of race, are treated worse than richer patients. S. Trawalter, K. M. Hoffman, and A. Waytz, "Racial Bias in Perceptions of Others' Pain," *PLOS One* 7, no. 11 (2012), doi.org/10.1371 /journal.pone.0048546; Hoffman et al., "Racial Bias in Pain Assessment." See also Michelle van Ryn and Jane Burke, "The Effect of Patient Race and Socio-Economic Status on Physicians' Perceptions of Patients," *Social Science and Medicine* 50, no. 6 (2000), doi.org/10.1016/S0277-9536(99)00338-X.

76. Kathleen S. Murphy, "Collecting Slave Traders: James Petiver, Natural History, and the British Slave Trade," *The William and Mary Quarterly* 70, no. 4 (2013), doi.org/10.5309/willmaryquar.70.4.0637.

77. Murphy, "Collecting Slave Traders."

78. Sasha Turner, "Slavery and the Production, Circulation and Practice of Medicine," *Social History of Medicine* 31, no. 4 (2018), doi.org/10.1093/shm/hky086.

79. Yue-Yung Hu et al., "Discrimination, Abuse, Harassment, and Burnout in Surgical Residency Training," *New England Journal of Medicine* 381, no. 18 (2019), doi.org/10.1056/nejmsa1903759.

80. Joseph Mpalirwa et al., "Patients, Pride, and Prejudice: Exploring Black Ontarian Physicians' Experiences of Racism and Discrimination," *Academic Medicine* 95, no. 11S (2020), journals.lww.com/academicmedicine/Fulltext /2020/11001/Patients,_Pride,_and_Prejudice_Exploring_Black.13.aspx. See also "How the Health Care System Has Racial Biases," *Now This Politics,* 2018, www.facebook.com/NowThisPolitics/videos/1985138634850950.

81. *Diversity in Medicine: Facts and Figures 2019* (Washington, DC: Association of American Medical Colleges, 2018), tinyurl.com/dyg3vkc8.

82. *Diversity and Disparities: A Benchmarking Study of US Hospitals in 2015* (American Hospital Association, 2015).

83. D. R. Williams and T. D. Rucker, "Understanding and Addressing Racial Disparities in Health Care," *Health Care Financing Review* 21, no. 4 (2000), ncbi .nlm.nih.gov/pubmed/11481746.

84. Hoffman et al., "Racial Bias in Pain Assessment."

85. V. Grubbs, "Precision in GFR Reporting: Let's Stop Playing the Race Card," *Clinical Journal of the American Society of Nephrology* 15, no. 8 (2020), doi.org/10.2215/CJN.00690120.

86. Leila R. Zelnick et al., "Association of the Estimated Glomerular Filtration Rate with vs Without a Coefficient for Race with Time to Eligibility for Kidney Transplant," *JAMA Network Open* 4, no. 1 (2021), doi.org/10.1001/jamanetworkopen.2020.34004.

87. Philip E. Bickler, John R. Feiner, and John W. Severinghaus, "Effects of Skin Pigmentation on Pulse Oximeter Accuracy at Low Saturation," *Anesthesiology* 102, no. 4 (2005), doi.org/10.1097/00000542-200504000-00004.

88. Eboni G. Price-Haywood et al., "Hospitalization and Mortality Among Black Patients and White Patients with Covid-19," *New England Journal of Medicine* 382, no. 26 (2020), doi.org/10.1056/nejmsa2011686.

89. R. G. Wilkerson et al., "Silent Hypoxia: A Harbinger of Clinical Deterioration in Patients with Covid-19," *American Journal of Emergency Medicine* 38, no. 10 (2020), doi.org/10.1016/j.ajem.2020.05.044.

90. Michael W. Sjoding et al., "Racial Bias in Pulse Oximetry Measurement," *New England Journal of Medicine* 383, no. 25 (2020), doi.org/10.1056/nejmc2029240.

91. Richard D. Granstein, Lynn Cornelius, and Kanade Shinkai, "Diversity in Dermatology—A Call for Action," *JAMA Dermatology* 153, no. 6 (2017), doi.org/10.1001/jamadermatol.2017.0296.

92. Kesha J. Buster, Erica I. Stevens, and Craig A. Elmets, "Dermatologic Health Disparities," *Dermatologic Clinics* 30, no. 1 (2012), doi.org/10.1016/j.det.2011.08.002.

93. J. C. Lester, S. C. Taylor, and M.-M. Chren, "Under-Representation of Skin of Colour in Dermatology Images: Not Just an Educational Issue," *British Journal of Dermatology* 180, no. 6 (2019), doi.org/10.1111/bjd.17608.

94. J. C. Lester et al., "Absence of Images of Skin of Colour in Publications of Covid-19 Skin Manifestations," *British Journal of Dermatology* 183, no. 3 (2020), doi.org/10.1111/bjd.19258.

95. Lester, Taylor, and Chren, "Under-Representation of Skin of Colour."

96. P. S. Chan et al., "Racial Differences in Survival after In-Hospital Cardiac Arrest," *JAMA* 302, no. 11 (2009), doi.org/10.1001/jama.2009.1340.

97. Marcella Alsan, Owen Garrick, and Grant Graziani, "Does Diversity Matter for Health? Experimental Evidence from Oakland," *American Economic Review* 109, no. 12 (2019), doi.org/10.1257/aer.20181446.

98. Ibid.

99. Abraham Flexner, *The American College: A Criticism* (New York: Century, 1908); T. N. Bonner, "Searching for Abraham Flexner," *Academic Medicine* 73, no. 2 (1998), journals.lww.com/academicmedicine/Fulltext/1998/02000/Searching_for_Abraham_Flexner.14.aspx.

100. Molly Cooke et al., "American Medical Education 100 Years after the Flexner Report," *New England Journal of Medicine* 355, no. 13 (2006), doi.org/10.1056/nejmra055445.

101. Abraham Flexner, *Medical Education in the United States and Canada* (Princeton, NJ: Carnegie Foundation for the Advancement of Teaching, 1910), chap. 14.

102. T. Savitt, "Abraham Flexner and the Black Medical Schools. 1992," *Journal*

of the National Medical Association 98, no. 9 (2006), www.ncbi.nlm.nih.gov /pubmed/17019906.

103. Frank W. Stahnisch and Marja Verhoef, "The Flexner Report of 1910 and Its Impact on Complementary and Alternative Medicine and Psychiatry in North America in the 20th Century," *Evidence-Based Complementary and Alternative Medicine* (2012), doi.org/10.1155/2012/647896.

104. Flexner, *Medical Education*, 158.

105. Tiffany Willoughby-Herard, *Waste of a White Skin: The Carnegie Corporation and the Racial Logic of White Vulnerability* (Oakland: University of California Press, 2015).

106. Marcella Alslan, *Does Diversity Matter for Health? Experimental Evidence from Oakland* (Cambridge, MA: National Bureau of Economic Research, 2018).

107. *Diversity in Medicine: Facts and Figures 2019* (Washington, DC: Association of American Medical Colleges, 2018), tinyurl.com/dyg3vkc8.

108. C. T. Laurencin and M. Murray, "An American Crisis: The Lack of Black Men in Medicine," *Journal of Racial and Ethnic Health Disparities* 4, no. 3 (2017), doi .org/10.1007/s40615-017-0380-y.

109. Samir Gandesha, "The Spectre of the 1930s," in *Back to the '30s? Recurring Crises of Capitalism, Liberalism, and Democracy*, ed. Jeremy Rayner et al. (Cham, Switzerland: Springer International, 2020); Cedric J. Robinson, *Black Marxism: The Making of the Black Radical Tradition* (Chapel Hill: University of North Carolina Press, 2000).

110. Patel and Moore, *A History of the World in Seven Cheap Things*, 187; Keith E. Sealing, "Blood Will Tell: Scientific Racism and the Legal Prohibitions against Miscegenation," *Michigan Journal of Race and Law* 5, no. 2 (1999), 610, heinonline.org/HOL/P?h = hein.journals/mjrl5&i = 567.

111. Carl Linnaeus, *Systema Naturae*, 10th ed. (Holmiae: Salvius, 1758), 20–22.

112. Larry Barsness, *Heads, Hides and Horns: The Complete Buffalo Book* (Fort Worth: Texas Christian University Press, 2000), 243, 240, 251.

113. Nicole Vogelzangs et al., "Association of Depressive Disorders, Depression Characteristics and Antidepressant Medication with Inflammation," *Translational Psychiatry* 2, no. 2 (2012), doi.org/10.1038/tp.2012.8; Kathryn E. Wellen and Gökhan S. Hotamisligil, "Inflammation, Stress, and Diabetes," *Journal of Clinical Investigation* 115, no. 5 (2005), doi.org/10.1172/JCI25102.

114. Nick Estes, "The Empire of All Maladies," *Baffler*, July 2020.

115. K. Wienski, "Leading Health Challenges Pine Ridge Reservation, South Dakota Oglala Lakota Sioux," *Juniper Online Journal of Public Health* 1, no. 5 (2017).

116. K. W. Bauer et al., "High Food Insecurity and Its Correlates Among Families Living on a Rural American Indian Reservation," *American Journal of Public Health* 102, no. 7 (2012), doi.org/10.2105/AJPH.2011.300522.

117. Alison Bashford, "'Is White Australia Possible?' Race, Colonialism and Tropical Medicine," *Ethnic and Racial Studies* 23, no. 2 (2000), doi.org/10.1080 /014198700329042.

118. W. Anderson, "Geography, Race and Nation: Remapping 'Tropical' Australia, 1890–1930," *Medical History. Supplement*, no. 20 (2000), pubmed.ncbi.nlm.nih .gov/11769929.

119. Francis Galton, *Hereditary Genius: An Inquiry into Its Laws and Consequences* (London: Macmillan, 1869).

120. Ibid., 72.

121. Christine B. Hickman, "The Devil and the One Drop Rule: Racial Categories, African Americans, and the U.S. Census," *Michigan Law Review* 95, no. 5 (1997), doi.org/10.2307/1290008; David A. Hollinger, "Amalgamation and Hypodescent: The Question of Ethnoracial Mixture in the History of the United States," *American Historical Review* 108, no. 5 (2003), doi.org/10.1086/ahr/108.5.1363.

122. Nicholas W. Gillham, "Cousins: Charles Darwin, Sir Francis Galton and the Birth of Eugenics," *Significance* 6, no. 3 (2009), doi.org/10.1111/j.1740-9713.2009.00379.x.

123. Charles Darwin, *The Descent of Man and Selection in Relation to Sex* (New York: D. Appleton, 1876).

124. Galton, *Hereditary Genius*, 340.

125. Philippa Levine, "Anthropology, Colonialism, and Eugenics," in *The Oxford Handbook of the History of Eugenics,* ed. Alison Bashford and Philippa Levine (New York: Oxford University Press, 2010), 46.

126. Jennifer Robertson, "Eugenics in Japan: Sanguinous Repair," in Bashford and Levine, *The Oxford Handbook;* Gilberto Hochman, Nísia Trindade Lima, and Marcos Chor Maio, "The Path of Eugenics in Brazil: Dilemmas of Miscegenation," ibid.

127. Harry H. Laughlin, *The Second International Exhibition of Eugenics* (Baltimore: Williams & Wilkins, 1923), wellcomecollection.org/works/cf72yps9.

128. David M. Pressel, "Nuremberg and Tuskegee: Lessons for Contemporary American Medicine," *Journal of the National Medical Association* 95, no. 12 (2003), pubmed.ncbi.nlm.nih.gov/14717481.

129. Allan M. Brandt, "Racism and Research: The Case of the Tuskegee Syphilis Study," *Hastings Center Report* 8, no. 6 (1978): 24, doi.org/10.2307/3561468.

130. Daniel Z. Buchman, Anita Ho, and Daniel S. Goldberg, "Investigating Trust, Expertise, and Epistemic Injustice in Chronic Pain," *Journal of Bioethical Inquiry* 14 (2017), doi.org/10.1007/s11673-016-9761-x.

131. Miranda Fricker, *Epistemic Injustice: Power and the Ethics of Knowing* (New York: Oxford University Press, 2009), 97.

132. Olúfẹ́mi O. Táíwò, "Being-in-the-Room Privilege: Elite Capture and Epistemic Deference," *Philosopher* 108, no. 4 (2020), www.thephilosopher1923.org/essay-taiwo.

133. Alexandra Kalev and Frank Dobbin, *Does Diversity Training Increase Corporate Diversity? Regulation Backlash and Regulatory Accountability* (Cambridge, MA: Kennedy School, 2020), tinyurl.com/3g48fpov.

134. Kevin J. Gutierrez, "The Performance of 'Antiracism' Curricula," *New England Journal of Medicine* 383 (2020), doi.org/10.1056/nejmpv2025046.

135. Howard I. Maibach and Albert M. Kligman, "The Micrometer Syringe for Quantitative Skin Testing," *Archives of Dermatology* 87, no. 6 (1963), doi.org/10.1001/archderm.1963.01590180071015.

136. Robert J. Feldmann and Howard I. Maibach, "Percutaneous Penetration of Some Pesticides and Herbicides in Man," *Toxicology and Applied Pharmacology* 28, no. 1 (1974), doi.org/10.1016/0041-008x(74)90137-9; Allen M. Hornblum, *Acres of Skin: Human Experiments at Holmesburg Prison: A Story of Abuse and Exploitation in the Name of Medical Science* (New York: Routledge, 1998).

137. Danielle Echeverria, "UCSF Group Demands 'Anti-Racist' Changes," *San Francisco Chronicle,* August 4, 2020, tinyurl.com/4qsf983v.

138. Jeph Herrin et al., "Hospital Leadership Diversity and Strategies to Advance

Health Equity," *Joint Commission Journal on Quality and Patient Safety* 44, no. 9 (2018), doi.org/10.1016/j.jcjq.2018.03.008.

139. B. Brecht, "Theatre for Learning," *Tulane Drama Review* 6, no. 1 (1961): 24.

140. Gilmore, *Golden Gulag*, 242; Sandra Wexler et al., "We're Not the Enemy and We're Not Asking for the World: Low-Wage Hospital Service Workers' Advocacy for Fair Wages," *Journal of Sociology and Social Welfare* 47, no. 1 (2020): 148, scholarworks.wmich.edu/jssw/vol47/iss1/7.

141. Timothy Snyder, *Bloodlands: Europe Between Hitler and Stalin* (New York: Basic Books, 2010), 160.

142. Claudio Saunt, *Unworthy Republic: The Dispossession of Native Americans and the Road to Indian Territory* (New York: Norton, 2020). On Tocqueville, see Melvin Richter, "Tocqueville on Algeria," *Review of Politics* 25, no. 3 (1963), www.jstor.org/stable/1405738.

143. William B. Cohen, "The Algerian War, the French State and Official Memory," *Historical Reflections / Réflexions Historiques* 28, no. 2 (2002), www.jstor.org/stable/41299235.

144. Lewis R. Gordon, *What Fanon Said: A Philosophical Introduction to His Life and Thought* (New York: Fordham University Press, 2015).

145. Richard C. Keller, "Clinician and Revolutionary: Frantz Fanon, Biography, and the History of Colonial Medicine," *Bulletin of the History of Medicine* 81, no. 4 (2007): 827, www.jstor.org/stable/44452161.

146. V. Campuzano et al., "Friedreich's Ataxia: Autosomal Recessive Disease Caused by an Intronic GAA Triplet Repeat Expansion," *Science* 271, no. 5254 (1996), doi.org/10.1126/science.271.5254.1423.

147. Frantz Fanon and Asselah Slimane, "The Phenomenon of Agitation in the Psychiatric Milieu: General Considerations, Psychopathological Meaning," in *Alienation and Freedom*, ed. Jean Khalfa and Robert J. C. Young, trans. Steven Corcoran (London: Bloomsbury, 2018).

148. Jean Khalfa, "Fanon and Psychiatry," *Nottingham French Studies* 54, no. 1 (2015): 66, doi.org/10.3366/nfs.2015.0106.

149. Frantz Fanon, *Studies in a Dying Colonialism* (New York: Monthly Review Press, 1965), 133.

150. Mahmood Mamdani's argument for decolonization doesn't engage with Fanon and, in presenting a post-apartheid South Africa as the political embodiment of decolonization, would, we suspect, have been a finding with which Fanon would have disagreed. Mahmood Mamdani, *Neither Settler nor Native: The Making and Unmaking of Permanent Minorities* (Cambridge, MA: Belknap Press, 2020).

151. "End the War on Black Migrants," End the War on Black People, 2021, accessed January 29, 2021, m4bl.org/policy-platforms/end-the-war-on-migrants/.

152. Catherine A. Okoro et al., "Prevalence of Disabilities and Health Care Access by Disability Status and Type Among Adults—United States, 2016," *Morbidity and Mortality Weekly Report* 67, no. 32 (2018).

153. Alicia Garza, "A Herstory of the #Blacklivesmatter Movement," in *Are All the Women Still White? Rethinking Race, Expanding Feminisms*, ed. Janell Hobson (Albany: State University of New York Press, 2016), 25.

154. See, e.g., Alondra Nelson, *Body and Soul: The Black Panther Party and the Fight Against Medical Discrimination* (Minneapolis: University of Minnesota Press, 2011).

155. Michel Foucault, *The Birth of Biopolitics: Lectures at the Collège de France, 1978–79*, ed. Michel Senellart (Basingstoke, UK: Palgrave Macmillan, 2008).

156. Lola Olufemi, *Feminism, Interrupted: Disrupting Power* (London: Pluto Press, 2020); Akwugo Emejulu, "Revolution Is Not a One Time Event," *White Review*, June 2020, www.thewhitereview.org/feature/revolution-is-not-a-one-time-event-2.

157. "Defund OPD," 2020, www.defundopd.org.

158. Michael Rosen, Eric Ting, and Katie Dowd, "'Defund the Police'? Here's How Much Bay Area Cities Spend on Police Departments," *SF Gate*, June 15, 2020, tinyurl.com/2tzpu5yt.

159. Tim J. Wise, *White Like Me: Reflections on Race from a Privileged Son*, rev. and updated. ed. (Brooklyn: Soft Skull Press, 2008).

160. Stefano Harmey and Fred Moten, *The Undercommons: Fugitive Planning and Black Study* (New York: Minor Compositions, 2013).

161. David E. Alexander, "Ecotone," in *Environmental Geology* (Dordrecht: Springer Netherlands, 1999).

162. Salit Kark, "Ecotones and Ecological Gradients," in *Ecological Systems: Selected Entries from the Encyclopedia of Sustainability Science and Technology*, ed. Rik Leemans (New York: Springer, 2013).

163. Larry Harris, "Edge Effects and Conservation of Biotic Diversity," *Conservation Biology* 2 (1988), doi.org/10.2307/2386291.

164. Menno Schilthuizen, "Ecotone: Speciation-Prone," *Trends in Ecology and Evolution* 15, no. 4 (2000), doi.org/10.1016/s0169-5347(00)01839-5.

165. Paul G Risser, "The Status of the Science Examining Ecotones: A Dynamic Aspect of Landscape Is the Area of Steep Gradients Between More Homogeneous Vegetation Associations," *BioScience* 45, no. 5 (1995), doi.org/10.2307/1312492.

166. T. B. Smith, "A Role for Ecotones in Generating Rainforest Biodiversity," *Science* 276, no. 5320 (1997), doi.org/10.1126/science.276.5320.1855.

167. Martin Stokes, *Ethnicity, Identity and Music* (Oxford: Berg, 1994), 8.

168. Rolf Lidskog, "The Role of Music in Ethnic Identity Formation in Diaspora: A Research Review," *International Social Science Journal* 66, no. 219–20 (2017), doi.org/10.1111/issj.12091.

169. Gerald Horne, *Jazz and Justice: Racism and the Political Economy of the Music* (New York: NYU Press, 2019), 8.

170. Ibid.

171. Ibid.

172. "Bulbancha Is Still a Place," 2020, accessed December 1, 2020, bulbanchaisstillaplace.org/resources.

173. Case Watkins, "Essential Geographies of New Orleans Music," *American Association of Geographers Newsletter*, August 31, 2017, news.aag.org/2017/08/essential-geographies-of-new-orleans-music/.

174. Ibid., 2.

175. Ted Gioia, *The History of Jazz* (Oxford: Oxford University Press, 1998), 3.

176. Charles B. Hersch, "Review: Jazz and the Boundaries of Race," *Perspectives on Politics* 10, no. 3 (2012): 704, www.jstor.org/stable/23260189.

177. Ibid.

178. Horne, *Jazz and Justice*, 9.

179. Andre Kimo Stone Guess, "For Wynton Marsalis, Forgetting the Roots of Jazz

Is Forgetting the History of Race in America," *The Undefeated*, January 12, 2018, theundefeated.com/features/for-wynton-marsalis-forgetting-the-roots -of-jazz-is-forgetting-the-history-of-race-in-america/.

180. Ted Gioia, *Music: A Subversive History* (New York: Basic Books, 2019).
181. "Black American Music and the Jazz Tradition," 2014, accessed February 3, 2021, nicholaspayton.wordpress.com/2014/04/30/black-american-music-and-the-jazz -tradition.
182. Nat Hentoff, "The Devil's Music," *The Washington Post*, August 23, 1985, tinyurl .com/ur2izgxi.
183. Lawrence Tedder, *Jazz and Blues on Edison* vol. 2, 1917–1929, CD, Edison Collection.
184. Horne, *Jazz and Justice*, 14.
185. William H. Youngren, "Black and White Intertwined," *Atlantic*, February 1999, tinyurl.com/pwjdxv5o.
186. Horne, *Jazz and Justice*, 18.
187. Dasum Allah, "NYPD Admits to Rap Intelligence Unit," *Village Voice*, March 16, 2004, tinyurl.com/yst6dk3k.
188. Horne, *Jazz and Justice*.

7. ENDOCRINE SYSTEM

1. Paulo Freire, *Pedagogy of the Oppressed*, trans. Myra Ramos Bergman (New York: Continuum, 2005), 88–93.
2. E. S. Epel et al., "Meditation and Vacation Effects Have an Impact on Disease-Associated Molecular Phenotypes," *Translational Psychiatry* 6, no. 8 (2016), doi.org/10.1038/tp.2016.164.
3. Jessica de Bloom et al., "Effects of Vacation from Work on Health and Well-Being: Lots of Fun, Quickly Gone," *Work and Stress* 24, no. 2 (2010), doi.org /10.1080/02678373.2010.493385.
4. Ksenia Kirillova and Dan Wang, "Smartphone (Dis)Connectedness and Vaca-tion Recovery," *Annals of Tourism Research* 61 (2016), doi.org/10.1016/j.annals .2016.10.005.
5. Epel et al., "Meditation and Vacation Effects."
6. Richard Louv, *Last Child in the Woods: Saving Our Children from Nature-Deficit Disorder* (Chapel Hill, NC: Algonquin Books, 2005).
7. Emily J. Hadgkiss et al., "Health-Related Quality of Life Outcomes at 1 and 5 Years After a Residential Retreat Promoting Lifestyle Modification for People with Multiple Sclerosis," *Neurological Sciences* 34, no. 2 (2013), doi.org/10 .1007/s10072-012-0982-4
8. Richard J. Ellis, "'I Know for Certain . . . That These Are Bad People': The Intrac-table Problem of Guantánamo," *Comparative American Studies: An International Journal* 8, no. 3 (2010): 179, doi.org/10.1179/147757010X12773889525740.
9. The British were at the time, as Ellis points out, fighting Spain for the right to maintain the exclusive right to supply slaves for Spanish colonies.
10. *Experiments in Torture: Evidence of Human Subject Research and Experimenta-tion in the "Enhanced" Interrogation Program* (Cambridge, MA: Physicians for Human Rights, 2010).
11. "Young Guantanamo Afghan to Sue US," *BBC News*, August 27, 2009, news .bbc.co.uk/2/hi/south_asia/8224357.stm.
12. Vincent Iacopino and Stephen N. Xenakis, "Neglect of Medical Evidence of

Torture in Guantánamo Bay: A Case Series," *PLOS Medicine* 8, no. 4 (2011): 2, doi.org/10.1371/journal.pmed.1001027.

13. Josh White, "Tactic Used After It Was Banned: Detainees at Guantanamo Were Moved Often, Documents Say," *The Washington Post*, August 8, 2008, tinyurl.com/467ua6bc.

14. Jane Sutton, "Guantanamo Prisoner Cites 2-Week Sleep Deprivation," *Reuters*, June 19, 2008, tinyurl.com/giqu7odc.

15. The Guantanamo detention facility remains open, twenty years after 9/11. At the time of writing, forty people are still incarcerated there. Jawad returned to Afghanistan in 2009, after the US military agreed that it didn't have enough evidence to bring him to trial. Andrei Scheinkman et al., "The Guantanamo Docket," *The New York Times*, January 21, 2021, www.nytimes.com/interactive/projects/guantanamo.

16. Russel J. Reiter et al., "Melatonin as an Antioxidant: Under Promises but Over Delivers," *Journal of Pineal Research* 61, no. 3 (2016), doi.org/10.1111/jpi.12360; Jimo Borjigin, L. Samantha Zhang, and Anda-Alexandra Calinescu, "Circadian Regulation of Pineal Gland Rhythmicity," *Molecular and Cellular Endocrinology* 349, no. 1 (2012), doi.org/10.1016/j.mce.2011.07.009.

17. Yvan Touitou, Alain Reinberg, and David Touitou, "Association Between Light at Night, Melatonin Secretion, Sleep Deprivation, and the Internal Clock: Health Impacts and Mechanisms of Circadian Disruption," *Life Sciences* 173 (2017), doi.org/10.1016/j.lfs.2017.02.008; Reiter et al., "Melatonin as Antioxidant."

18. Matthew P. Walker, *Why We Sleep: Unlocking the Power of Sleep and Dreams* (New York: Scribner, 2017); A. Carrillo-Vico et al., "The Modulatory Role of Melatonin on Immune Responsiveness," *Current Opinion in Investigational Drugs* 7, no. 5 (2006), www.ncbi.nlm.nih.gov/pubmed/16729718.

19. Carrillo-Vico et al., "Modulatory Role of Melatonin."

20. M. N. Mead, "Benefits of Sunlight: A Bright Spot for Human Health," *Environmental Health Perspectives* 116, no. 4 (2008), doi.org/10.1289/ehp.116-a160; Joann E. Manson et al., "Vitamin D Supplements and Prevention of Cancer and Cardiovascular Disease," *New England Journal of Medicine* 380, no. 1 (2019), doi.org/10.1056/nejmoa1809944.

21. Christos C. Zouboulis, "The Skin as an Endocrine Organ," *Dermato-Endocrinology* 1, no. 5 (2009), doi.org/10.4161/derm.1.5.9499.

22. Anthony R. Mawson, "Breast Cancer in Female Flight Attendants," *The Lancet* 352, no. 9128 (1998); Vilhjálmur Rafnsson et al., "Risk of Breast Cancer in Female Flight Attendants: A Population-Based Study (Iceland)," *Cancer Causes and Control* 12, no. 2 (2001), doi.org/10.1023/A:1008983416836.

23. Gaia Favero, "Melatonin as an Anti-Inflammatory Agent Modulating Inflammasome Activation," *International Journal of Endocrinology* 2017 (2017), doi.org/10.1155/2017/1835195.

24. Andrzej Slominski et al., "Melatonin in the Skin: Synthesis, Metabolism and Functions," *Trends in Endocrinology and Metabolism* 19, no. 1 (2008), doi.org/10.1016/j.tem.2007.10.007; Jung Goo Lee et al., "The Neuroprotective Effects of Melatonin: Possible Role in the Pathophysiology of Neuropsychiatric Disease," *Brain Sciences* 9, no. 10 (2019), doi.org/10.3390/brainsci9100285; Katherine M. Evely et al., "Melatonin Receptor Activation Increases Gluta-

matergic Synaptic Transmission in the Rat Medial Lateral Habenula," *Synapse* 70, no. 5 (2016), doi.org/10.1002/syn.21892.

25. Lee et al., "Neuroprotective Effects of Melatonin."

26. José L. Mauriz et al., "A Review of the Molecular Aspects of Melatonin's Anti-Inflammatory Actions: Recent Insights and New Perspectives," *Journal of Pineal Research* 54, no. 1 (2013), doi.org/10.1111/j.1600-079x.2012.01014.x.

27. Zhang et al., "Melatonin Alleviates Acute Lung Injury."

28. N. Rohleder, "Stimulation of Systemic Low-Grade Inflammation by Psychosocial Stress," *Psychosomatic Medicine* 76, no. 3 (2014), doi.org/10.1097/PSY .0000000000000049.

29. Yadi Zhou et al., "A Network Medicine Approach to Investigation and Population-Based Validation of Disease Manifestations and Drug Repurposing for Covid-19," *PLOS Biology* 18, no. 11 (2020), doi.org/10.1371/journal .pbio.3000970.

30. Ruben Manuel Luciano Colunga Biancatelli et al., "Melatonin for the Treatment of Sepsis: The Scientific Rationale," *Journal of Thoracic Disease* 12, no. S1 (2020), doi.org/10.21037/jtd.2019.12.85.

31. Reiter et al., "Melatonin as Antioxidant."

32. Janet M. Mullington et al., "Sleep Loss and Inflammation," *Best Practice and Research Clinical Endocrinology and Metabolism* 24, no. 5 (2010), doi.org/10 .1016/j.beem.2010.08.014.

33. Judith E. Carroll et al., "Partial Sleep Deprivation Activates the DNA Damage Response (DDR) and the Senescence-Associated Secretory Phenotype (SASP) in Aged Adult Humans," *Brain, Behavior, and Immunity* 51 (2016), doi.org/10 .1016/j.bbi.2015.08.024.

34. Carol A. Everson, Bernard M. Bergmann, and Allan Rechtschaffen, "Sleep Deprivation in the Rat: III. Total Sleep Deprivation," *Sleep* 12, no. 1 (1989), doi.org/10.1093/sleep/12.1.13.

35. A. Vaccaro et al., "Sleep Loss Can Cause Death Through Accumulation of Reactive Oxygen Species in the Gut," *Cell* 181, no. 6 (2020), doi.org/10.1016 /j.cell.2020.04.049.

36. Marta Jackowska et al., "Short Sleep Duration Is Associated with Shorter Telomere Length in Healthy Men: Findings from the Whitehall II Cohort Study," *PLOS One* 7, no. 10 (2012), doi.org/10.1371/journal.pone.0047292.

37. Edward O. Wilson, *Sociobiology: The New Synthesis* (Cambridge, MA.: Belknap Press, 1975), 6.

38. Saul L. Miller and Jon K. Maner, "Scent of a Woman," *Psychological Science* 21, no. 2 (2010), doi.org/10.1177/0956797609357733.

39. Y. Martins et al., "Preference for Human Body Odors Is Influenced by Gender and Sexual Orientation," *Psychological Science* 16, no. 9 (2005), doi.org/10 .1111/j.1467-9280.2005.01598.x.

40. R. H. Porter and J. Winberg, "Unique Salience of Maternal Breast Odors for Newborn Infants," *Neuroscience and Biobehavioral Reviews* 23, no. 3 (1999), doi.org/10.1016/s0149-7634(98)00044-x.

41. S. Gelstein et al., "Human Tears Contain a Chemosignal," *Science* 331, no. 6014 (2011), doi.org/10.1126/science.1198331.

42. David T. Hughes and Vanessa Sperandio, "Inter-Kingdom Signalling: Communication Between Bacteria and Their Hosts," *Nature Reviews Microbiology* 6, no. 2 (2008), doi.org/10.1038/nrmicro1836.

43. H. Ueda, Y. Kikuta, and K. Matsuda, "Plant Communication: Mediated by Individual or Blended Vocs?," *Plant Signaling and Behavior* 7, no. 2 (2012), doi .org/10.4161/psb.18765.

44. Jessa H. Thurman, Tobin D. Northfield, and William E. Snyder, "Weaver Ants Provide Ecosystem Services to Tropical Tree Crops," *Frontiers in Ecology and Evolution* 7 (2019), doi.org/10.3389/fevo.2019.00120.

45. M. Gagliano et al., "Tuned In: Plant Roots Use Sound to Locate Water," *Oecologia* 184, no. 1 (2017), doi.org/10.1007/s00442-017-3862-z.

46. Alexandra E. Proshchina et al., "Ontogeny of Neuro-Insular Complexes and Islets Innervation in the Human Pancreas," *Frontiers in Endocrinology*, April 22, 2014, doi.org/10.3389/fendo.2014.00057.

47. L. Gwei-Djen and J. Needham, "Medieval Preparations of Urinary Steroid Hormones," *Nature* 200 (1963), doi.org/10.1038/2001047a0.

48. Kaviraj Kunjlal Bhishagratna, *An English Translation of the Sushruta Samhita, Based on Original Sansrkit Text* (Calcutta: Kaviraj Kunjlal Bhishagratna, 1911), vol. 2.

49. Perry Jones, "The History of Women's Liberation in Choral Music," *Choral Journal* 16, no. 6 (1976).

50. J. S. Jenkins, "The Lost Voice: A History of the Castrato," *Journal of Pediatric Endocrinology and Metabolism* 13, suppl. 6 (2000), doi.org/10.1515/jpem-2000-s625.

51. D. Nugent, "Transplantation in Reproductive Medicine: Previous Experience, Present Knowledge and Future Prospects," *Human Reproduction Update* 3, no. 3 (1997), doi.org/10.1093/humupd/3.3.267; M. Borell, "Brown-Sequard's Organotherapy and Its Appearance in America at the End of the Nineteenth Century," *Bulletin of the History of Medicine* 50, no. 3 (1976), www.ncbi.nlm .nih.gov/pubmed/791406.

52. W. M. Bayliss and E. H. Starling, "The Mechanism of Pancreatic Secretion," *Journal of Physiology* 28, no. 5 (1902), doi.org/10.1113/jphysiol.1902.sp000920.

53. René Descartes, *Selected Correspondence of Descartes,* ed. Jonathan Bennett, 108, www.earlymoderntexts.com/assets/pdfs/descartes1619_2.pdf.

54. Syeda Afroze, "The Physiological Roles of Secretin and Its Receptor," *Annals of Translational Medicine* 1, no. 3 (2012), doi.org/10.3978/j.issn.2305-5839 .2012.12.01.

55. E. H. Starling, "The Croonian Lectures on the Chemical Correlation of the Functions of the Body," *The Lancet* 166, no. 4276 (1905): 340, doi.org/10.1016 /s0140-6736(01)62437-1.

56. Eugen Steinach and Josef Löbel, *Sex and Life; Forty Years of Biological and Medical Experiments* (New York: Viking, 1940). Such treatments continue around the world: Joo Yong Lee and Kang Su Cho, "Chemical Castration for Sexual Offenders: Physicians' Views," *Journal of Korean Medical Science* 28, no. 2 (2013), synapse.koreamed.org/DOIx.php?id = 10.3346%2Fjkms.2013.28 .2.171.

57. Tyler M. Adamson et al., "The Global State of Conversion Therapy—A Preliminary Report and Current Evidence Brief," *SocArXiv Papers* (2020), doi.org /10.31235/osf.io/9ew78.

58. William H. Welch, "The General Pathology of Fever," *New England Journal of Medicine* 118, no. 15 (1888), doi.org/10.1056/nejm188804121181501.

59. Guido Majno, *The Healing Hand: Man and Wound in the Ancient World* (Cambridge, MA: Harvard University Press, 1975).

60. Hilaire J. Thompson, "Fever: A Concept Analysis," *Journal of Advanced Nursing* 51, no. 5 (2005), doi.org/10.1111/j.1365-2648.2005.03520.x.

61. E. Atkins, "Fever: Its History, Cause, and Function," *Yale Journal of Biology and Medicine* 55, no. 3–4 (1982), www.ncbi.nlm.nih.gov/pubmed/6758374.

62. Welch, "General Pathology of Fever."

63. Atkins, "Fever: Its History, Cause."

64. Charles A. Dinarello, "Biology of Interleukin 1," *FASEB Journal* 2, no. 2 (1988), doi.org/10.1096/fasebj.2.2.3277884.

65. Paul Young et al., "Acetaminophen for Fever in Critically Ill Patients with Suspected Infection," *New England Journal of Medicine* 373, no. 23 (2015), doi.org/10.1056/nejmoa1508375.

66. Juliet J. Ray, "Fever: Suppress or Let It Ride?," *Journal of Thoracic Disease* (2015), doi.org/10.3978/j.issn.2072-1439.2015.12.28.

67. M. Shibata, "Hypothalamic Neuronal Responses to Cytokines," *Yale Journal of Biology and Medicine* 63, no. 2 (1990), www.ncbi.nlm.nih.gov/pubmed/2205055.

68. Inbal Goshen and Raz Yirmiya, "Interleukin-1 (IL-1): A Central Regulator of Stress Responses," *Frontiers in Neuroendocrinology* 30, no. 1 (2009), doi.org/10.1016/j.yfrne.2008.10.001.

69. T. Mandrup-Poulsen et al., "Affinity-Purified Human Interleukin I Is Cytotoxic to Isolated Islets of Langerhans," *Diabetologia* 29, no. 1 (1986), doi.org/10.1007/BF02427283.

70. Louise J. Maple-Brown and Denella Hampton, "Indigenous Cultures in Countries with Similar Colonisation Histories Share the Challenge of Intergenerational Diabetes," *Lancet Global Health* 8, no. 5 (2020), doi.org/10.1016/s2214-109x(20)30072; Britt Voaklander et al., "Prevalence of Diabetes in Pregnancy Among Indigenous Women in Australia, Canada, New Zealand, and the USA: A Systematic Review and Meta-Analysis," *Lancet Global Health* 8, no. 5 (2020), doi.org/10.1016/s2214-109x(20)30046-2.

71. Bruce S. McEwen, "Stress, Adaptation, and Disease: Allostasis and Allostatic Load," *Annals of the New York Academy of Sciences* 840, no. 1 (1998), doi.org/10.1111/j.1749-6632.1998.tb09546.x.

72. Josiemer Mattei, Sabrina E. Noel, and Katherine L. Tucker, "A Meat, Processed Meat, and French Fries Dietary Pattern Is Associated with High Allostatic Load in Puerto Rican Older Adults," *Journal of the American Dietetic Association* 111, no. 10 (2011), doi.org/10.1016/j.jada.2011.07.006; Michelle Christian and Gary Gereffi, "The Marketing and Distribution of Fast Food," in *Pediatric Obesity: Etiology, Pathogenesis, and Treatment*, ed. Michael Freemark (New York: Springer, 2010).

73. Errol M. Thomson, "Air Pollution, Stress, and Allostatic Load: Linking Systemic and Central Nervous System Impacts," *Journal of Alzheimer's Disease* 69, no. 3 (2019), doi.org/10.3233/JAD-190015.

74. Ana Isabel Ribeiro et al., "Neighbourhood Socioeconomic Deprivation and Allostatic Load: A Multi-Cohort Study," *Scientific Reports* 9, no. 1 (2019), doi.org/10.1038/s41598-019-45432-4.

75. Lianne Tomfohr et al., "Everyday Discrimination and Nocturnal Blood Pressure Dipping in Black and White Americans," *Psychosomatic Medicine* 72, no. 3 (2010), doi.org/10.1097/psy.0b013e3181d0d8b2.

76. O. Kenrik Duru et al., "Allostatic Load Burden and Racial Disparities in

Mortality," *Journal of the National Medical Association* 104, no. 1 (2012), doi .org/10.1016/S0027-9684(15)30120-6.

77. Joseph Eyer, "Hypertension as a Disease of Modern Society," *International Journal of Health Services* 5, no. 4 (1975), doi.org/10.2190/ut72-3rtx-v0kn-64af; S. Blumenthal and S. L. Kamisar, "The National Heart, Lung, and Blood Institute: Its Commitment to Hypertension," *Pediatric Annals* 6, no. 6 (1977), www .ncbi.nlm.nih.gov/pubmed/865914.

78. Michael Gurven et al., "Does Blood Pressure Inevitably Rise with Age?," *Hypertension* 60, no. 1 (2012), doi.org/10.1161/hypertensionaha.111.189100.

79. Evanthia Diamanti-Kandarakis et al., "Endocrine-Disrupting Chemicals: An Endocrine Society Scientific Statement," *Endocrine Reviews* 30, no. 4 (2009), doi.org/10.1210/er.2009-0002; Cristina Casals-Casas and Béatrice Desvergne, "Endocrine Disruptors: From Endocrine to Metabolic Disruption," *Annual Review of Physiology* 73, no. 1 (2011), doi.org/10.1146/annurev-physiol-012110 -142200.

80. Teresa M. Attina et al., "Exposure to Endocrine-Disrupting Chemicals in the USA: A Population-Based Disease Burden and Cost Analysis," *The Lancet Diabetes and Endocrinology* 4, no. 12 (2016), doi.org/10.1016/s2213 -8587(16)30275-3.

81. Åke Bergman et al., *State of the Science of Endocrine Disrupting Chemicals 2012* (Geneva: World Health Organization, 2013).

82. Barbara Casassus, "Hormone Disrupting Chemicals: Slow Progress to Regulation," *BMJ* 361 (2018), doi.org/10.1136/bmj.k1876.

83. Stéphane Horel, *A Toxic Affair: How the Chemical Lobby Blocked Action on Hormone Disrupting Chemicals* (Paris: Corporate Europe Observatory, 2015), corporateeurope.org/sites/default/files/toxic_lobby_edc.pdf.

84. Casassus, "Hormone Disrupting Chemicals."

85. Yan Zheng, Sylvia H. Ley, and Frank B. Hu, "Global Aetiology and Epidemiology of Type 2 Diabetes Mellitus and Its Complications." *Nature Reviews Endocrinology* 14, no. 2 (2018), doi.org/10.1038/nrendo.2017.151; E. C. Rhodes, U. P. Gujral, and K. M. Narayan, "Mysteries of Type 2 Diabetes: The Indian Elephant Meets the Chinese Dragon," *European Journal of Clinical Nutrition* 71, no. 7 (2017), doi.org/10.1038/ejcn.2017.93.

86. Bernard Srour et al., "Ultraprocessed Food Consumption and Risk of Type 2 Diabetes Among Participants of the Nutrinet-Santé Prospective Cohort," *JAMA Internal Medicine* 180, no. 2 (2020), doi.org/10.1001/jamainternmed .2019.5942.

87. Robin Anderson, "Diabetes in Gitxaala: Colonization, Assimilation and Economic Change," M.A. thesis, University of British Colombia, 2007; Kristen M. Jacklin et al., "Health Care Experiences of Indigenous People Living with Type 2 Diabetes in Canada," *CMAJ: Canadian Medical Association Journal* 189, no. 3 (2017), doi.org/10.1503/cmaj.161098; Odette R. Gibson and Leonie Segal, "Limited Evidence to Assess the Impact of Primary Health Care System or Service Level Attributes on Health Outcomes of Indigenous People with Type 2 Diabetes: A Systematic Review," *BMC Health Services Research* 15, no. 1 (2015), doi.org/10.1186/s12913-015-0803-6.

88. Jennifer L. Harris et al., *Sugary Drink Advertising to Youth: Continued Barrier to Public Health Progress*, (Storrs, CT: Rudd Center for Food Policy and Obesity, 2020), tinyurl.com/33xrkp67.

89. Hector Balcazar and Ana Bertha Perez Lizaur, "Sugar-Sweetened Soda Consumption in Mexico: The Translation of Accumulating Evidence for an Increasing Diabetes Risk in Mexican Women," *Journal of Nutrition* 149, no. 5 (2019), doi.org/10.1093/jn/nxz007.

90. Elisabeth Donaldson, *Advocating for Sugar-Sweetened Beverage Taxation: A Case Study of Mexico* (Baltimore: Johns Hopkins Bloomberg School of Public Health, 2015).

91. Luz Maria Sánchez-Romero et al., "Projected Impact of Mexico's Sugar-Sweetened Beverage Tax Policy on Diabetes and Cardiovascular Disease: A Modeling Study," *PLOS Medicine* 13, no. 11 (2016), doi.org/10.1371/journal .pmed.1002158.

92. John Scott-Railton et al., "Bitter Sweet: Supporters of Mexico's Soda Tax Targeted with NSO Exploit Links," University of Toronto, 2017, tspace.library.utoronto.ca /bitstream/1807/96730/1/Report%2389—bittersweet.pdf; Nicole Perlroth, "Spyware's Odd Targets: Backers of Mexico's Soda Tax," *The New York Times*, February 12, 2017, A1. tinyurl.com/10cuyah6.

93. Cristin E. Kearns, Stanton A. Glantz, and Laura A. Schmidt, "Sugar Industry Influence on the Scientific Agenda of the National Institute of Dental Research's 1971 National Caries Program: A Historical Analysis of Internal Documents," *PLOS Medicine* 12, no. 3 (2015), doi.org/10.1371/journal.pmed .1001798; Robert Proctor, *Golden Holocaust: Origins of the Cigarette Catastrophe and the Case for Abolition* (Berkeley: University of California Press, 2011); D. Stuckler et al., "The Health Effects of the Global Financial Crisis: Can We Reconcile the Differing Views? A Network Analysis of Literature Across Disciplines," *Health Economics, Policy and Law* 10, no. 1 (2015), doi.org/10 .1017/S1744133114000255; and in particular Marion Nestle, *Unsavory Truth: How Food Companies Skew the Science of What We Eat* (New York: Basic Books, 2018).

94. Stéphane Foucart and Stéphane Horel, "Perturbateurs endocriniens: Ces experts contestés qui jouent ses semeurs de doute," *Le Monde*, June 22, 2020, tinyurl.com/3a5v2mns.

95. Legal threats are among the tactics deployed. Happily, the tobacco and soda industries are running into a losing streak, though this doesn't seem to have prevented the threats against government around litigation. Soraya Boudia and Nathalie Jas, *Powerless Science?: Science and Politics in a Toxic World* (New York: Berghahn Books, 2014); Eric Crosbie, Angela Carriedo, and Laura A. Schmidt, "Hollow Threats: Transnational Food and Beverage Companies' Use of International Agreements to Fight Front-of-Pack Nutrition Labeling in Mexico and Beyond," *International Journal of Health Policy and Management* (forthcoming), doi.org/10.34172/ijhpm.2020.146.

96. Susan Y. Euling et al., "Examination of US Puberty-Timing Data from 1940 to 1994 for Secular Trends: Panel Findings," *Pediatrics* 121, suppl. 3 (2008), doi .org/10.1542/peds.2007-1813D.

97. Alexandra M. Binder et al., "Childhood and Adolescent Phenol and Phthalate Exposure and the Age of Menarche in Latina Girls," *Environmental Health* 17, no. 1 (2018), doi.org/10.1186/s12940-018-0376-z; Ji Hyun Kim and Jung Sub Lim, "Early Menarche and Its Consequence in Korean Female: Reducing Fructose Intake Could Be One Solution," *Clinical and Experimental Pediatrics* 64, no. 1 (2020), doi.org/10.3345/cep.2019.00353; G. M. Skutsch, "Role of

Artificial Lighting in Decreasing the Age of Menarche," *The Lancet* 2, no. 7672 (1970), doi.org/10.1016/s0140-6736(70)91379-6.

98. *World Urbanization Prospects: The 2009 Revision* (New York: United Nations, 2009).

99. C. M. Law, "The Growth of Urban Population in England and Wales, 1801–1911," *Transactions of the Institute of British Geographers*, no. 41 (1967), doi.org/10.2307/621331.

100. Mark J. Bouman, "Luxury and Control: The Urbanity of Street Lighting in Nineteenth-Century Cities," *Journal of Urban History* 14, no. 1 (1987). While the Chinese figured out how to use bamboo to pipe in natural gas to light up homes as early as AD 347, it took Europeans till the eighteenth century to start illuminating their public lives with gas lamps. Peter James, *Ancient Inventions* (New York: Ballantine Books, 1994). In the 1600s in Paris, streetlamps consisted of candles enclosed by glass on iron posts, lit each night by a lamplighter. Thousands of these lamps, which covered all of Paris's 912 streets, were a policing technology. During that era in France, the perception of police shifted from general administrators to their modern authoritarian identity, "seen as the executors of absolutist power, control, and repression." Woflgang Schivelbusch, "The Policing of Street Lighting," *Yale French Studies* no. 73 (1987), doi.org/10.2307/2930197. The public lighting system as carried out by the police in Paris became a symbol of that oppressive presence and the change of the streets from a place that extended conviviality from one's home into public to a space to be kept lawful and orderly.

101. William Rowan, "Light and Seasonal Reproduction in Animals," *Biological Reviews* 13, no. 4 (1938), doi.org/10.1111/j.1469-185x.1938.tb00523.x.

102. Kristen J. Navara and Randy J. Nelson, "The Dark Side of Light at Night: Physiological, Epidemiological, and Ecological Consequences," *Journal of Pineal Research* 43, no. 3 (2007), doi.org/10.1111/j.1600-079X.2007.00473.x.

103. Kathleen E. West et al., "Blue Light from Light-Emitting Diodes Elicits a Dose-Dependent Suppression of Melatonin in Humans," *Journal of Applied Physiology* 110, no. 3 (2010), doi.org/10.1152/japplphysiol.01413.2009.

104. Jenny Q. Ouyang, Scott Davies, and Davide Dominoni, "Hormonally Mediated Effects of Artificial Light at Night on Behavior and Fitness: Linking Endocrine Mechanisms with Function," *Journal of Experimental Biology* 221, no. 6 (2018), doi.org/10.1242/jeb.156893.

105. Mathieu Troïanowski et al., "Effects of Traffic Noise on Tree Frog Stress Levels, Immunity, and Color Signaling," *Conservation Biology* 31, no. 3 (2017), doi.org/10.1111/cobi.12893.

106. Demian Halperin, "Environmental Noise and Sleep Disturbances: A Threat to Health?," *Sleep Science* 7, no. 4 (2014), doi.org/10.1016/j.slsci.2014.11.003.

107. Mette Sørensen et al., "Long-Term Exposure to Road Traffic Noise and Incident Diabetes: A Cohort Study," *Environmental Health Perspectives* 121, no. 2 (2013), doi.org/doi:10.1289/ehp.1205503.

108. Charlotte Hurtley, *Night Noise Guidelines for Europe* (Copenhagen: WHO Regional Office Europe, 2009).

109. Joan A. Casey et al., "Race/Ethnicity, Socioeconomic Status, Residential Segregation, and Spatial Variation in Noise Exposure in the Contiguous United States," *Environmental Health Perspectives* 125, no. 7 (2017), doi.org/doi:10.1289/EHP898.

110. Wazir Alam, "GIS Based Assessment of Noise Pollution in Guwahati City of

Assam, India," *International Journal of Environmental Sciences* 2, no. 2 (2011), tinyurl.com/1tjxzvtm; N. Garg et al., "A Pilot Study on the Establishment of National Ambient Noise Monitoring Network across the Major Cities of India," *Applied Acoustics* 103, pt. A (2016), doi.org/10.1016/j.apacoust.2015.09.010.

111. Miller McPherson, Lynn Smith-Lovin, and Matthew E. Brashears, "Social Isolation in America: Changes in Core Discussion Networks over Two Decades," *American Sociological Review* 71, no. 3 (2006), doi.org/10.1177/000312240607100301.

112. John T. Cacioppo, Stephanie Cacioppo, and Dorret I. Boomsma, "Evolutionary Mechanisms for Loneliness," *Cognition and Emotion* 28, no. 1 (2014), doi.org/10.1080/02699931.2013.837379.

113. Oliver Gruebner, "Cities and Mental Health," *Deutches Ärtzeblatt International* 114 (2017), doi.org/10.3238/arztebl.2017.0121.

114. V. H. Menec et al., "Examining Individual and Geographic Factors Associated with Social Isolation and Loneliness Using Canadian Longitudinal Study on Aging (CLSA) Data," *PLOS One* 14, no. 2 (2019), doi.org/10.1371/journal.pone.0211143.

115. Pamela Qualter et al., "Loneliness Across the Life Span," *Perspectives on Psychological Science* 10, no. 2 (2015), doi.org/10.1177/1745691615568999.

116. John T. Cacioppo et al., "The Neuroendocrinology of Social Isolation," *Annual Review of Psychology* 66, no. 1 (2015), doi.org/10.1146/annurev-psych-010814-015240; Inbal Goshen and Raz Yirmiya, "Interleukin-1 (IL-1): A Central Regulator of Stress Responses," *Frontiers in Neuroendocrinology* 30, no. 1 (2009), doi.org/10.1016/j.yfrne.2008.10.001.

117. A. Cheema et al., "Urbanization and Prevalence of Type 2 Diabetes in Southern Asia: A Systematic Analysis," *Journal of Global Health* 4, no. 1 (2014), doi.org/10.7189/jogh.04.010404; Matthew J. Salois, "Obesity and Diabetes, the Built Environment, and the 'Local' Food Economy in the United States, 2007," *Economics and Human Biology* 10, no. 1 (2012), doi.org/10.1016/j.ehb.2011.04.001; John E. Stewart et al., "Diabetes and the Socioeconomic and Built Environment: Geovisualization of Disease Prevalence and Potential Contextual Associations Using Ring Maps," *International Journal of Health Geographics* 10, no. 1 (2011), doi.org/10.1186/1476-072x-10-18.

118. H. Tilg and A. R. Moschen, "Adipocytokines: Mediators Linking Adipose Tissue, Inflammation and Immunity," *Nature Reviews Immunology* 6, no. 10 (2006), doi.org/10.1038/nri1937.

119. Rajita Sinha, "Chronic Stress, Drug Use, and Vulnerability to Addiction," *Annals of the New York Academy of Sciences* 1141, no. 1 (2008), doi.org/10.1196/annals.1441.030.

120. A. Verdejo-Garcia et al., "Negative Emotion-Driven Impulsivity Predicts Substance Dependence Problems," *Drug and Alcohol Dependence* 91, no. 2–3 (2007), doi.org/10.1016/j.drugalcdep.2007.05.

121. M. D. Anestis, E. A. Selby, and T. E. Joiner, "The Role of Urgency in Maladaptive Behaviors," *Behaviour Research and Therapy* 45, no. 12 (2007), doi.org/10.1016/j.brat.2007.08.012.

122. C. S. Li and R. Sinha, "Inhibitory Control and Emotional Stress Regulation: Neuroimaging Evidence for Frontal-Limbic Dysfunction in Psycho-Stimulant Addiction," *Neuroscience and Biobehavioral Reviews* 32, no. 3 (2008), doi.org/10.1016/j.neubiorev.2007.10.003.

123. David T. Courtwright, *The Age of Addiction: How Bad Habits Became Big Business* (Cambridge, MA: Belknap Press, 2019).

124. Frederik Stjernfelt and Anne Mette Lauritzen, *Your Post Has Been Removed: Tech Giants and Freedom of Speech* (Cham, Switzerland: Springer International, 2020), 48.

125. Tim Wu, *The Attention Merchants: The Epic Scramble to Get Inside Our Heads* (New York: Vintage, 2017).

126. A. Danese et al., "Adverse Childhood Experiences and Adult Risk Factors for Age-Related Disease: Depression, Inflammation, and Clustering of Metabolic Risk Markers," *Archives of Pediatrics and Adolescent Medicine* 163, no. 12 (2009), doi.org/10.1001/archpediatrics.2009.214; M. Chen and R. E. Lacey, "Adverse Childhood Experiences and Adult Inflammation: Findings from the 1958 British Birth Cohort," *Brain, Behavior and Immunity* 69 (2018), doi.org/10.1016/j.bbi .2018.02.007; N. A. John-Henderson et al., "Adverse Childhood Experiences and Immune System Inflammation in Adults Residing on the Blackfeet Reservation: The Moderating Role of Sense of Belonging to the Community," *Annals of Behavioral Medicine* (2019), doi.org/10.1093/abm/kaz029; E. Flouri et al., "Prenatal and Childhood Adverse Life Events, Inflammation and Depressive Symptoms Across Adolescence," *Journal of Affective Disorders* 260 (2019), doi .org/10.1016/j.jad.2019.09.024; E. Vasquez et al., "Association Between Adverse Childhood Events and Multimorbidity in a Racial and Ethnic Diverse Sample of Middle-Aged and Older Adults," *Innovation in Aging* 3, no. 2 (2019), doi.org /10.1093/geroni/igz016; J. P. Gouin et al., "Resilience Resources Moderate the Association of Adverse Childhood Experiences with Adulthood Inflammation," *Annals of Behavioral Medicine* 51, no. 5 (2017), doi.org/10.1007/s12160-017-9891 -3; T. W. McDade, "Early Environments and the Ecology of Inflammation," *Proceedings of the National Academy of Sciences of the United States of America* 109, suppl. 2 (2012), doi.org/10.1073/pnas.1202244109.

127. S. E. Nennig and J. R. Schank, "The Role of NFKB in Drug Addiction: Beyond Inflammation," *Alcohol and Alcoholism* 52, no. 2 (2017), doi.org/10.1093/alcalc /agw098.

128. M. R. Lashkarizadeh et al., "Impact of Opium Addiction on Levels of Pro- and Anti-Inflammatory Cytokines After Surgery," *Addiction and Health* 8, no. 1 (2016), www.ncbi.nlm.nih.gov/pubmed/27274788; Nennig and Schank, "Role of NFKB in Drug Addiction."

129. W. Kim et al., "The Effect of Cognitive Behavior Therapy-Based Psychotherapy Applied in a Forest Environment on Physiological Changes and Remission of Major Depressive Disorder," *Psychiatry Investigation* 6, no. 4 (2009), doi.org/10.4306/pi.2009.6.4.245.

130. Jeffrey M. Craig, Alan C. Logan, and Susan L. Prescott, "Natural Environments, Nature Relatedness and the Ecological Theater: Connecting Satellites and Sequencing to Shinrin-Yoku," *Journal of Physiological Anthropology* 35, no. 1 (2016), doi.org/10.1186/s40101-016-0083-9; Margaret M. Hansen, Reo Jones, and Kirsten Tocchini, "Shinrin-Yoku (Forest Bathing) and Nature Therapy: A State-of-the-Art Review," *International Journal of Environmental Research and Public Health* 14, no. 8 (2017), doi.org/10.3390/ijerph14080851.

131. G. Gimpl and F. Fahrenholz, "The Oxytocin Receptor System: Structure, Function, and Regulation," *Physiological Reviews* 81, no. 2 (2001), doi.org/10 .1152/physrev.2001.81.2.629.

132. R. Hurlemann et al., "Oxytocin Enhances Amygdala-Dependent, Socially Reinforced Learning and Emotional Empathy in Humans," *Journal of Neuroscience* 30, no. 14 (2010), doi.org/10.1523/jneurosci.5538-09.2010.

133. H. Shen, "Neuroscience: The Hard Science of Oxytocin," *Nature* 522, no. 7557 (2015), doi.org/10.1038/522410a.

134. D. Wei et al., "Endocannabinoid Signaling Mediates Oxytocin-Driven Social Reward," *Proceedings of the National Academy of Sciences of the United States of America* 112, no. 45 (2015), doi.org/10.1073/pnas.1509795112.

135. Gimpl and Fahrenholz, "Oxytocin Receptor System."

136. V. Morhenn, L. E. Beavin, and P. J. Zak, "Massage Increases Oxytocin and Reduces Adrenocorticotropin Hormone in Humans," *Alternative Therapies in Health and Medicine* 18, no. 6 (2012), www.ncbi.nlm.nih.gov/pubmed/23251939.

137. Markus Heinrichs et al., "Social Support and Oxytocin Interact to Suppress Cortisol and Subjective Responses to Psychosocial Stress," *Biological Psychiatry* 54, no. 12 (2003), doi.org/10.1016/s0006-3223(03)00465-7; Kerstin Uvnäs-Moberg and Maria Petersson, "Oxytocin, a Mediator of Anti-Stress, Well-Being, Social Interaction, Growth and Healing," *Zeitschrift für Psychosomatische Medizin und Psychotherapie* 51, no. 1 (2005), doi.org/10.13109/zptm.2005.51.1.57; Lauren M. Sippel et al., "Oxytocin and Stress-Related Disorders: Neurobiological Mechanisms and Treatment Opportunities," *Chronic Stress* 1 (2017), doi.org/10.1177/2470547016687996.

138. M. Clodi et al., "Oxytocin Alleviates the Neuroendocrine and Cytokine Response to Bacterial Endotoxin in Healthy Men," *American Journal of Physiology-Endocrinology and Metabolism* 295, no. 3 (2008), doi.org/10.1152/ajpendo.90263.2008; Tong Li et al., "Approaches Mediating Oxytocin Regulation of the Immune System," *Frontiers in Immunology* 7 (2017), doi.org/10.3389/fimmu.2016.00693.

139. C. K. W. De Dreu et al., "Oxytocin Promotes Human Ethnocentrism," *Proceedings of the National Academy of Sciences of the United States of America* 108, no. 4 (2011), doi.org/10.1073/pnas.1015316108; Simone G. Shamay-Tsoory et al., "Giving Peace a Chance: Oxytocin Increases Empathy to Pain in the Context of the Israeli–Palestinian Conflict," *Psychoneuroendocrinology* 38, no. 12 (2013), doi.org/10.1016/j.psyneuen.2013.09.015.

140. Paul J. Zak, Angela A. Stanton, and Sheila Ahmadi, "Oxytocin Increases Generosity in Humans," *PLOS One* 2, no. 11 (2007), doi.org/10.1371/journal.pone.0001128; Michael Kosfeld et al., "Oxytocin Increases Trust in Humans," *Nature* 435, no. 7042 (2005), doi.org/10.1038/nature03701; Gregor Domes et al., "Oxytocin Improves 'Mind-Reading' in Humans," *Biological Psychiatry* 61, no. 6 (2007), doi.org/10.1016/j.biopsych.2006.07.015.

141. Carolyn H. Declerck, Christopher Boone, and Toko Kiyonari, "Oxytocin and Cooperation Under Conditions of Uncertainty: The Modulating Role of Incentives and Social Information," *Hormones and Behavior* 57, no. 3 (2010), doi.org/10.1016/j.yhbeh.2010.01.006.

142. Yina Ma et al., "Opposing Oxytocin Effects on Intergroup Cooperative Behavior in Intuitive and Reflective Minds," *Neuropsychopharmacology* 40, no. 10 (2015), doi.org/10.1038/npp.2015.87.

143. Mona Lisa Chanda and Daniel J. Levitin, "The Neurochemistry of Music," *Trends in Cognitive Sciences* 17, no. 4 (2013), doi.org/10.1016/j.tics.2013.02.007.

144. J. R. Keeler et al., "The Neurochemistry and Social Flow of Singing: Bonding

and Oxytocin," *Frontiers in Human Neuroscience* 9 (2015), doi.org/10.3389/fnhum .2015.00518.

145. Constantina Theofanopoulou, "A Hypothesis on a Role of Oxytocin in the Social Mechanisms of Speech and Vocal Learning," *Proceedings of the Royal Society B: Biological Sciences* 284, no. 1861 (2017), doi.org/10.1098/rspb.2017.0988.

146. Kerstin Uvnäs-Moberg, Linda Handlin, and Maria Petersson, "Self-Soothing Behaviors with Particular Reference to Oxytocin Release Induced by Non-Noxious Sensory Stimulation," *Frontiers in Psychology* 5 (2015), doi.org/10 .3389/fpsyg.2014.01529.

147. Shen, "Neuroscience."

148. Gideon Nave, Colin Camerer, and Michael McCullough, "Does Oxytocin Increase Trust in Humans? A Critical Review of Research," *Perspectives on Psychological Science* 10, no. 6 (2015), doi.org/10.1177/1745691615600138.

149. Peter Singer, *Animal Liberation: A New Ethics for Our Treatment of Animals* (New York: New York Review, 1975).

150. Lucette Flandroy et al., "The Impact of Human Activities and Lifestyles on the Interlinked Microbiota and Health of Humans and of Ecosystems," *Science of the Total Environment* 627 (2018), doi.org/10.1016/j.scitotenv.2018.01.288.

151. Brenda M. Restoule, *The Soul Wounds of the Anishinabek People* (2013), issuu .com/anishinabeknews/docs/soul_wounds_booklet.

152. Richard Henry Pratt, "The Advantages of Mingling Indians with Whites" (1892), in *Americanizing the American Indians: Writings by "Friends of the Indian" 1800–1900*, ed. Francis Paul Prucha (Cambridge, MA: Harvard University Press, 1973).

153. Restoule, *Soul Wounds of Anishinabek People*.

154. Katherine Pettipas, *Severing the Ties That Bind: Government Repression of Indigenous Religious Ceremonies on the Prairies* (Winnipeg: University of Manitoba Press, 1994).

155. D. H. Whalen, Margaret Moss, and Daryl Baldwin, "Healing Through Language: Positive Physical Health Effects of Indigenous Language Use," *F1000Research* 5 (2016), doi.org/10.12688/f1000research.8656.1.

156. Constantina Theofanopoulou, Cedric Boeckx, and Erich D. Jarvis, "A Hypothesis on a Role of Oxytocin in the Social Mechanisms of Speech and Vocal Learning," *Proceedings of the Royal Society B: Biological Sciences* 284, no. 1861 (2017), doi.org/10.1098/rspb.2017.0988.

157. R. T. Oster et al., "Cultural Continuity, Traditional Indigenous Language, and Diabetes in Alberta First Nations: A Mixed Methods Study," *International Journal for Equity in Health* 13 (2014), doi.org/10.1186/s12939-014-0092-4.

158. Darcy Hallett, Michael J. Chandler, and Christopher E. Lalonde, "Aboriginal Language Knowledge and Youth Suicide," *Cognitive Development* 22, no. 3 (2007), doi.org/10.1016/j.cogdev.2007.02.001.

159. Oster et al., "Cultural Continuity," 6.

160. Kandice Grossman, "Tigerswan at Standing Rock: Ethics of Private Military Use Against an Environmental-Justice Movement," *Case Studies in the Environment* 3, no. 1 (2019), doi.org/10.1525/cse.2019.002139.

8. NERVOUS SYSTEM

1. Lisa Kemmerer, *Sister Species: Women, Animals, and Social Justice* (Chicago: University of Illinois Press, 2011), 16.

2. Scott F. Gilbert, Jan Sapp, and Alfred I. Tauber, "A Symbiotic View of Life: We Have Never Been Individuals," *Quarterly Review of Biology* 87, no. 4 (2012), doi.org/10.1086/668166.

3. René Dietrich, "'Pando/Pando' Across the Americas: Transnational Settler Territorialities and Decolonial Pluralities," *Journal of Transnational American Studies* 11, no. 1 (2020), escholarship.org/uc/item/6g60x78r.

4. Bret Gustafson, "Bolivia 9/11: Bodies and Power on a Feudal Frontier," *Caterwaul Quarterly*, July 14, 2009, tinyurl.com/1uu4giuq.

5. The US media were, of course, involved. Glenn Greenwald, "*The New York Times* Admits Key Falsehoods That Drove Last Year's Coup in Bolivia: Falsehoods Peddled by the U.S., Its Media, and the *Times*," *The Intercept*, June 8, 2020, tinyurl.com/5gon2y67.

6. Lucien Chauvin and Anthony Faiola, "As the U.S.-Backed Government in Bolivia Unleashes a Wave of Political Persecution, the Trump Administration Remains Silent," *The Washington Post*, March 6 2020, tinyurl.com/slmd5nmc.

7. Maribel Aponte-García, "Bolivia: A World Power in Lithium, the Coup d'État and the Dispute for Technological Supremacy Between the USA and China 1," *Journal of Applied Business and Economics* 22, no. 3 (2020); Thea N. Riofrancos, *Resource Radicals: From Petro-Nationalism to Post-Extractivism in Ecuador* (Durham, NC: Duke University Press, 2020).

8. Kate Aronoff, "The Socialist Win in Bolivia and the New Era of Lithium Extraction," *New Republic*, October 19, 2020, tinyurl.com/d05eofgq.

9. Jennifer DeWoody et al., "'Pando' Lives: Molecular Genetic Evidence of a Giant Aspen Clone in Central Utah," *Western North American Naturalist* 68, no. 4 (2008), tinyurl.com/i1us3dj3; Paul C. Rogers and Jody A. Gale, "Restoration of the Iconic Pando Aspen Clone: Emerging Evidence of Recovery," *Ecosphere* 8, no. 1 (2017), doi.org/10.1002/ecs2.1661; Paul C. Rogers and Darren J. McAvoy, "Mule Deer Impede Pando's Recovery: Implications for Aspen Resilience from a Single-Genotype Forest," *PLOS One* 13, no. 10 (2018), doi.org/10.1371/journal.pone.0203619.

10. Sherwin Bitsui and Allison Adelle Hedge Coke, "A Couple of Poets Passing Time, December," Association of Writers and Writing Programs, 2021, www.awpwriter.org/community_calendar/spotlight_view/bitsui_hedgecoke.

11. The timeline is still being debated. Birger Rasmussen et al., "Reassessing the First Appearance of Eukaryotes and Cyanobacteria," *Nature* 455, no. 7216 (2008), doi.org/10.1038/nature07381.

12. Lawrence A. David and Eric J. Alm, "Rapid Evolutionary Innovation During an Archaean Genetic Expansion," *Nature* 469, no. 7328 (2011), doi.org/10.1038/nature09649.

13. K. Luby-Phelps, "Cytoarchitecture and Physical Properties of Cytoplasm: Volume, Viscosity, Diffusion, Intracellular Surface Area," *International Review of Cytology* 192 (2000), doi.org/10.1016/s0074-7696(08)60527-6.

14. Eugene V. Koonin, "Origin of Eukaryotes from Within Archaea, Archaeal Eukaryome and Bursts of Gene Gain: Eukaryogenesis Just Made Easier?," *Philosophical Transactions of the Royal Society B: Biological Sciences* 370, no. 1678 (2015), doi.org/10.1098/rstb.2014.0333.

15. Verena Zimorski et al., "Endosymbiotic Theory for Organelle Origins," *Current Opinion in Microbiology* 22 (2014), doi.org/10.1016/j.mib.2014.09.008.

16. Y. M. Bar-On, R. Phillips, and R. Milo, "The Biomass Distribution on Earth,"

Proceedings of the National Academy of Sciences of the United States of America 115, no. 25 (2018): 6506–11. doi.org/10.1073/pnas.1711842115.

17. A. Pietryczuk et al., "Abundance and Species Diversity of Fungi in Rivers with Various Contaminations," *Current Microbiology* 75 (2017), doi.org/10.1007 /s00284-017-1427-3; Katja Sterflinger, Donatella Tesei, and Kristina Zakharova, "Fungi in Hot and Cold Deserts with Particular Reference to Microcolonial Fungi," *Fungal Ecology* 5, no. 4 (2012), doi.org/10.1016/j.funeco.2011.12.007; R. S. Redman et al., "Thermotolerance Generated by Plant/Fungal Symbiosis," *Science* 298, no. 5598 (2002), doi.org/10.1126/science.1072191; M. Ivarsson, S. Bengtson, and A. Neubeck, "The Igneous Oceanic Crust—Earth's Largest Fungal Habitat?," *Fungal Ecology* 20 (2016), doi.org/10.1016/j.funeco.2016.01.009.

18. Jennifer Frazer, "The World's Largest Mining Operation Is Run by Fungi," *Scientific American*, November 5, 2015, blogs.scientificamerican.com/artful -amoeba/the-world-s-largest-mining-operation-is-run-by-fungi/.

19. Lynn Margulis and Eva Barreno, "Looking at Lichens," *BioScience* 53, no. 8 (2003), doi.org/10.1641/0006-3568(2003)053[0776:LAL]2.0.CO;2.

20. David Griffiths, "Queer Theory for Lichens," *UnderCurrents: Journal of Critical Environmental Studies* 19 (2015).

21. Brian D. Fath, Carly A. Dean, and Harald Katzmair, "Navigating the Adaptive Cycle: An Approach to Managing the Resilience of Social Systems," *Ecology and Society* 20, no. 2 (2015), doi.org/10.5751/es-07467-200224.

22. Michael S. A. Graziano and Sabine Kastner, "Human Consciousness and Its Relationship to Social Neuroscience: A Novel Hypothesis," *Cognitive Neuroscience* 2, no. 2 (2011), doi.org/10.1080/17588928.2011.565121.

23. Eric Kandel, James Schwartz, and Thomas Jessell, *Principles of Neural Science*, 4th ed. (New York: McGraw-Hill Medical, 2000).

24. Frederico A. C. Azevedo et al., "Equal Numbers of Neuronal and Nonneuronal Cells Make the Human Brain an Isometrically Scaled-up Primate Brain," *Journal of Comparative Neurology* 513, no. 5 (2009), doi.org/10.1002/cne.21974.

25. Kandel, Schwartz, and Jessell, *Principles of Neural Science*.

26. Douglass Godwin, Robert L. Barry, and René Marois, "Breakdown of the Brain's Functional Network Modularity with Awareness," *Proceedings of the National Academy of Sciences of the United States of America* 112, no. 12 (2015), doi.org/10.1073/pnas.1414466112; Todd E. Feinberg and Jon Mallatt, "Phenomenal Consciousness and Emergence: Eliminating the Explanatory Gap," *Frontiers in Psychology* 11 (2020), doi.org/10.3389/fpsyg.2020.01041; Francis Crick and Christof Koch, "Consciousness and Neuroscience," *Cerebral Cortex* 8 (1998), authors.library.caltech.edu/40355/1/feature_article.pdf ; S. Dehaene, "Towards a Cognitive Neuroscience of Consciousness: Basic Evidence and a Workspace Framework," *Cognition* 79, no. 1–2 (2001), doi.org/10.1016/s0010 -0277(00)00123-2.

27. Graziano and Kastner, "Human Consciousness and Its Relationship."

28. Kandel, Schwartz, and Jessell, *Principles of Neural Science*; Geoffrey Hinton, "Neural Networks Learn from Experience," *Scientific American* 267, no. 3 (1992), jstor.org/stable/24939221.

29. Olaf Sporns and Richard F. Betzel, "Modular Brain Networks," *Annual Review of Psychology* 67, no. 1 (2016), doi.org/10.1146/annurev-psych-122414-033634.

30. Hinton, "Neural Networks Learn."

31. Jeffrey L. Elman, "Learning and Development in Neural Networks: The Im-

portance of Starting Small," *Cognition* 48, no. 1 (1993), doi.org/10.1016/0010
-0277(93)90058-4.

32. Johan Mårtensson et al., "Growth of Language-Related Brain Areas after
    Foreign Language Learning," *NeuroImage* 63, no. 1 (2012), doi.org/10.1016/j
    .neuroimage.2012.06.043

33. Matúš Adamkovič and Marcel Martončik, "A Review of Consequences of Pov-
    erty on Economic Decision-Making: A Hypothesized Model of a Cognitive
    Mechanism," *Frontiers in Psychology* 8 (2017), doi.org/10.3389/fpsyg.2017.01784;
    A. K. Shah, S. Mullainathan, and E. Shafir, "Some Consequences of Having Too
    Little," *Science* 338, no. 6107 (2012), doi.org/10.1126/science.1222426.

34. Mark Neocleous, "Resisting Resilience," *Radical Philosophy* 178, no. 6 (2013).

35. Elif Eyigoz et al., "Linguistic Markers Predict Onset of Alzheimer's Disease,"
    EClinicalMedicine 28 (2020), doi.org/10.1016/j.eclinm.2020.100583.

36. Henry W. Querfurth and Frank M. Laferla, "Alzheimer's Disease," *New En-
    gland Journal of Medicine* 362, no. 4 (2010), doi.org/10.1056/nejmra0909142.

37. *Alzheimer's Facts and Figures* (Chicago: Alzheimer's Association, 2020), www
    .alz.org/media/Documents/alzheimers-facts-and-figures_1.pdf.

38. Wilfred F. A. Den Dunnen et al., "No Disease in the Brain of a 115-Year-Old
    Woman," *Neurobiology of Aging* 29, no. 8 (2008), doi.org/10.1016/j.neurobiolaging
    .2008.04.010.

39. Kelly Del Tredici and Heiko Braak, "Neurofibrillary Changes of the Alzheimer
    Type in Very Elderly Individuals: Neither Inevitable nor Benign," *Neurobiology
    of Aging* 29, no. 8 (2008), doi.org/10.1016/j.neurobiolaging.2008.04.016.

40. J. A. Hardy and G. A. Higgins, "Alzheimer's Disease: The Amyloid Cascade
    Hypothesis," *Science* 256, no. 5054 (1992), doi.org/10.1126/science.1566067.

41. Michel Goedert, "Tau Protein and the Neurofibrillary Pathology of Alzhei-
    mer's Disease," *Trends in Neurosciences* 16, no. 11 (1993), doi.org/10.1016
    /0166-2236(93)90078-z.

42. Michael F. Egan et al., "Randomized Trial of Verubecestat for Mild-to-
    Moderate Alzheimer's Disease," *New England Journal of Medicine* 378, no. 18
    (2018), doi.org/10.1056/nejmoa1706441.

43. Rachelle S. Doody et al., "A Phase 3 Trial of Semagacestat for Treatment of
    Alzheimer's Disease," *New England Journal of Medicine* 369, no. 4 (2013), doi
    .org/10.1056/nejmoa1210951.

44. Ole Isacson, "The Consequences of Coronavirus-Induced Cytokine Storm
    Are Associated with Neurological Diseases, Which May Be Preventable,"
    Frontiers in Neurology 11 (2020), doi.org/10.3389/fneur.2020.00745.

45. Pam Belluck, "'I Feel Like I Have Dementia': Brain Fog Plagues Covid Survi-
    vors," *The New York Times*, October 11, 2020, tinyurl.com/yb43fdfc.

46. Stephanie J. Soscia et al., "The Alzheimer's Disease-Associated Amyloid B-
    Protein Is an Antimicrobial Peptide," *PLOS One* 5, no. 3 (2010), doi.org/10
    .1371/journal.pone.0009505; Seong-Cheol Park et al., "Functional Character-
    ization of Alpha-Synuclein Protein with Antimicrobial Activity," *Biochemical
    and Biophysical Research Communications* 478, no. 2 (2016), doi.org/10.1016/j
    .bbrc.2016.08.052.

47. Lesley Jones et al., "Genetic Evidence Implicates the Immune System and
    Cholesterol Metabolism in the Aetiology of Alzheimer's Disease," *PLOS One*
    5, no. 11 (2010), doi.org/10.1371/journal.pone.0013950.

48. Donata M. Paresce, Richik N. Ghosh, and Frederick R. Maxfield, "Microglial

Cells Internalize Aggregates of the Alzheimer's Disease Amyloid B-Protein via a Scavenger Receptor," *Neuron* 17, no. 3 (1996), doi.org/10.1016/s0896 -6273(00)80187-7.

49. Melinda E. Lull and Michelle L. Block, "Microglial Activation and Chronic Neurodegeneration," *Neurotherapeutics* 7, no. 4 (2010), doi.org/10.1016/j.nurt .2010.05.014; Florent Ginhoux and Marco Prinz, "Origin of Microglia: Current Concepts and Past Controversies," *Cold Spring Harbor Perspectives in Biology* 7, no. 8 (2015), doi.org/10.1101/cshperspect.a020537.

50. Helmut Kettenmann and Alexei Verkhratsky, "Neuroglia: The 150 Years After," *Trends in Neurosciences* 31, no. 12 (2008), doi.org/10.1016/j.tins.2008.09 .003.

51. Simon Makin, "The Amyloid Hypothesis on Trial," *Nature* 559, no. 7715 (2018), doi.org/10.1038/d41586-018-05719-4; Georg W. Kreutzberg, "Microglia: A Sensor for Pathological Events in the CNS," *Trends in Neurosciences* 19, no. 8 (1996), doi.org/10.1016/0166-2236(96)10049-7.

52. Paresce, Ghosh, and Maxfield, "Microglial Cells Internalize Aggregates"; Ginhoux and Prinz, "Origin of Microglia"; Makin, "Amyloid Hypothesis on Trial."

53. Marc Fakhoury, "Microglia and Astrocytes in Alzheimer's Disease: Implications for Therapy," *Current Neuropharmacology* 16, no. 5 (2018), doi.org/10 .2174/1570159x15666170720095240.

54. Antero Salminen et al., "Astrocytes in the Aging Brain Express Characteristics of Senescence-Associated Secretory Phenotype," *European Journal of Neuroscience* 34, no. 1 (2011), doi.org/10.1111/j.1460-9568.2011.07738.x.

55. Lull and Block, "Microglial Activation"; T. Wyss-Coray and L. Mucke, "Inflammation in Neurodegenerative Disease—A Double-Edged Sword," *Neuron* 35, no. 3 (2002), doi.org/10.1016/s0896-6273(02)00794-8; Christopher K. Glass et al., "Mechanisms Underlying Inflammation in Neurodegeneration," *Cell* 140, no. 6 (2010), doi.org/10.1016/j.cell.2010.02.016.

56. Shigeru Watanabe, "Chapter Five—Social Modification of Amphetamine Reward," *International Review of Neurobiology* 140 (2018), doi.org/10.1016/bs.irn .2018.07.023

57. Michael D. Weber, Jonathan P. Godbout, and John F. Sheridan, "Repeated Social Defeat, Neuroinflammation, and Behavior: Monocytes Carry the Signal," *Neuropsychopharmacology* 42, no. 1 (2017), doi.org/10.1038/npp.2016 .102.

58. Vivian Wang, "Erica Garner, Activist and Daughter of Eric Garner, Dies at 27," *The New York Times*, December 30, 2017, nytimes.com/2017/12/30 /nyregion/erica-garner-dead.html.

59. S. Mackenzie et al., "From Science to Action: The Trauma of Police Killings in the US," paper presented at the American Public Health Association National Conference, Atlanta, 2019.

60. B. S. McEwen, "Sex, Stress and the Hippocampus: Allostasis, Allostatic Load and the Aging Process," *Neurobiology of Aging* 23, no. 5 (2002), doi.org/10.1016 /s0197-4580(02)00027-1; Carmen Sandi, "Stress, Cognitive Impairment and Cell Adhesion Molecules," *Nature Reviews Neuroscience* 5, no. 12 (2004), doi.org/10 .1038/nrn1555; J. Douglas Bremner, "Does Stress Damage the Brain?," *Biological Psychiatry* 45, no. 7 (1999), doi.org/10.1016/s0006-3223(99)00009-8; Bruce S. McEwen et al., "Mechanisms of Stress in the Brain," *Nature Neuroscience* 18, no. 10 (2015), doi.org/10.1038/nn.4086.

61. Megan Zuelsdorff, "Lifetime Stressful Experiences, Racial Disparities, and Cognitive Performance: Findings from the Wisconsin Registry for Alzheimer's Prevention (WRAP) Study," *Alzheimer's and Dementia*, July 1, 2017, doi .org/10.1016/j.jalz.2017.07.085; Claudio Fiocchi, "Lifetime Stress May Boost Dementia Risk for Blacks," *Medpage Today*, 2017, www.alzinfo.org/articles /midlife-stress-may-increase-dementia-risk.

62. Megan Zuelsdorff et al., "Stressful Life Events and Racial Disparities in Cognition Among Middle-Aged and Older Adults," *Journal of Alzheimer's Disease* 73 (2020), doi.org/10.3233/JAD-190439.

63. Anthony S. Zannas et al., "Lifetime Stress Accelerates Epigenetic Aging in an Urban, African American Cohort: Relevance of Glucocorticoid Signaling," *Genome Biology* 16, no. 1 (2015), doi.org/10.1186/s13059-015-0828-5.

64. Hugo D. Critchley, "Review: Electrodermal Responses: What Happens in the Brain," *Neuroscientist* 8, no. 2 (2002), doi.org/10.1177/107385840200800209.

65. Glen Cook and Charles Mitschow, "Beyond the Polygraph: Deception Detection and the Autonomic Nervous System," *Federal Practitioner* 36, no. 7 (2019), pubmed.ncbi.nlm.nih.gov/31384120.

66. In their paper, researchers from the University of Nebraska and the University of Texas did not disclose the name of this university. Jacob E. Cheadle et al., "Race and Ethnic Variation in College Students' Allostatic Regulation of Racism-Related Stress," *Proceedings of the National Academy of Sciences of the United States of America* 117, no. 49 (2020), doi.org/10.1073/pnas.1922025117. The experiment used the twentieth-century technologies of the galvanic response, a lie detector, to measure the nervous system's response to white supremacy. It tracked the testimony of young people of color about racism in the twenty-first century, corroborating it with a measure of stress. As if their testimony weren't enough.

67. McEwen, "Sex, Stress and the Hippocampus"; McEwen et al., "Mechanisms of Stress in the Brain."

68. Elizabeth Rose Mayeda et al., "Inequalities in Dementia Incidence Between Six Racial and Ethnic Groups over 14 years," *Alzheimer's and Dementia* 12, no. 3 (2016), doi.org/10.1016/j.jalz.2015.12.007.

69. Zuelsdorff et al., "Stressful Life Events."

70. Megan L. Zuelsdorff et al., "Stressful Events, Social Support, and Cognitive Function in Middle-Aged Adults with a Family History of Alzheimer's Disease," *Journal of Aging and Health* 25, no. 6 (2013), doi.org/10.1177 /0898264313498416.

71. Keenan Walker, "Systemic Inflammation During Midlife and Cognitive Change over 20 Years," *Neurology* 92, no. 11 (2019), doi.org/10.1212/WNL .0000000000007094.

72. C. Holmes et al., "Systemic Inflammation and Disease Progression in Alzheimer Disease," *Neurology* 73, no. 10 (2009), doi.org/10.1212/wnl.0b013e3181b6bb95; V. H. Perry, C. Cunningham, and C. Holmes, "Systemic Infections and Inflammation Affect Chronic Neurodegeneration," *Nature Reviews Immunology* 7, no. 2 (2007), doi.org/10.1038/nri2015.

73. Holmes et al., "Systemic Inflammation."

74. H. Akiyama et al., "Inflammation and Alzheimer's Disease," *Neurobiology of Aging* 21, no. 3 (2000), doi.org/10.1016/s0197-4580(00)00124-x; John V. Forrester, Paul G. McMenamin, and Samantha J. Dando, "CNS Infection and

Immune Privilege," *Nature Reviews Neuroscience* 19, no. 11 (2018), doi.org/10.1038/s41583-018-0070-8.

75. B. H. Mullish, "Letter: Improvements in Mental Health after Faecal Microbiota Transplantation—An Underexplored Treatment-Related Benefit?," *Alimentary Pharmacology and Therapeutics* 47, no. 11 (2018), doi.org/10.1111/apt.14626.

76. G. B. Rogers et al., "From Gut Dysbiosis to Altered Brain Function and Mental Illness: Mechanisms and Pathways," *Molecular Psychiatry* 21, no. 6 (2016), doi.org/10.1038/mp.2016.50.

77. Edward T. Bullmore, *The Inflamed Mind: A Radical New Approach to Depression* (New York: Picador, 2019).

78. Jessica M. Yano et al., "Indigenous Bacteria from the Gut Microbiota Regulate Host Serotonin Biosynthesis," *Cell* 161, no. 2 (2015), doi.org/10.1016/j.cell.2015.02.047

79. Efrain C. Azmitia, "Evolution of Serotonin: Sunlight to Suicide," *Handbook of Behavioral Neuroscience* 31 (2020), doi.org/10.1016/B978-0-444-64125-0.00001-3.

80. Efrain C. Azmitia, "Serotonin and Brain: Evolution, Neuroplasticity, and Homeostasis," *International Review of Neurobiology* 77 (2007), doi.org/10.1016/S0074-7742(06)77002-7 .

81. I. P. Lapin and G. F. Oxenkrug, "Intensification of the Central Serotoninergic Processes as a Possible Determinant of the Thymoleptic Effect," *The Lancet* 293, no. 7586 (1969), doi.org/10.1016/s0140-6736(69)91140-4; A. Coppen et al., "5-Hydroxytryptamine (5-HT) in the Whole-Blood of Patients with Depressive Illness," *Postgraduate Medical Journal* 52, no. 605 (1976), doi.org/10.1136/pgmj.52.605.156.

82. Steven H. Zeisel, "Nutritional Importance of Choline for Brain Development," *Journal of the American College of Nutrition* 23, no. sup6 (2004), doi.org/10.1080/07315724.2004.10719433.

83. Jane A. Foster and Karen-Anne McVey Neufeld, "Gut-Brain Axis: How the Microbiome Influences Anxiety and Depression," *Trends in Neurosciences* 36, no. 5 (2013), doi.org/10.1016/j.tins.2013.01.005.

84. Gil Sharon et al., "The Central Nervous System and the Gut Microbiome," *Cell* 167, no. 4 (2016), doi.org/10.1016/j.cell.2016.10.027.

85. Ibid.

86. Richard Daneman and Alexandre Prat, "The Blood-Brain Barrier," *Cold Spring Harbor Perspectives in Biology* 7, no. 1 (2015), doi.org/10.1101/cshperspect.a020412; Giuliani and Alessandro Peri, "Effects of Hyponatremia on the Brain," *Journal of Clinical Medicine* 3, no. 4 (2014), doi.org/10.3390/jcm3041163.

87. Sharon et al., "Central Nervous System and Gut Microbiome."

88. J. Ochoa-Repáraz et al., "A Polysaccharide from the Human Commensal Bacteroides Fragilis Protects against CNS Demyelinating Disease," *Mucosal Immunology* 3, no. 5 (2010), doi.org/10.1038/mi.2010.29.

89. Sharon et al., "Central Nervous System and Gut Microbiome."

90. Nicholas M. Vogt et al., "Gut Microbiome Alterations in Alzheimer's Disease," *Scientific Reports* 7, no. 1 (2017), doi.org/10.1038/s41598-017-13601-y.

91. Alfonsina D'Amato et al., "Faecal Microbiota Transplant from Aged Donor Mice Affects Spatial Learning and Memory Via Modulating Hippocampal Synaptic Plasticity and Neurotransmission-Related Proteins in Young Recipients," *Microbiome* 8, no. 1 (2020), doi.org/10.1186/s40168-020-00914-w.

92. R. C. E. Bowyer et al., "Socioeconomic Status and the Gut Microbiome: A Twinsuk Cohort Study," *Microorganisms* 7, no. 1 (2019), doi.org/10.3390/microorganisms7010017.

93. Rogers et al., "From Gut Dysbiosis to Altered Brain Function"; Foster and Neufeld, "Gut–Brain Axis."

94. Athena Athanasiou, *Agonistic Mourning: Political Dissidence and the Women in Black* (Edinburgh: Edinburgh University Press, 2017).

95. Nora Amalia Femenía and Carlos Ariel Gil, "Argentina's Mothers of Plaza de Mayo: The Mourning Process from Junta to Democracy," *Feminist Studies* 13, no. 1 (1987), doi.org/10.2307/3177832.

96. J. A. du Pisani, M. Broodryk, and P. W. Coetzer, "Protest Marches in South Africa," *Journal of Modern African Studies* 28, no. 4 (1990), doi.org/10.1017/S0022278X00054744.

97. Federico Morelli et al., "The Vulture in the Sky and the Hominin on the Land: Three Million Years of Human–Vulture Interaction," *Anthrozoös* 28, no. 3 (2015), doi.org/10.1080/08927936.2015.1052279.

98. Meera Subramanian, "Towering Silence: For Millennia Zoroastrians Have Used Vultures to Dispose of Their Dead. What Will Happen When the Birds Disappear?," *Science and Spirit* 19, no. 3 (2008), doi.org/10.3200/SSPT.19.3.34-39.

99. Bruno Bonaz, Valérie Sinniger, and Sonia Pellissier, "Anti-Inflammatory Properties of the Vagus Nerve: Potential Therapeutic Implications of Vagus Nerve Stimulation," *Journal of Physiology* 594, no. 20 (2016), doi.org/10.1113/jp271539.

100. G. R. Johnston and N. R. Webster, "Cytokines and the Immunomodulatory Function of the Vagus Nerve," *British Journal of Anaesthesia* 102, no. 4 (2009), doi.org/10.1093/bja/aep037.

101. Cora Stefanie Weber et al., "Low Vagal Tone Is Associated with Impaired Post Stress Recovery of Cardiovascular, Endocrine, and Immune Markers," *European Journal of Applied Physiology* 109, no. 2 (2010), doi.org/10.1007/s00421-009-1341-x.

102. Sigrid Breit et al., "Vagus Nerve as Modulator of the Brain-Gut Axis in Psychiatric and Inflammatory Disorders," *Frontiers in Psychiatry* 9 (2018), doi.org/10.3389/fpsyt.2018.00044.

103. Bonaz, Sinniger, and Pellissier, "Anti-Inflammatory Properties of Vagus Nerve."

104. B. Rael Cahn et al., "Yoga, Meditation and Mind-Body Health: Increased BDNF, Cortisol Awakening Response, and Altered Inflammatory Marker Expression After a 3-Month Yoga and Meditation Retreat," *Frontiers in Human Neuroscience* 11 (2017), doi.org/10.3389/fnhum.2017.00315.

105. Roderik J. S. Gerritsen and Guido P. H. Band, "Breath of Life: The Respiratory Vagal Stimulation Model of Contemplative Activity," *Frontiers in Human Neuroscience* 12 (2018), doi.org/10.3389/fnhum.2018.00397.

106. Jing Kang, Austin Scholp, and Jack J. Jiang, "A Review of the Physiological Effects and Mechanisms of Singing," *Journal of Voice* 32, no. 4 (2018), doi.org/10.1016/j.jvoice.2017.07.008.

107. Leroy Vail and Landeg White, "Forms of Resistance: Songs and Perceptions of Power in Colonial Mozambique," *American Historical Review* 88, no. 4 (1983), doi.org/10.2307/1874024.

108. Gregory M. Filip and Lisa M. Ganio, "Early Thinning in Mixed-Species Plantations of Douglas-Fir, Hemlock, and True Fir Affected by Armillaria Root

Disease in Westcentral Oregon and Washington: 20 Year Results," *Western Journal of Applied Forestry* 19, no. 1 (2004), doi.org/10.1093/wjaf/19.1.25.

109. Anne Casselman, "Strange but True: The Largest Organism on Earth Is a Fungus," *Scientific American*, October 4, 2007, tinyurl.com/36gr6mln.

110. György Sipos, James B Anderson, and László G Nagy, "Armillaria," *Current Biology* 28, no. 7 (2018), doi.org/10.1016/j.cub.2018.01.026.

111. J. W. Hanna et al., "Maximum Entropy-Based Bioclimatic Models Predict Areas of Current and Future Suitable Habitat for *Armillaria* Species in Western Oregon and Western Washington," paper presented at the 66th Western International Forest Disease Work Conference, June 3–7, 2019, Estes Park, CO, www.fs.fed.us/rm/pubs_journals/2020/rmrs_2020_hanna_j003.pdf; Tomáš Větrovský et al., "A Meta-Analysis of Global Fungal Distribution Reveals Climate-Driven Patterns," *Nature Communications* 10, no. 1 (2019), doi.org/10.1038/s41467-019-13164-88. Mycorrhizal fungi that effectively sink carbon dioxide in forests can tolerate a much narrower range of temperatures than plant pathogens. As global temperatures increase, the fates of these fungi and the forests—not to mention the people—that depend upon them are at stake.

112. Martin Parniske, "Arbuscular Mycorrhiza: The Mother of Plant Root Endosymbioses," *Nature Reviews Microbiology* 6, no. 10 (2008), doi.org/10.1038/nrmicro1987.

113. Mark C. Brundrett, "Coevolution of Roots and Mycorrhizas of Land Plants," *New Phytologist* 154, no. 2 (2002), doi.org/10.1046/j.1469-8137.2002.00397.x.

114. Parniske, "Arbuscular Mycorrhiza."

115. Ibid.

116. Meena Kapahi and Sarita Sachdeva, "Bioremediation Options for Heavy Metal Pollution," *Journal of Health and Pollution* 9, no. 24 (2019), doi.org/10.5696/2156-9614-9.24.191203.

117. Fariba Mohsenzadeh et al., "Phytoremediation of Petroleum-Polluted Soils: Application of Polygonum Aviculare and Its Root-Associated (Penetrated) Fungal Strains for Bioremediation of Petroleum-Polluted Soils," *Ecotoxicology and Environmental Safety* 73, no. 4 (2010), doi.org/10.1016/j.ecoenv.2009.08.020.

118. Michael Phillips, *Mycorrhizal Planet* (White River Junction, VT: Chelsea Green, 2017).

119. Ibid.; Parniske, "Arbuscular Mycorrhiza."

120. Parniske, "Arbuscular Mycorrhiza."

121. Ibid.

122. Merlin Sheldrake, *Entangled Life: How Fungi Make Our Worlds, Change Our Minds and Shape Our Futures* (New York: Random House, 2020), 127.

123. Sabine C. Jung et al., "Mycorrhiza-Induced Resistance and Priming of Plant Defenses," *Journal of Chemical Ecology* 38, no. 6 (2012), doi.org/10.1007/s10886-012-0134-6.

124. Diane Toomey, "Exploring How and Why Trees 'Talk' to Each Other," *Yale Environment 360*, 2016, e360.yale.edu/features/exploring_how_and_why_trees_talk_to_each_other; Suzanne W. Simard and Daniel M. Durall, "Mycorrhizal Networks: A Review of Their Extent, Function, and Importance," *Canadian Journal of Botany* 82, no. 8 (2004), doi.org/10.1139/b04-116.

125. François P. Teste et al., "Access to Mycorrhizal Networks and Roots of Trees: Importance for Seedling Survival and Resource Transfer," *Ecology* 90, no. 10 (2009), doi.org/10.1890/08-1884.1.

126. Michael Winkelman, "Introduction: Evidence for Entheogen Use in Prehistory and World Religions," *Journal of Psychedelic Studies* 3, no. 2 (2019), doi .org/10.1556/2054.2019.024.

127. Elisa Guerra-Doce, "Psychoactive Substances in Prehistoric Times: Examining the Archaeological Evidence," *Time and Mind* 8, no. 1 (2015), doi.org/10 .1080/1751696x.2014.993244; H. R. El-Seedi et al., "Prehistoric Peyote Use: Alkaloid Analysis and Radiocarbon Dating of Archaeological Specimens of Lophophora from Texas," *Journal of Ethnopharmacology* 101, no. 1–3 (2005), doi.org/10.1016/j.jep.2005.04.022.

128. Weston La Barre, "Old and New World Narcotics: A Statistical Question and an Ethnological Reply," *Economic Botany* 24, no. 1 (1970), doi.org/10.1007 /bf02860640.

129. M. D. Merlin, "Archaeological Evidence for the Tradition of Psychoactive Plant Use in the Old World," *Economic Botany* 57, no. 3 (2003), www.jstor.org /stable/4256701.

130. Ibid.

131. Evgenia Fotiou, "The Globalization of Ayahuasca Shamanism and the Erasure of Indigenous Shamanism," *Anthropology of Consciousness* 27, no. 2 (2016), doi .org/10.1111/anoc.12056.

132. The psychedelic lysergic acid diethylamide (LSD) was first synthesized in 1938 from ergotamine, a substance derived from the fungus ergot or *Claviceps purpura,* which grows on rye. Ergot features in a physiological hypothesis of the Salem witch trials of 1692, put forth by then graduate student Linnda Caporael. From her analysis, she concluded that instead of the devil, it was the fungus who induced the symptoms attributed to witchcraft. Seasonal weather patterns at the time of the witch trials would have been optimal for the fungus to thrive on the rye harvest. Acting on the central nervous system, ergot can cause mania, psychosis, and the sensation that bugs are crawling all over one's body—all symptoms experienced by the young people accused of witchcraft. Shortly after Carporael's paper came out in *Science,* the same journal published a long rebuttal by two psychologists, Nicholas P. Spanos and Jack Gottlieb, trying to disprove the hypothesis. A few years later the historian Mary Matossian, who specializes in social behavior caused by fungal outbreaks, upheld Carporael's analysis: a modern-day tug-of-war between men and women over who gets to narrate the history of witch hunts. Linnda R. Caporael, "Ergotism: The Satan Loosed in Salem," *Science* 192, no. 4234 (1976), doi.org/10.1126/science.769159 ; M. R. Lee, "The History of Ergot of Rye (*Claviceps purpurea*) III: 1940–80," *Journal of the Royal College of Physicians of Edinburgh* 40, no. 1 (2010), doi.org/10.4997/jrcpe.2010.115.

133. Juan F. López-Giménez and Javier González-Maeso, "Hallucinogens and Serotonin 5-HT$_{2A}$ Receptor-Mediated Signaling Pathways," in *Behavioral Neurobiology of Psychedelic Drugs,* vol. 36, *Current Topics in Behavioral Neurosciences,* ed. A. L. Halberstadt, F. X. Vollenweider, and D.E. Nichols (Berlin: Springer, 2017), doi.org/10.1007/7854_2017_478.

134. M. Kometer et al., "Activation of Serotonin 2A Receptors Underlies the Psilocybin-Induced Effects on α Oscillations, N170 Visual-Evoked Potentials, and Visual Hallucinations," *Journal of Neuroscience* 33, no. 25 (2013), doi.org /10.1523/jneurosci.3007-12.2013.

135. Efrain C. Azmitia, "Evolution of Serotonin: Sunlight to Suicide," *Handbook*

of Behavioral Neuroscience 31 (2020), doi.org/10.1016/B978-0-444-64125-0.00001-3.

136. Bangning Yu et al., "Serotonin 5-Hydroxytryptamine$_{2A}$ Receptor Activation Suppresses Tumor Necrosis Factor-α-Induced Inflammation with Extraordinary Potency," *Journal of Pharmacology and Experimental Therapeutics* 327, no. 2 (2008), doi.org/10.1124/jpet.108.143461.

137. Peter S. Hendricks et al., "Classic Psychedelic Use Is Associated with Reduced Psychological Distress and Suicidality in the United States Adult Population," *Journal of Psychopharmacology* 29, no. 3 (2015), doi.org/10.1177/0269881114565653; J. W. Murrough et al., "Ketamine for Rapid Reduction of Suicidal Ideation: A Randomized Controlled Trial," *Psychological Medicine* 45, no. 16 (2015), doi.org/10.1017/s0033291715001506; Thomas J. Riedlinger and June E. Riedlinger, "Psychedelic and Entactogenic Drugs in the Treatment of Depression," *Journal of Psychoactive Drugs* 26, no. 1 (1994), doi.org/10.1080/02791072.1994.10472600; Vitor Caiaffo et al., "Anti-Inflammatory, Antiapoptotic, and Antioxidant Activity of Fluoxetine," *Pharmacology Research and Perspectives* 4, no. 3 (2016), doi.org/10.1002/prp2.231.

138. H. G. Ruhé, N. S. Mason, and A. H. Schene, "Mood Is Indirectly Related to Serotonin, Norepinephrine and Dopamine Levels in Humans: A Meta-Analysis of Monoamine Depletion Studies," *Molecular Psychiatry* 12, no. 4 (2007), doi.org/10.1038/sj.mp.4001949.

139. Andrea I. Luppi et al., "LSD Alters Dynamic Integration and Segregation in the Human Brain," *NeuroImage* 227 (2021), doi.org/10.1016/j.neuroimage.2020.117653.

140. N. L. Mason et al., "Me, Myself, Bye: Regional Alterations in Glutamate and the Experience of Ego Dissolution with Psilocybin," *Neuropsychopharmacology* 45, no. 12 (2020), doi.org/10.1038/s41386-020-0718-8.

141. A. A. Feduccia, J. Holland, and M. C. Mithoefer, "Progress and Promise for the MDMA Drug Development Program," *Psychopharmacology (Berlin)* 235, no. 2 (2018), doi.org/10.1007/s00213-017-4779-2.

142. Alan K. Davis et al., "Psychedelic Treatment for Trauma-Related Psychological and Cognitive Impairment Among US Special Operations Forces Veterans," *Chronic Stress* 4 (2020), doi.org/10.1177/2470547020939564.

143. Marcela Ot'alora G. et al., "3,4-Methylenedioxymethamphetamine-Assisted Psychotherapy for Treatment of Chronic Posttraumatic Stress Disorder: A Randomized Phase 2 Controlled Trial," *Journal of Psychopharmacology* 32, no. 12 (2018), doi.org/10.1177/0269881118806297.

144. Riedlinger and Riedlinger, "Psychedelic and Entactogenic Drugs"; Collin M. Reiff et al., "Psychedelics and Psychedelic-Assisted Psychotherapy," *American Journal of Psychiatry* 177, no. 5 (2020), doi.org/10.1176/appi.ajp.2019.19010035.

145. Rafael Guimarães dos Santos, José Carlos Bouso, and Jaime E. C. Hallak, "Serotonergic Hallucinogens/Psychedelics Could Be Promising Treatments for Depressive and Anxiety Disorders in End-Stage Cancer," *BMC Psychiatry* 19, no. 1 (2019), doi.org/10.1186/s12888-019-2288-z.

146. Stephen Ross et al., "Rapid and Sustained Symptom Reduction Following Psilocybin Treatment for Anxiety and Depression in Patients with Life-Threatening Cancer: A Randomized Controlled Trial," *Journal of Psychopharmacology* 30, no. 12 (2016), doi.org/10.1177/0269881116675512.

147. Gabrielle I. Agin-Liebes et al., "Long-Term Follow-up of Psilocybin-Assisted Psychotherapy for Psychiatric and Existential Distress in Patients with Life-Threatening Cancer," *Journal of Psychopharmacology* 34, no. 2 (2020), doi.org/10.1177/0269881119897615.

148. Mellody Hayes, "Psychedelics in Palliative Care," *Scientific American,* March 20, 2020, blogs.scientificamerican.com/observations/psychedelics-in-palliative-care/.

149. Nicole Leite Galvão-Coelho et al., "Changes in Inflammatory Biomarkers Are Related to the Antidepressant Effects of Ayahuasca," *Journal of Psychopharmacology* 34, no. 10 (2020), doi.org/10.1177/0269881120936486.

150. Evgenia Fotiou, "The Role of Indigenous Knowledges in Psychedelic Science," *Journal of Psychedelic Studies* 4, no. 1 (2019), doi.org/10.1556/2054.2019.031.

151. M. Keith Chen, Judith A. Chevalier, and Elisa F. Long, "Nursing Home Staff Networks and Covid-19," *Proceedings of the National Academy of Sciences of the United States of America* 118, no. 1 (2021), doi.org/10.1073/pnas.2015455118.

152. Liat Ayalon et al., "Long-Term Care Settings in the Times of Covid-19: Challenges and Future Directions," *International Psychogeriatrics* 32, no. 10 (2020), doi.org/10.1017/s1041610220001416. One reason for the unusually low number of nursing home deaths from Covid in India may be that residents were returned to their families at the beginning of the outbreak. Jallavi Panchamia et al., "Low Covid-19 Mortality in Old Age Homes in Western India: An Empirical Study," *medRxiv* (2020), doi.org/10.1101/2020.12.08.20245134.

153. Eva Boodman, "Nursing Home Abolition: Prisons and the Institutionalization of Older Adult Care," *Details: Journal of Ethical Urban Living* 2, no. 1 (2019), jeul.cognethic.org/jeulv2i1_Boodman.pdf; Ai-jen Poo, *The Age of Dignity: Preparing for the Elder Boom in a Changing America* (New York: New Press, 2015). Just as prisons were part of a fix for deindustrializing California in the 1990s, care homes have become a site of Keynesian stimulus for the Rust Belt. See Gabriel Winant, "'Hard Times Make for Hard Arteries and Hard Livers': Deindustrialization, Biopolitics, and the Making of a New Working Class," *Journal of Social History* 53, no. 1 (2019), doi.org/10.1093/jsh/shy11; Gabriel Winant, *The Next Shift: The Fall of Industry and the Rise of Health Care in Rust Belt America* (Boston: Harvard University Press, 2021).

154. L. Calderon-Garciduenas et al., "Quadruple Abnormal Protein Aggregates in Brainstem Pathology and Exogenous Metal-Rich Magnetic Nanoparticles: The Substantia Nigrae Is a Very Early Target in Young Urbanites and the Gastrointestinal Tract Likely a Key Brainstem Portal," *Environmental Research* 191 (2020), doi.org/10.1016/j.envres.2020.110139.

155. Anamika Dubey et al., "Soil Microbiome: A Key Player for Conservation of Soil Health Under Changing Climate," *Biodiversity and Conservation* 28, no. 8–9 (2019), doi.org/10.1007/s10531-019-01760-5; Erik Verbruggen et al., "Positive Effects of Organic Farming on Below-Ground Mutualists: Large-Scale Comparison of Mycorrhizal Fungal Communities in Agricultural Soils," *New Phytologist* 186, no. 4 (2010), doi.org/10.1111/j.1469-8137.2010.03230.x.

156. Jonathan Watts and John Vidal, "Environmental Defenders Being Killed in Record Numbers Globally, New Research Reveals," *The Guardian*, July 13, 2017, tinyurl.com/ljom8ps9.

157. Varshini Prakash and Guido Girgenti, *Winning the Green New Deal: Why We Must, How We Can* (New York: Simon & Schuster, 2020), 208.

158. Naomi Klein, "Care and Repair: Left Politics in the Age of Climate Change," *Dissent* 67, no. 1 (2020), doi.org/10.1353/dss.2020.0008.

159. Joel Millward-Hopkins et al., "Providing Decent Living with Minimum Energy: A Global Scenario," *Global Environmental Change* 65 (2020), doi.org/10.1016/j.gloenvcha.2020.102168.

160. U.S. House of Representatives, "H. Res. 109: Recognizing the Duty of the Federal Government to Create a Green New Deal," February 7, 2019 www.congress.gov/116/bills/hres109/BILLS-116hres109ih.pdf.

161. Thomas Wiedmann et al., "Scientists' Warning on Affluence," *Nature Communications* 11, no. 1 (2020), doi.org/10.1038/s41467-020-16941-y.

162. Stan Cox, *The Green New Deal and Beyond: Ending the Climate Emergency While We Still Can* (San Francisco: City Lights, 2020).

163. Zak Colman, "Green New Deal Won't Call for End to Fossil Fuels," *Politico*, February 4, 2019, www.politico.com/story/2019/02/04/green-new-deal-fossil-fuels-1142544.

164. Ruth Wilson Gilmore, "Fatal Couplings of Power and Difference: Notes on Racism and Geography," *Professional Geographer* 54, no. 1 (2002): 18, doi.org/10.1111/0033-0124.00310.

165. Zaragosa Vargas, "Tejana Radical: Emma Tenayuca and the San Antonio Labor Movement During the Great Depression," *Pacific Historical Review* 66, no. 4 (1997), doi.org/10.2307/3642237; Douglas F. Cannon and Laura E. Cannon, "Headlines vs. History," *Media History* 25, no. 2 (2019), doi.org/10.1080/13688804.2016.1262248; D. H. Dinwoodie, "Deportation: The Immigration Service and the Chicano Labor Movement in the 1930s," *New Mexico Historical Review* 52, no. 3 (1977); Francisco E. Balderrama and Raymond Rodriguez, *Decade of Betrayal: Mexican Repatriation in the 1930s* (Albuquerque: University of New Mexico Press, 1995).

166. Howard Kester, *Revolt Among the Sharecroppers* (New York: Covici, 1936), 26.

167. Donald Parman, "Twentieth-Century Indian History: Achievements, Needs, and Problems," *OAH Magazine of History* 9, no. 1 (1994), www.jstor.org/stable/25162997. The 1934 Indian Reorganization Act consolidated the Dawes Act and, under the administration of John Collier, allowed the Bureau of Indian Affairs to continue its self-regard of benevolent patriarchy. Richard O. Clemmer, "Hopis, Western Shoshones, and Southern Utes: Three Different Responses to the Indian Reorganization Act of 1934," *American Indian Culture and Research Journal* 10, no. 2 (2007), doi.org/10.17953/aicr.10.2.b60q70g353272087.

168. Matthias Neumann and Gabriele Winker, "Fighting for Care Work Resources," in *Degrowth in Movement(s)*, ed. Corinna Burkhart, Matthias Schmelzer, and Nina Treu (Hampshire, UK: Zero Books, 2020); Gabriele Winker, *Care Revolution: Schritte in eine solidarische Gesellschaft* (transcript Verlag, 2015), doi.org/10.14361/transcript.9783839430408; Friederike Habermann, *Ecommony: UmCARE zum Miteinander* (Königstein im Taunus, Germany: Ulrike Helmer Verlag, 2016).

9. DEEP MEDICINE

1. Frantz Fanon, *The Wretched of the Earth*, trans. Constance Farrington (London: Penguin, 1965), 35.

2. Barbara Alice Mann, *Iroquoian Women: The Gantowisas* (New York: P. Lang, 2000), 7.

3. Stefano Harmey and Fred Moten, *The Undercommons: Fugitive Planning and Black Study* (New York: Minor Compositions, 2013), 140.

4. Mayra Quirindongo et al., *Lost and Found: Missing Mercury from Chemical Plants Pollutes Air and Water* (New York: Natural Resources Defense Council, 2006).

5. Beth Schwartzapfel, "1 in 5 Prisoners in the U.S. Has Had Covid-19," *Marshall Project* 2020, tinyurl.com/5axqk7xh.

6. Heather Kovich, "Rural Matters—Coronavirus and the Navajo Nation," *New England Journal of Medicine* 383, no. 2 (2020), doi.org/10.1056/nejmp2012114.

7. Hong Zhou et al., "A Novel Bat Coronavirus Closely Related to SARS-CoV-2 Contains Natural Insertions at the S1/S2 Cleavage Site of the Spike Protein," *Current Biology* 30, no. 11 (2020), doi.org/10.1016/j.cub.2020.05.023; Peng Zhou et al., "A Pneumonia Outbreak Associated with a New Coronavirus of Probable Bat Origin," *Nature* 579, no. 7798 (2020), doi.org/10.1038/s41586-020-2012-7.

8. Adrienne Murray, "Coronavirus: Denmark Shaken by Cull of Millions of Mink," *BBC News*, November 11, 2020, www.bbc.com/news/world-europe-54890229.

9. Jon Henley, "Decomposing Mink in Denmark 'May Have Contaminated Groundwater,'" *The Guardian*, December 10, 2020, tinyurl.com/y7g7unxf.

10. Elizabeth Imbert et al., "Coronavirus Disease 2019 Outbreak in a San Francisco Homeless Shelter," *Clinical Infectious Diseases*, August 3, 2020, doi.org/10.1093/cid/ciaa1071.

11. Jennifer Jett, "Restrictions Continue to Ease, but Not for Migrant Workers," *The New York Times*, December 18, 2020, tinyurl.com/1t3j4y1v.

12. Fred Moten, *Stolen Life* (Durham, NC: Duke University Press, 2018), 131.

13. Jack Halberstam, "The Wild Beyond: With and for the Undercommons," in *The Undercommons: Fugitive Planning and Black Study*, ed. Stefano Harmey and Fred Moten (New York: Minor Compositions, 2013), 11.

14. Angela Y. Davis, *Are Prisons Obsolete?* (Toronto: Publishers Group Canada, 2003), 107.

15. Angela Y. Davis, "Incarcerated Women: Transformative Strategies," *Black Renaissance* 1, no. 1 (1996); Angela Y. Davis, *If They Come in the Morning: Voices of Resistance* (New York: Third Press, 1971).

16. Angela Y. Davis and Dylan Rodriguez, "The Challenge of Prison Abolition: A Conversation," *Social Justice* 27, no. 3 (2000), www.jstor.org/stable/29767244; George Jackson, *Blood in My Eye* (New York: Random House, 1972); George Jackson, *Soledad Brother: The Prison Letters of George Jackson* (New York: Coward-McCann, 1970).

17. Chris Joyner and Nick Thieme, "Police Killings More Likely in Agencies That Get Military Gear, Data Shows," *Atlanta Journal-Constitution*, October 8, 2020, tinyurl.com/yv6cufmw.

18. Rachel Kushner, "Is Prison Necessary? Ruth Wilson Gilmore Might Change Your Mind," *The New York Times*, April 17, 2019, tinyurl.com/uymt7l2i.

19. Simon N. Williams and Marion Nestle, "'Big Food': Taking a Critical Perspective on a Global Public Health Problem," *Critical Public Health* 25, no. 3 (2015), doi.org/10.1080/09581596.2015.1021298.

20. Ruth Wilson Gilmore, "Abolition Geography and the Problem of Innocence," in *Futures of Black Radicalism*, ed. Gaye Theresa Johnson and Alex Lubin (London: Verso, 2017); Nik Heynen and Megan Ybarra, "On Abolition Ecologies and Making "Freedom as a Place," *Antipode* (2020), doi.org/10.1111/anti .12666.

21. Michel Foucault, *Power/Knowledge: Selected Interviews and Other Writings, 1972–1977*, ed. Colin Gordon (New York: Pantheon, 1980), 151.

22. Yan Dhyansky, "The Indus Valley Origin of Yoga Practice," *Artibus Asiae* 48, no. 1–2 (1987).

23. Jim Butcher, "Mindfulness as a Management Technique Goes Back to at Least the 1970s," *Harvard Business Review*, May 2, 2018, tinyurl.com/yml3eoqh; Madhav Goyal et al., "Meditation Programs for Psychological Stress and Well-Being," *JAMA Internal Medicine* 174, no. 3 (2014), doi.org/10.1001 /jamainternmed.2013.13018.

24. Janice M. Zeller and Pamela F. Levin, "Mindfulness Interventions to Reduce Stress Among Nursing Personnel," *Workplace Health and Safety* 61, no. 2 (2013), doi.org/10.1177/216507991306100207.

25. Kate Aronoff, *Overheated: How Capitalism Broke the Planet—and How We Fight Back* (New York: Bold Type Books, 2021).

26. Eve Tuck and K. Wayne Yang, "Decolonization Is Not a Metaphor," *Decolonization: Indigeneity, Education and Society* 1, no. 1 (2012): 3, jps.library.utoronto .ca/index.php/des/article/view/18630.

27. Melanie Yazzie and Cutcha Risling Baldy, "Indigenous People and the Politics of Water," *Decolonization: Indigeneity, Education and Society* 7, no. 1 (2018).

28. Tuck and Yang, "Decolonization," 3.

29. Alicia Elliott, *A Mind Spread Out on the Ground* (Toronto: Doubleday Canada, 2019), 55.

30. Gilmore, "Abolition Geography"; Heynen and Ybarra, "On Abolition Ecologies."

31. Committee on Land Acknowledgment, *UT Land Acknowledgement* (Austin: University of Texas Program in Native American and Indigenous Studies, 2021), liberalarts.utexas.edu/nais/land-acknowledgement/index.php.

32. Oleg Simakov et al., "Hemichordate Genomes and Deuterostome Origins," *Nature* 527, no. 7579 (2015), doi.org/10.1038/nature16150.

33. Richard B. Hovey et al., "Enhancing Indigenous Health Promotion Research Through Two-Eyed Seeing: A Hermeneutic Relational Process," *Qualitative Health Research* 27, no. 9 (2017), doi.org/10.1177/1049732317697948.

34. Tuck and Yang, "Decolonization."

35. Alleen Brown, Will Parrish, and Alice Speri, "Leaked Documents Reveal Counterterrorism Tactics Used at Standing Rock to 'Defeat Pipeline Insurgencies,'" *The Intercept*, May 27, 2017, tinyurl.com/yhshw75w.

36. "To envision a society as democratic and caring is to envision a society whose account of justice balances how the burdens and joys of caring are equalized so as to leave every citizen with as much freedom as possible. Such a vision requires that citizens see clearly how they care with others, that is, how they think about responsibilities for care." Joan Tronto, *Caring Democracy: Markets, Equality and Justice* (New York: NYU Press, 2013), 43.

37. "Care, V," Oxford English Dictionary (Oxford: Oxford University Press). www .oed.com/view/Entry/27902?rskey=Ia7tkj&result=4.

38. Roberta Waite and Deena Nardi, "Nursing Colonialism in America: Implications for Nursing Leadership," *Journal of Professional Nursing* 35, no. 1 (2019), doi.org/10.1016/j.profnurs.2017.12.013; Elizabeth McGibbon et al., "Toward Decolonizing Nursing: The Colonization of Nursing and Strategies for Increasing the Counter-Narrative," *Nursing Inquiry* 21, no. 3 (2014), doi .org/10.1111/nin.12042.

39. Priscilla M. Wehi, Jacqueline R. Beggs, and Tara G. McAllister, "Ka Mua, Ka Muri: The Inclusion of Mātauranga Māori in New Zealand Ecology," *New Zealand Journal of Ecology* 43, no. 3 (2019), doi.org/10.20417/nzjecol.43.40.

40. Natalie Kurashima, Jason Jeremiah, and Tamara Ticktin, "I Ka Wā Ma Mua: The Value of a Historical Ecology Approach to Ecological Restoration in Hawai'i," *Pacific Science* 71, no. 4 (2017), doi.org/10.2984/71.4.4.

41. Fanon, *Wretched of the Earth*, 36.

42. "Because settler colonialism is built upon an entangled triad structure of settler-native-slave, the decolonial desires of white, nonwhite, immigrant, postcolonial and oppressed people can similarly be entangled in resettlement, reoccupation, and rehabilitation that actually further settler colonialism. The metaphorization of decolonization makes possible a set of evasions, or 'settler moves to innocence,' that problematically attempt to reconcile settler guilt and complicity, and rescue settler futurity." Tuck and Yang, "Decolonization," 1.

ACKNOWLEDGMENTS

This book took generations and years to bring about. We are deeply grateful to our ancestors and to those whose shared knowledge made this book possible: Alison Ehara Brown, Allison Hedge Coke, Amita Bhaviskar, Anita Chitaya, Ann Marie Sayers, Aoife O'Donovan, Ashanté M. Reese, Aude Bouagnon, Beth Karlin, Boots Riley, Braden Tierney, Brock Dollman, Candace Ducheneaux, Carroll Fife and Dominique Walker of Moms 4 Housing, Cat Brooks and the crew at Anti-Police Terror Project, Charlene Vasquez-Gomez, Chief Caleen Sisk, Chief Twinkle Borge, Corrina Gould, Crystal Wahpepah, Desirae Harp, Dr. Cleavon Gilman, Dr. Coleen Kivlahan, Dr. David Kingfisher, Dr. Heather Certain, Dr. Jesse Turner, Dr. Josh Connor, Dr. Juliana Morris, Dr. Kalama O Ka'aina, Dr. Keolu Fox, Dr. Leigh Kimberg, Dr. Madhavi Dandu, Dr. Olivia Park, Dr. Phuoc Le, Dr. Ramona Tascoe, Dr. Sara Jumping Eagle, Dr. Simon Ma, Dr. Sri Shamasunder, Dr. Wayne Yang, Dr. Yakira Teitel, Elizabeth Hoover, Eoin Brodie, Fabian Fernandez, Fergus Shanahan, Fuifuilupe Niumeitolu, Geri Pettus, Gina Madrid, Gregg Castro, Guillermo Gómez-Peña, Gwen Woods, Hawane Rios, Hi'ilei Julia Hobart, James Koshiba, Jason McLennan Jo Love Cruz, Johnella LaRose, Jonathan Cordero, Joseph Kunkel, Kanyon Sayers-Roods, Kaveri Gill, Kim DeOCampo, L. Frank Manriquez, Leet Killer, Leroy Moore, Linda Black Elk, Lisa Tiny Garcia and the family of POOR Magazine, Louis Ungaro, Lyla June Johnston, Malik Yakini, Marcus Shelby, Marsha Wibowo, Martin Reinhardt, Melissa Rose, Meredith Alberta Palmer, Mia Maltz, Michael

Painter, Michael Travis Laub, Miles Allard, Mqapheli Bonono, Muteado Silencio, Nancy Turner, Nicolle Gonzales of Changing Woman Initiative, Niria Alicia Garcia, Nitanis Desjarlais, Noah Morris, Nomusa Sizani, Olowan Martinez, Patricia St. Onge, Pennie Opal Plant, Peter Mazunda, Peter Sterling, Pua Case, Rachel Bezner Kerr, Rachel Wexler, Rani Mukherjee, Red Warrior Society Refugio and Elvira Niet, Rowen White, Rudy Reddog, S'bu Zikode, Shalmali Guttal, Sharon Jinkerson-Brass, Solomon Reese, Stephanie Redmond, Sue Lynch, Tasha Peltier and Alayna Eagleshield of Mni Wiconi Clinic and Farm, The Frisco 5 (Cristina Gutierrez, Ike Ali Pinkston, Ilych "Equipto" Sato, Edwin Lindo, Averi Sellasie Blackwell), Tim Horsburgh, Tim LaSalle, Tipiziwin Tollman, Uncle Bobby X and Aunt B, Val Segrest, Vanessa Bolin, Walter Riley, Wounded Knee DeOCampo, Yolanda Banks Reed, Zak Piper, Félix Kury and all the students and patients of Clinica Martín-Baró, Mordecai Ettinger and the Health Justice Commons, The Do No Harm Coalition, and the patients and students who are our lifelong teachers.

We offer our deep thanks to those who supported us while we wrote: Aaron Kierbel, Adrian Arias, Alexis Tatarsky, Annie Droste, Avi Lewis, Ben Hirsch, Caro Mueller, Carol Park, Charlotte María Sáenz, Christine Lam, Cooper Freeman, David Hochschild, Dr. Alexandra Gottlieb, Dr. Andy Lai, Dr. Bradley Monash, Dr. Bradley Sharpe, Dr. Carmen Cobb, Dr. Cynthia Fenton, Dr. David Arboleda, Dr. Deborah Cohan, Dr. Cynthia Li, Dr. Feifei Xue, Dr. Francisco Alvarez, Dr. Kiran Gupta, Dr. Meghna Motiani, Dr. Muharrem Yunce, Dr. Priyanka Agarwal, Dr. Robert Wachter, Dr. Sajan Patel, Dr. Sara Murray, Dr. Tim Judson, Eric Tang, Erin Lentz, Eugene Sepulveda, ill weaver, Jason Cons, Jena King, John Eichenseer, John Fossum, Karen and Mattie Gold, Kat Steele, Kavi Marya, Kendra Garrett, Laura Harnish, Leah Lamdin, María Fernanda Valecillos Felice, Mario Alberto Silva, Mark Lipson, Mia Rallow, Mike Painter, Moise Velasquez-Manoff, Mona Caron, Nancy Schaub, Naomi Klein, Nassim Assefi, Nell Scott, Nuna Teal, Rebecca McInroy, Rich Reddick, Richard Pithouse, Roxanne Dunbar Ortiz, Rucha Chitnis, Sharmila

Rudrappa, Sofia Pablo-Hirano, Stacey Liane Lippincott, Steven Porter, Susana Aragon, Tarun Marya, the four generations of the Jimenez family, The Mesa Refuge, Tom Philpott, and Vashna Jagarnath.

We are grateful to those whose knowledge brought this book to the world: Carina Imbornone, Caitlin O'Beirne, Chloe Texier-Rose, Debra Helfand, Daniel del Valle, Emily DeHuff, Hillary Tisman, Janet Biehl, Janet Evans-Scanlon, Jonathan Woollen, Juliana Froggatt, Klee Benally, Laura Starrett, Mitzi Angel, Nancy Elgin, Nina Frieman, Sarita Varma, Sheila O'Shea, Stephanie Umeda, Thomas Colligan, Tamara Kawar, and, deeply, Kris Dahl, Karolina Sutton, Eric Chinski, and Deborah Ghim for their care and accompaniment.

We mourn our loved ones and teachers who passed along our journey: Alex Nieto, Amigo Bob Cantisano, Amilcar Perez Lopez, Bharat Kumar Marya, Charles Hill, Debra White Plume, Gil Scott-Heron, Hank Herrera, Jessica Nelson Williams, LaDonna Bravebull Allard, Lindley Dodson, Luis Gongora Pat, Mario Woods, Oscar Grant, Peter Bissegger, Rene Yañez, Sahleem Tindle, Snodumo Luvela, Varsha Patel, Verne Bryant, all the ones who have lost their lives to police violence, and the people, healers, and carers who have died during the Covid pandemic.

And finally, we are deeply grateful for those whose love made everything possible: Radhesh Marya, Debra Ferreboeuf and John Ferreboeuf, Charles Patel, Pratima Patel, Livleen Kahlon and Swarn Kahlon, Mini Kahlon, the universe and the butterfly, Benjamin Fahrer, the buzzing bees, and our children.

INDEX

Page numbers in *italics* refer to illustrations

A NOTE ABOUT THE AUTHORS

Dr. Rupa Marya is a physician, an activist, a mother, and a composer. She is an associate professor of medicine at the University of California, San Francisco, where she practices and teaches internal medicine. She is a cofounder of the Do No Harm Coalition, a collective of health workers committed to addressing disease through structural change. At the invitation of Lakȟóta health leaders, she is helping to set up the Mni Wiconi Health Clinic and Farm at Standing Rock to decolonize medicine and food. She is a cofounder of the Deep Medicine Circle, an organization committed to healing the wounds of colonialism through food, medicine, story, and learning. Working with her husband, the agroecological farmer Benjamin Fahrer, and the Association of Ramaytush Ohlone, she is a part of the Farming Is Medicine project, where farmers are recast as ecological stewards of rematriated land and food is liberated from the market economy. She has toured twenty-nine countries with her band, Rupa and the April Fishes, whose music was described by the legend Gil Scott-Heron as "Liberation Music."

Raj Patel is a research professor at the University of Texas at Austin's Lyndon B. Johnson School of Public Affairs, a professor in the university's department of nutrition, and a research associate at Rhodes University, South Africa. He is the author of *Stuffed and Starved* and the *New York Times* bestselling *The Value of Nothing*, and the coauthor of *A History of the World in Seven Cheap Things*. A James Beard Foundation Leadership Award winner, he is the codirector of a groundbreaking documentary on climate change and the global food system, *The Ants and the Grasshopper*. He serves on the International Panel of Experts on Sustainable Food Systems and has advised governments worldwide on the causes of and solutions to crises of sustainability.